Modern Management of Perinatal Psychiatric Disorder

Carol Henshaw

John Cox

Joanne Barton

RCPsych Publications

© The Royal College of Psychiatrists 2009
Reprinted 2013

RCPsych Publications is an imprint of the Royal College of Psychiatrists,
17 Belgrave Square, London SW1X 8PG
http://www.rcpsych.ac.uk

British Library Cataloguing-in-Publication Data.
A catalogue record for this book is available from the British Library.
ISBN 978 1 904671 36 7

Distributed in North America by Publishers Storage and Shipping Company.

The views presented in this book do not necessarily reflect those of the Royal College
of Psychiatrists, and the publishers are not responsible for any error of omission or fact.

Cover artwork © Joanne Savill 2009.

Printed by Bell & Bain Limited, Glasgow, UK.

Contents

Abbreviations

ADHD	attention-deficit hyperactivity disorder
BDI	Beck Depression Inventory
CBT	cognitive–behavioural therapy
CEMD	Confidential Enquiry into Maternal Deaths
CI	confidence interval
CNS	central nervous system
DSM	Diagnostic and Statistical Manual for Mental Disorders
ECT	electroconvulsive therapy
EPDS	Edinburgh Postnatal Depression Scale
GP	general practitioner
HPA	hypothalamic–pituitary–adrenal
HRSD	Hamilton Rating Scale for Depression
ICD	International Classification of Diseases
LSD	lysergic acid diethylamide
MAOI	monoamine oxidase inhibitor
MDI	Mental Developmental Index
NHS	National Health Service
NICE	National Institute for Health and Clinical Excellence
NOS	not otherwise specified
OR	odds ratio
PDSS	Postpartum Depression Screening Scale
PTSD	post-traumatic stress disorder
RCT	randomised controlled trial
RR	relative risk
SNRI	serotonin noradrenaline reuptake inhibitor
SSRI	selective serotonin reuptake inhibitor

STAI   Spielberger State–Trait Anxiety Inventory
WHO   World Health Organization
YBOCS   Yale–Brown Obsessive Compulsive Scale

Tables

Boxes

Figures

The authors

Carol Henshaw was Consultant Psychiatrist with Cheshire and Wirral Partnership National Health Service (NHS) Trust and Senior Lecturer at Keele University from 1996 to 2008. She is now Honorary Visiting Fellow at Staffordshire University. Her interest in perinatal mental health began during a research project investigating the relationship between postpartum blues and depression which eventually led to her MD. During higher clinical training she became a member of the Marcé Society, a scientific society devoted to mental illness related to childbearing, of which she was Pesident from 2004 to 2006. She sits on the Executive Committee of the Royal College of Psychiatrists' Perinatal Section and is chairing the revision of the College Report 'Patients as Parents: Addressing the Needs, Including the Safety of Children whose Parents have Mental Illness'.

John Cox is Professor Emeritus at Keele University and part time Professor of Mental Health at the University of Gloucestershire. He is immediate Past Secretary General of the World Psychiatric Association and Past President of the Royal College of Psychiatrists. He has been an active researcher and clinician in perinatal psychiatry since his first work in Uganda over three decades ago. At Keele he developed the first day-hospital for parents with perinatal mental health problems and previously worked in Edinburgh where he developed with colleagues the Edinburgh Postnatal Depression Scale. He is a committed advocate for an integrative approach.

Joanne Barton is Consultant Child and Adolescent Psychiatrist who works for North Staffordshire Combined Healthcare NHS Trust, providing psychiatric input to a community-based child and adolescent mental health service. Her day-to-day work with children, young people and their families is a constant reminder of the importance of parental mental health to the well-being and development of children. Her interest in the impact of parental mental illness during the perinatal period developed during research for her PhD that examined the role of maternal expressed emotion in the development and maintenance of child disruptive behavioural problems.

Acknowledgements

We are enormously grateful to Ilana Crome and Khaled Ismail for their help with writing Chapter 5 and to Margaret Oates for writing the Introduction. Karin Cox deserves thanks for her help over the years with research, clinical work and writing. We are indebted to our spouses and families for tolerating our labours and to all the parents and children who have trusted in our care and whose needs continue to inspire our work.

Preface

Carol Henshaw, John Cox and Joanne Barton

The impetus for this book arose from our recognition that psychiatric trainees and mental health professionals need to acquire up-to-date knowledge about the diagnosis and management of mental disorders related to childbearing and the impact on the family, a topic that so often barely appears at all in major psychiatric textbooks and other educational resources. We hope that this book will also prove useful to other practitioners and researchers in the field and that our fruitful academic and clinical collaboration as adult and child psychiatrists will promote greater collaboration between these two specialities which would better serve our patients and their families.

There is clear evidence that maternal depression is a risk factor for stunted growth and impairment of cognitive development in children not only in Western countries but also in low- and middle-income countries (Walker *et al*, 2007). Maternal suicide has been the most common cause of maternal death in the UK in recent years (Lewis & Drife, 2001, 2004), so it is essential that clinicians are aware of the disorders that may lead to maternal suicides and that women who suffer from them or are at risk of doing so are identified, assessed and treated.

Although the majority of new onset and recurrent disorders related to childbirth are mood disorders, we also seek to address the growing realisation that anxiety disorders are both prominent and have an adverse effect on child development (O'Connor *et al*, 2002). In addition, women with other psychotic, non-psychotic and personality disorders will become pregnant and require managing throughout pregnancy and after delivery.

We have avoided specifically the use of the acronym 'PND' for the reasons outlined in Chapter 11 of Lewis & Drife (2001). This acronym was intended to refer to a non-psychotic unipolar depressive disorder occurring after childbirth (postnatal depression) but has in fact been misused and even become shorthand for almost any psychiatric condition following delivery. As a consequence, women with a history of serious mental illness may have unrecognised postnatal depression, with potentially serious consequences. Hence, we have been careful to specify in full, without this abbreviation, which disorder we are discussing.

In our experience, it is essential to approach the management of women with perinatal psychiatric disorders from a bio-psychosocial perspective and for health professionals to be fully aware of the sociocultural context and the 'meaning' of this illness for the mother and her family. It is our opinion that the optimal management of women with childbearing-related mental disorders requires clinical judgement of a high order and a full awareness that psychiatry is both an art and a science, and that its evidence base incorporates research-based evidence as well as the accumulated wisdom of a fully trained practitioner. We hope that this approach and its inherent values are reflected adequately in this book.

References

Lewis, G. & Drife, J. (2001) *Why Mothers Die 1997–1999. The Fifth Report of the Confidential Enquiries into Maternal Deaths in the United Kingdom.* RCOG Press.

Lewis, G. & Drife, J. (2004) *Why Mothers Die 2000–2002. The Sixth Report of the Confidential Enquiries into Maternal Deaths in the United Kingdom.* RCOG Press.

O'Connor, T. G., Heron, J., Glover, V., *et al* (2002) Antenatal anxiety predicts child behavioral/emotional problems independently of postnatal depression. *Journal of the American Academy of Child and Adolescent Psychiatry*, **41**, 1470–1477.

Walker, S. P., Wachs, T. D., Gardner, J. M., *et al* (2007) Child development: risk factors for adverse outcomes in developing countries. *Lancet*, **369**, 145–157.

Foreword

This book is a testament to the increasing recognition that maternal mental health problems are the core business of both psychiatry and maternity care.

'Perinatal psychiatry' is now the internationally accepted term for conditions complicating pregnancy and the postpartum year. These include not only new-onset conditions following delivery such as postnatal depression and puerperal psychosis but also pre-existing conditions which may relapse, recur or continue during pregnancy and the postpartum period. It is concerned not only with the medical and psychosocial management of the mother but also the impact of the disorder and its treatments on the developing infant before and after birth. Although in the UK perinatal psychiatry is a sub-specialty of adult psychiatry, it overlaps and shares common goals with child psychiatry and those concerned with infant development.

Why is perinatal psychiatry so important and why has it achieved such recent prominence in national policy and practice guidelines?

Postpartum psychiatric disorders have long been of great interest to psychiatric researchers. Childbirth offers a unique research paradigm: a clearly defined cohort, a mixture of neuroendocrine, psychosocial, anthropological, sociological and epidemiological factors that can be studied across time and cultures, of interest to both psychiatrists and obstetricians, to adult and child workers. It poses and answers questions that are not only relevant to present life events but can also inform the aetiology and treatment of disorders, particularly affective disorders, at other times.

Although there has been prominent research interest in perinatal psychiatric disorders for over 40 years with individual centres of excellence for the provision of care, in general, services have been patchy, inequitable and at a national level, inadequate. Only recently has this been recognised and a number of national policies and practice guidelines issued to rectify the problem (Royal College of Psychiatrists, 2000; Lewis & Drife, 2001; Scottish Executive, 2001; Department of Health, 2002; Scottish Intercollegiate Guidelines Network, 2002; Department of Health, 2004; Lewis & Drife, 2004; Lewis, 2007; National Institute for Health and Clinical

Excellence, 2007). The result is that in the UK all mental health providers and commissioners will be seeking to establish services for pregnant and postpartum women with psychiatric disorders.

These policies are underpinned by a number of factors. Pregnancy and childbirth is associated with a considerable psychiatric morbidity. A small but significant number of women will develop a profound psychotic illness in the early weeks following childbirth requiring specialist skills and resources for their and their infant's proper care. Although the number is small, it represents a substantial increase in risk of developing a psychotic illness following childbirth compared with other times. A larger number of women will develop a severe non-psychotic affective disorder and an even larger number mild to moderate affective disorder popularly known as postnatal depression. Overall, at least 10% of delivered women will experience a psychiatric disorder following childbirth. The more severe conditions will require the attention of specialised mental health services. The less severe conditions, although probably no more common than at other times, pose a major public health problem, with chronic maternal depression, particularly if associated with socio-economic adversity, having adverse effects on infant and child development. The perinatal period is also very important because of the risk of recurrence in women with pre-existing serious mental illness, particularly bipolar disorder. Childbirth is unique in psychiatry as a major provoker of mental illness that comes with 9 months warning. The perinatal period poses particular problems for the management of psychiatric disorders. Many psychotropic medications, particularly mood stabilisers, are problematic in pregnancy. Acute psychotic episodes in pregnancy compromise maternal and infant health. The distinctive clinical presentation, rapid onset and deterioration can demand a different response from psychiatric services than at other times. Throughout the perinatal period psychiatric professionals have to deal with two patients, both mother and infant. All of these factors consistently revealed by research over the years have been reinforced by the findings of the last four maternal deaths enquiries in the UK (Department of Health, 1998; Lewis & Drife, 2001, 2004; Lewis, 2007).

Pregnancy and the early postpartum period is exceptional for its level of surveillance by health professionals. This provides an opportunity not only for the early detection and prompt treatment of women who are ill but also for the identification in early pregnancy of those at risk of developing an illness following delivery and for secondary and perhaps primary prevention.

The Confidential Enquiry into Maternal Deaths

Most of the UK national policies for perinatal mental health have been strongly influenced by the UK maternal mortality enquiries over the past 4 years. These reveal that suicide in particular and psychiatric causes of maternal deaths in general are a leading cause of maternal mortality. This is also likely to be true internationally. It is generally accepted that maternal mortality is the 'tip of the iceberg' and it is therefore reasonable to assume that psychiatric disorder is also a leading cause of maternal morbidity.

In its current form, the Confidential Enquiry into Maternal Deaths (CEMD) is over 50 years old. In the UK, suicide has always been included as an indirect cause of maternal death; however, it is only since 1994 that suicide and other psychiatric causes of maternal death has been separately analysed and presented in the written report and a psychiatrist has been appointed as one of the central assessors to the CEMD. The CEMD combines both a maternal mortality surveillance and quantitative data analysis with an enquiry into individual cases revealing a description of the pathways of care and circumstances that were associated with an individual death. This combination of methods allows for the identification of themes and factors associated with poor outcome that in its turn has led to the development of practice guidelines with demonstrable impact on the quality of maternity care. In addition, it allows for the emergence of new themes which reflect not only changes in reproductive epidemiology and technology (e.g. increasing maternal age, rise in Caesarean sections, *in vitro* fertilisation) but also rapid societal changes such as the impact of asylum seekers and immigrants.

For the purposes of international comparison, it is important to understand how maternal mortality data is expressed. The maternal mortality rate refers to maternal deaths from 24 weeks of pregnancy to 42 days post-delivery. The causes are defined as direct (e.g. haemorrhage, pre-eclampsia) and indirect (e.g. pregnancy exacerbated conditions including suicide). The maternal mortality ratio is the number of maternal deaths compared with the number of births. International Classification of Diseases 10th edition (ICD–10) pregnancy-related deaths are all deaths that occur during pregnancy and the postpartum year. The UK CEMD includes all deaths up to 1 year but describes the data in such a way as to allow international comparison.

With each enquiry, the case ascertainment increases and is generally regarded as being more complete than in other countries. This factor needs to be taken into account when comparing findings from the UK with other countries. Since 1997, case ascertainment has been enhanced by an Office of National Statistics Linkage Study which identifies maternal deaths not reported directly to the CEMD. These deaths have been in the majority late indirect and coincidental deaths but have included a substantial number of suicides. Until the 2003–2005 CEMD, suicide was the second leading cause of indirect death (pregnancy and up to 42 days after delivery of the infant) but the leading cause of maternal death overall (up to 1 year) (Lewis & Drife, 2001, 2004). In the latest CEMD (2003–2005; Lewis, 2007), there has been a significant reduction in the numbers of suicides so that suicide is now the third leading cause of indirect deaths and the second leading cause of maternal death up to 1 year. Despite this reduction, a number of features of maternal suicide have remained constant over the last three CEMDs, reflected in the recommendations of the enquiry and its implications for both psychiatric and maternity practice. The overwhelming majority (over

80%) of maternal suicides had a previous psychiatric history. In the 1997–2002 CEMDs (Lewis & Drife, 2001, 2004), 50% of maternal suicides had a previous history of serious mental illness, contact with psychiatric services or admission to a psychiatric unit. In the main, women had either bipolar disorder or puerperal psychosis. These identifiable risk factors had not been detected in early pregnancy nor had proactive management plans been put in place. The postpartum recurrence seemed to have taken all by surprise and there was a delayed response to the women's rapidly deteriorating illness. The majority of these women died within the first 3 months following childbirth. None had been admitted to a mother and baby unit or cared for by specialised perinatal psychiatric services in either their current or previous maternities. In the latest CEMD (Lewis, 2007), a smaller proportion (37%) of maternal suicides had these characteristics. The reduction in maternal suicides was accounted for by a reduction in the number of women who died in late pregnancy or within the first 3 months postpartum. However, the majority of women who died from suicide within 3 months of delivery had the same characteristics as previously reported, that is to say a past history of serious mental illness, a failure to identify and manage their risk, a serious and rapidly deteriorating postpartum illness and a lack of management by specialised services. The recommendations of the CEMD therefore remain the same: women should be asked at early pregnancy assessment for a previous psychiatric history and those with a history of serious mental illness should have a plan in place for the management of that risk. All women with serious mental illness in late pregnancy and the postpartum period should be managed by specialised perinatal psychiatric teams and if admission is necessary, be admitted to a specialised mother and baby unit. In addition, the latest CEMD recommends in its 'top 10 recommendations' that women with serious mental illness should be counselled prior to conception about the associated risks with pregnancy. Sadly, a constant finding of the CEMD since 1994 has been the violent method of suicide. In contrast to the method of female suicide at other times, 80% of maternal suicides used violent methods. The most common was hanging followed by jumping from a height. Very few women died from an intentional overdose of prescribed or over-the-counter medication.

Suicide is not the only psychiatric cause of maternal death. The CEMD found that women also died from intentional or accidental overdoses of recreational drugs. A substantial number of women died from medical conditions that were either the consequence of their substance misuse exacerbated by pregnancy or because their psychiatric condition led to their medical conditions being missed or misattributed to psychiatric causes. These findings too have been constant over the last three CEMDs. A worrying theme to emerge from the last CEMD was the overall significant contribution of substance misuse to maternal mortality. Of all maternal deaths, 10% occurred in substance misusers, 57% of psychiatric deaths. Substance misuse was associated with avoiding antenatal care, high rates of removal of the infant into the care of local authorities and the subsequent absence of both psychiatric and maternity care for the mother. Very few of these women had had specialist care from drug addiction services during their pregnancies and this led to additional recommendations from the last CEMD. These include the provision of specialised 'one-stop shop' services for pregnant women who misuse substances which are nested within the maternity services with rapid access and active outreach as a principle of service provision.

The size and distinctive nature of perinatal psychiatric conditions and their consequences for the infant, as well as for the mother's future mental health justify educating all those involved in the care of women and the provision of specialised services for those who are seriously mentally ill. If all psychiatrists discussed with their patients the implications of their conditions and treatments for pregnancy, if all women at risk of serious mental illness following childbirth had proactive management plans in place and if those who became ill were treated by specialised services then it is likely that there could be a reduction in maternal mortality and morbidity from psychiatric causes and an improvement in infant mental health. The findings of the latest CEMD might suggest that the recommendations of previous enquiries are beginning to have an impact on maternal suicide. However, complacency is not justified and it sadly remains true that many maternal suicides were predictable and perhaps preventable.

Margaret Oates

References

Department of Health (1998) *Why Mothers Die. Report on Confidential Enquiries into Maternal Deaths in the United Kingdom 1994–96.* TSO (The Stationery Office).

Department of Health (2002) *Women's Mental Health: Into the Mainstream. Strategic Development of Mental Health Care for Women.* TSO (The Stationery Office).

Department of Health (2004) *National Service Framework for Children, Young People and Maternity Services: Maternity Services.* TSO (The Stationery Office).

Lewis, G. (ed.) (2007) *Saving Mothers' Lives. Reviewing Maternal Deaths to Make Motherhood Safer – 2003–2005. The Seventh Report on Confidential Enquiries into Maternal Deaths in the United Kingdom.* Confidential Enquiry into Maternal and Child Health.

Lewis, G. & Drife, J. (2001) *Why Mothers Die 1997–1999. The Fifth Report of the Confidential Enquiries into Maternal Deaths in the United Kingdom.* RCOG Press.

Lewis, G. & Drife, J. (2004) *Why Mothers Die 2000–2002. The Sixth Report of the Confidential Enquiries into Maternal Deaths in the United Kingdom.* RCOG Press.

National Institute for Health and Clinical Excellence (2007) *Antenatal and Postnatal Mental Health. Clinical Management and Service Guidance.* NICE.

Royal College of Psychiatrists (2000) *Perinatal Maternal Mental Health Services. Recommendations for Provision of Services for Childbearing Women* (Council Report CR88). Royal College of Psychiatrists.

Scottish Executive (2001) *Scottish Executive Framework for Maternity Services in Scotland.* Scottish Exceutive.

Scottish Intercollegiate Guidelines Network (2002) *Postnatal Depression and Puerperal Psychosis: a National Clinical Guideline.* Scottish Intercollegiate Guidelines Network.

CHAPTER 1

Historical perspectives and classification issues

French pioneers and current opinion

Louis Victor Marcé, a brilliant pupil of Jean-Étienne Dominique Esquirol in Paris, in his seminal thesis in 1858 regarded the mental illness that sometimes followed childbirth as a distinct disorder; he also anticipated the development of endocrinology by delineating a 'morbid sympathie' between the postnatal mental state and bodily functions. A further observation by this scholarly 'ancien intern' was to identify certain symptoms of childbearing mental disorder that were rarely found together in non-puerperal mental disorders. He was aware also of the specific forensic aspects of these case histories and in particular the risk of severe puerperal psychosis to both the infant and the mother.

In this way Marcé and Esquirol (who in 1838 reported on a large study of postnatal illness also in Paris) set the stage for further work in this field. It is regrettable, therefore, that their work was largely lost to English-speaking psychiatry until the 1970s when the Marcé Society was founded.

Thus, until the mid-20th century the various puerperal psychoses were regarded as conditions specific to childbirth. Numerous earlier papers (fully reviewed by Brockington, 1996) were published which described in detail the psychopathology of women with 'lactational psychosis', which often included delusions about the baby, sexual infidelity and religious themes. Confusion and perplexity were observed in women with non-infective psychoses; infections such as tuberculosis often contracted in the asylums, as well as pelvic infections, not uncommonly led to the death of the mother and to neglect of the baby.

Menzies (1893) provided an account of 140 women admitted to Rainhill Asylum in Lancashire and he used the then customary distinction between lactational and other psychoses.

In the Middle Ages, however, madness after childbirth was more likely to be primarily regarded as a religious rather than a medical problem: the mother was a witch and the 'possession' a punishment for misdemeanour. The postpartum mother was unclean, so the 'churching' ceremony was necessary, attended also by the midwife, before the mother could again attend Sunday services.

An autobiography by Margery Kempe, a medieval nun, provides a detailed account of her recurrent postpartum mental disorder; yet, despite her difficulties, this courageous woman travelled widely and exerted considerable influence for the good of others (Kempe, 1985).

In pre-Christian times, the Greek physicians from the school of Hippocrates on the island of Kos were more holistic in their approach. They regarded mental disorder, including postnatal mental disorder, as having a biological explanation (milk diverted from the breast to the brain or suppression of lochial discharge), yet they also offered prayers to gods such as Aesculapius or Apollo as a part of the healing process.

It is apparent, therefore, from this glimpse of history that postpartum mental disorders are regarded as different in their social implications from disorders at other times and that the provision of healthcare for women varies according to the prevailing opinions about causation – the choice of therapy being determined by the 'explanatory models' and beliefs about the cause of the illness as well as the prevalent scientific model; for example, 'hormones' in the mid-20th century (e.g. Dalton, 1980) and receptor sensitivity (Wieck *et al*, 1991) at the present time when biomedicine is the dominant paradigm for the explanation for most illnesses.

Present day international classifications

International classifications of mental and behavioural disorders (the International Classification of Diseases 10th edition (ICD–10) (World Health Organization, 1992) and the Diagnostic and Statistical Manual of Mental Disorders 4th edition (DSM–IV) (American Psychiatric Association, 1994)) will also reflect the dominant priorities of society, their implicit popular causal models and the search for a common language. In much recent research in mental health internationally there is an emphasis on the need to establish the reliability of psychiatric assessment, with less regard for their validity or for traditional folk categories.

Despite the plethora of papers describing puerperal psychoses published in the late 19th and early 20th century, this diagnosis was removed from ICD–9. Women with a postnatal onset of severe mental disorder were not therefore regarded as having any characteristics different from disorders at other times. This omission was partially corrected in ICD–10 when a 6-week postpartum onset specifier (4 weeks in DSM–IV) was introduced, but in DSM only for affective disorders.

Furthermore, in ICD–10 there is a specific and rather condescending instruction that the postpartum onset specifier should only be used when the condition cannot be characterised elsewhere, as might occur in a low-resource low- and middle-income country. Yet in several such countries (e.g. Uganda and Nigeria) there are indigenous folk classifications which include a specific postnatal mental disorder.

The limitations of ICD–10 for use in public health departments wishing to audit perinatal services or for use by researchers are all too apparent. A public inquiry following the suicide of a mother (a psychiatrist) with a postnatal bipolar mood disorder who had also killed her 3-month-old daughter recommendeds the establishment of specialist perinatal psychiatry services and improved screening for woman at high risk of developing a puerperal psychosis (North East London Strategic Health Authority, 2003). With existing classifications of perinatal mental disorder, and in particular the lack of a mandatory onset specifier, it is difficult to collect these statistics or to identify from hospital records women who are at risk of developing psychosis after childbirth.

Any revision of international classifications of mental disorder should therefore reflect these clinical and public health priorities, as well as the scientific evidence for the specificity of childbearing mental disorder and any new data on the genetic or other aetiology of bipolar puerperal mental illness.

Towards ICD–11

The World Health Organization (WHO) and the World Psychiatric Association (Mezzich, 2007) are both aware of these limitations of ICD–10 and for a decade at least have been undertaking a radical critique of existing classifications and proposed that they should be more integrative and take fully into account the quality of life and the relationship problems which may trigger mental disorder, as well as consider the protective factors.

International classifications of mental disorders should be a spur to creative thinking (e.g. Cox, 2002). Yet they can also restrict innovation if their claims for a scientific evidence base are accepted uncritically while ignoring values or if the disorders are diagnosed without regard to the social context and the meaning of the illness for the patient.

In Uganda in the early 1970s, when ICD–8 was being revised, the exclusion of puerperal psychosis was in stark contrast to the experience of local psychiatrists and contrary to the Kiganda classification of mental disorder used in the community (Orley, 1970). A traditional Kiganda postnatal illness, *Amakiro*, was openly described by the women: it was caused by promiscuity during pregnancy and characterised by a belief that the mother might eat her baby (Cox, 1979). *Amakiro* could be prevented by a change in behaviour or by taking herbal medicines available in the market.

An international classification of mental disorder, therefore, may need to consider the relevance of these local categories to understanding the causes and consequences of perinatal mental disorders, and in particular the cultural context in which the classification is to be used.

3

Western societies

Recent changes in the values and priorities of Western societies, which reflect the dominant values in society, may partially determine the frequency and the classification of perinatal mental disorder. These changes include:

- the impact of the user movement on the use and acceptability of psychiatric classifications
- the multi-professional context in which mental health services are delivered
- the levels of disability and quality of life associated with the mental health problem.

The dramatic reduction in birth rates in Western Europe has been construed by a journalist (Bunting, 2006) as being a consequence of the cultural changes in the roles of men and women: the desire of women to retain autonomy, financial independence and to avoid dependency. Increased awareness of antenatal as well as postnatal depression and greater concern to provide assistance during pregnancy may therefore be a result of this cultural shift and the breaks in the transmission of women's knowledge (Fitzgerald *et al*, 1988), as well as more widely dispersed families with grandparents less available to assist because of their greater mobility and improved health.

Updated classifications of mental disorders should therefore discourage a reductionist approach to clinical practice and reinstate the patient and the patient's relationship with the health professional as central to the diagnostic assessment process. Any classification should be valid as well as reliable.

The World Psychiatric Association International Guidelines for Diagnostic Assessment (Mezzich, 2007) innovatively includes a narrative and descriptive approach to patient assessment, and proposes that the quality of life and an individual's belief system, including their religious beliefs, be recorded.

The ICD–10 Classification of Mental and Behavioural Disorders (World Health Organization, 1992) concluded the preface with the apposite reflection that 'a classification is a way of seeing the world at a point in time'. As the world has changed and become globalised, the classification of mental disorders in general and the postnatal mental disorders in particular need now to be carefully reviewed (Box 1.1 and 1.2).

Although there is no specific category for puerperal psychosis in DSM–IV, the distinctive features of perinatal mental disorders are nevertheless listed in the accompanying text (Box 1.3).

What is special about postnatal disorders?

This important question was considered at an international workshop in Sweden held in 1996, when the following characteristics were agreed, and the revised classification was later endorsed by the Marcé Society.

Box 1.1 ICD–10 mental and behavioural disorders associated with the puerperium (F53. –)

This category is unusual and apparently paradoxical in carrying a recommendation that it should be used only when unavoidable. Its inclusion is recognition of the very real practical problems in many developing countries that make the gathering of details about many cases of puerperal illness virtually impossible. However, even in the absence of sufficient information to allow a diagnosis of some variety of affective disorder (or, more rarely, schizophrenia), there will usually be enough known to allow diagnosis of a mild (F53.0) or severe (F53.1) disorder; this subdivision is useful for estimations of workload, and when decisions are to be made about provision of services.

The inclusion of this category should not be taken to imply that, given adequate information, a significant proportion of cases of postpartum mental illness cannot be classified in other categories. Most experts in this field are of the opinion that a clinical picture of puerperal psychosis is so rarely (if ever) reliably distinguishable from affective disorder or schizophrenia that a special category is not justified. Any psychiatrist who is of the minority opinion that special postpartum psychoses do indeed exist may use this category, but should be aware of its real purpose.

Reproduced with permission from World Health Organization, 1992

- The birth context, which shapes experience and the expression of the perinatal disorder.
- The impact on the mother, which has the potential to damage self-image and sense of loss at a time of transition.
- The impact on the child, partner and family, which is greater at a sensitive period.
- Untreated perinatal mental disorder has high morbidity and a cascading effect.
- Readiness for help is raised in the postnatal period.
- Systems to help are more available because services are organised to ensure frequent contacts with maternity and primary care services.
- Lower stigma in some countries because of high-profile public figures.
- High yield for intervention because of the preceding circumstances.
- Birth can trigger mental disorders.
- Pregnancy and birth have distinctive biological components.
- Onset of perinatal mental disorder is contrary to cultural expectation.

However, problems with the current classifications of perinatal mental disorder include the following.

- Failure to include an obligatory specifier to cover a range of diagnoses, rather a category that can only be used in exceptional circumstances, or a limited specifier.

Box 1.2 ICD–10 F53 Mental and behavioural disorders associated with the puerperium, not elsewhere classified

F53.0   *Mild mental and behavioural disorders associated with the puerperium, not elsewhere classified*

Includes: postnatal depression NOS, postpartum depression NOS

F53.1   *Severe mental and behavioural disorders associated with the puerperium, not elsewhere classified*

Includes: puerperal psychosis NOS

F53.8   *Other mental and behavioural disorders associated with the puerperium, not elsewhere classified*

F53.9   *Puerperal mental disorder, unspecified*

This classification should be used only for mental disorders associated with the puerperium (commencing within 6 weeks of delivery) that do not meet the criteria for disorders classified elsewhere in this book, either because insufficient information is available, or because it is considered that special additional clinical features are present which make classification elsewhere inappropriate. It will usually be possible to classify mental disorders associated with the puerperium by using two other codes: the first is from elsewhere in Chapter V (F) and indicates the specific type of mental disorder (usually affective (F30–F39)), and the second is 099.3 (mental diseases and diseases of the nervous system complicating the puerperium) of ICD–10.

Reproduced with permission from World Health Organization, 1992

- Failure to use a research-supported time period for onset after delivery. The evidence from case register studies indicates that the majority of excess presentations over expected rates are within 3 months of delivery (Kendell *et al*, 1983).
- DSM does not allow easy coding for an acute mixed atypical psychosis commonly seen by those who treat severe postpartum disorders.

Non-psychotic unipolar postnatal depression

The DSM–IV does not deal well with the milder (sub-syndromal or sub-threshold) depressions that are increasingly recognised as very prevalent and of high-associated morbidity. These 'mild depressive disorders' (ICD–10) are of particular importance in the postnatal period. They may have an adverse impact on infant feeding, attachment and development, and may develop into a major depressive disorder with additional risk to mother and infant.

The term 'postnatal depression' is best considered therefore as a category for a group of mood disorders exacerbated or triggered by childbirth. These disorders may be sub-threshold or sub-syndromal because they do not fulfil

---

Box 1.3 DSM–IV postpartum onset specifier

Criteria for postpartum onset specifier

The specifier With Postpartum Onset can be applied to the current (or most recent) Major Depressive, Manic, or Mixed Episode of Major Depressive Disorder, Bipolar I Disorder, or Bipolar II Disorder or to Brief Psychotic Disorder (p. 302) if onset is within 4 weeks after delivery of a child. In general, the symptomatology of the postpartum Major Depressive, Manic, or Mixed Episode does not differ from the symptomatology in nonpostpartum mood episodes and may include psychotic features. A fluctuating course and mood lability may be more common in postpartum episodes. When delusions are present, they often concern the newborn infant (e.g. the newborn is possessed by the devil, has special powers, or is destined for a terrible fate). In both the psychotic and nonpsychotic presentations, there may be suicidal ideation, obsessional thought regarding violence to the child, lack of concentration, and psychomotor agitation. Women with postpartum Major Depressive Episodes often have severe anxiety, panic attacks, spontaneous crying long after the usual duration of 'baby blues' (i.e. 3–7 days postpartum), disinterest in their new infant, and insomnia (more likely to manifest a' difficulty falling asleep than as early morning awakening).

Many women feel especially guilty about having depressive feelings at a time when they believe they should be happy. They may be reluctant to discuss their symptoms or their negative feelings toward the child. Less-than-optimal development of the mother–infant relationship may result from the clinical condition itself or from separations from the infant. Infanticide is most often associated with postpartum psychotic episodes that are characterized by command hallucinations to kill the infant or delusions that the infant is possessed, but it can also occur in severe postpartum mood episodes without such specific delusions or hallucinations. Postpartum mood (Major Depressive, Manic or Mixed) episodes with psychotic features appear to occur in from 1 in 500 to 1 in 1000 deliveries and may be more common in primiparous women. The risk of postpartum episodes with psychotic features is particularly increased for women with prior postpartum mood episodes but is also elevated for those with a prior history of a Mood Disorder (especially Bipolar I Disorder). Once a woman has had a postpartum episode with psychotic features, the risk of recurrence with each subsequent delivery is between 30% and 50%. There is also some evidence of increased risk of postpartum psychotic mood episodes among women without a history of Mood Disorders with a family history of Bipolar Disorders. Postpartum episodes must be differentiated from delirium occurring in the postpartum period, which is distinguished by a decreased level of awareness or attention.

---

criteria for DSM–IV major depressive disorder, but in ICD–10 would be classified as depressive episodes (mild).

Because postnatal depression is a term used by public health departments and women themselves to advocate services, it should be retained in ICD–11 and DSM–IV and restricted to all depressive disorders present within 1 year of childbirth.

For research purposes, however, it is helpful to distinguish new-onset postnatal depression from depression also present throughout pregnancy. Systems to identify new onsets would be very desirable.

Puerperal psychoses

- The puerperal psychosis specifier should be limited only to onsets in the first 3 months after delivery.
- The ICD category 'Mental and behavioural disorders associated with the puerperium not elsewhere classified' should be omitted.
- A new category in DSM–V should be introduced not limited to postpartum onsets but permitting this qualifier, with the following criteria:
  - sudden onset, not on background of chronic disorder
  - two or more of the following:
    1. mood disorders with lability
    2. delusions not characteristic of mood disorder or schizophrenia
    3. rapid fluctuations
    4. perplexity
    5. confusion or disorientation.

Conclusion

The debate about the optimal classification of perinatal mental disorder has illustrated that the birth event, and its associated mental disorders, are fully understood only if there is a grasp of the wholeness of the individual within a cultural context, and that explanatory models that span the brain and the mind as well as the psyche and the soul are routinely considered.

It is our opinion, based on research and clinical work, that for the best interests of women with mental illness, who need skilled specialist help, a mandatory postpartum specifier in revised classifications for all mental disorders be included and a diagnostic category for the specific puerperal psychoses whose symptomatology and course may be different from non-puerperal mental disorders be retained.

References

American Psychiatric Association (1994) *Diagnostic and Statistical Manual of Mental Disorders (4th edn) (DSM–IV)*, pp. 386–387. APA.

American Psychiatric Association (2000) *Diagnostic and Statistical Manual of Mental Disorders Fourth Edition, Text Revision (4th edn) (DSM–IV–TR)*. American Psychiatric Publishing.

Brockington, I. (1996) *Motherhood and Mental Health*. Oxford University Press.

Bunting, M. (2006) Behind the baby gap lies a culture of contempt for parenthood. *The Guardian*, Tuesday 7 March.

Cox, J. L. (1979) Amakiro: a Ugandan puerperal psychosis? *Social Psychiatry and Psychiatric Epidemiology*, **14**, 49–52.

Cox, J. L. (2002) Commentary towards a more integrated international system of psychiatric classification. *Psychopathology*, **35**, 195–196.

Dalton, K. (1980) *Depression After Childbirth*. Oxford University Press.

Esquirol, E. (1838) *Des Maladies Mentales Considérées sous les Rapports Médical, Hygénique et Médico Légal*. Baillière.

Fitzgerald, M. H., Ing, M., Ya, T. H., *et al* (1988) *Hear Our Voices: Trauma, Birthing and Mental Health among Cambodian Women*. Transcultural Mental Health Centre.

Kempe, M. (1985) *The Book of Margery Kempe*. Penguin Books.

Kendell, R. E., Rennie, D., Clarke, J. A., *et al* (1983) The social and obstetric correlates of psychiatric admission in the puerperium. *Psychological Medicine*, **150**, 341–350.

Marcé, L. V. (1858) *Traité de la Folie des Femmes enceintes: des Nouvelles Accouchées et des Nourrices*. Baillière.

Menzies, W. F. (1893) Puerperal insanity. An analysis of 140 consecutive cases. *American Journal of Insanity*, 50, 148–185.

Mezzich, J. E. (2002) The WPA International Guidelines for Diagnostic Assessment. *World Psychiatry*, **1**, 36–39.

Mezzich, J. E. (2007) Psychiatry for the person: articulating medicine's science and humanism. *World Psychiatry*, **6**, 1–3.

North East London Strategic Health Authority (2003) *Report of an Independent Inquiry into the Care and Treatment of Daksha Emson MBBS, MRCPsych, MSc, and her Daughter Freya*. North East London Strategic Health Authority.

Orley, J. H. (1970) *Culture and Mental Illness. A Study from Uganda*. East African Publishing House.

Wieck, A., Kumar, R., Hirst, A. D., *et al* (1991) Increased sensitivity of dopamine receptors and recurrence of affective psychosis after childbirth. *BMJ*, **303**, 613–616.

World Health Organization (1992) *The ICD–10 Classification of Mental and Behavioural Disorders*. WHO.

9

CHAPTER 2

Perinatal depression, anxiety, stress and adjustment

Childbirth is a time of enormous upheaval and adjustment in biological, psychological and social terms. It is therefore not surprising that it is associated with a considerable amount of morbidity in terms of both depressive and anxiety disorders. This chapter looks at these disorders and their management.

Postnatal depression

In the year following childbirth, 13% of women experience depression (O'Hara & Swain, 1996) and a similar number become depressed during pregnancy (O'Hara et al, 1984). The distress to the mother and her family is obvious and some women who have experienced postnatal depression will change their plans for future pregnancies because of fears or recurrence, effects on the family or severity of the illness (Peindl et al, 1995). The consequences for partners and children are discussed in Chapter 6.

Both mothers with postnatal depression and their infants consume more community care services than mother–infant dyads not affected by depression (Petrou et al, 2002) and US data indicate that even one emergency department visit for their infant distinguished mothers with depression from those who were not depressed (Mandl et al, 1999). Mothers with depression stop breastfeeding earlier (Henderson et al, 2003), costs for community nursing, social care and paediatricians are higher (Roberts et al, 2001) and they are more impaired on more dimensions of the Short Form – 36 health survey (Boyce et al, 2000) than age-appropriate normative data and postpartum women without depression. Role limitations owing to physical problems are greater in primiparous than multiparous mothers (Boyce et al, 2000).

Postnatal depression is clearly a major public health problem.

Is postnatal depression a specific entity?

Whether or not postnatal depression is a specific concept still challenges researchers. In the late 1950s, researchers began to document non-psychotic illnesses that occurred after childbirth and observed that over a quarter of newly delivered women experienced emotional distress (e.g. Gordon & Gordon, 1959). Pitt's seminal paper in 1968 described many of the symptoms as atypical (Pitt, 1968). Subsequently, the general view became that if standardised rating scales and diagnostic interviews are employed, the symptomatic profile does not differ from unipolar depression occurring at other times (although the content of negative or intrusive thoughts may focus on the maternal role and the infant). However, a case-record review of women with postnatal major depression and those with major depression unrelated to childbearing found that women with depression after delivery were more likely to present with anxiety features and took longer to recover (Hendrick et al, 2000).

The prevalence appears to be no different to the prevalence of depression in non-puerperal women and between those who have adoptive and natural children and those who have only adoptive children (Cooper et al, 1988; Cox et al, 1993; Dean et al, 1995). However, onset of postnatal episodes cluster in the first few weeks after delivery. Women whose first episode of depression is postnatal have an increased risk of further postnatal episodes and not non-puerperal episodes in the ensuing 5 years, while those whose first postnatal episode was a recurrence of a prior disorder have an increased risk for non-puerperal but not puerperal recurrences. Postnatal episodes are shorter in duration (Cooper & Murray, 1995).

Epidemiology

Although prevalence rates are similar for much of the world, including culturally diverse communities in Western Europe, the USA, Australia, rural India and Africa, Turkey and Hong Kong, some variation is beginning to emerge. Malta (a very stable population where women have their extended families in close proximity) has a point prevalence at 8 weeks postpartum of 8.7% (Felice et al, 2004), whereas in Khayelitsha township outside Cape Town in South Africa (where there is enormous social adversity) the rate is 34.7% (Cooper et al, 1999).

High Edingurgh Postnatal Depression Scale (EPDS) scores have been found in women born in a non-English speaking country but now living in London (Onozawa et al, 2003). Halbreich & Karkun (2006), reviewing the available epidemiological studies, found rates ranging from almost 0 to 60%. Prevalence figures are higher where self-report scales are used to define caseness as opposed to diagnostic interviews, but there are likely to be many other cross-cultural factors at work (see Chapter 11).

Most untreated episodes will last for a few weeks to a few months but a third may last for up to a year and 10% into the second year of the infant's life (Feggetter et al, 1981; Watson et al, 1984). The social context is an important maintaining factor; persistent depression has been shown to be associated with poverty, having five or more children, an uneducated husband and no confidante (Rahman & Creed, 2007).

Between a third and a half of all depressions occurring after birth will be continuations of episodes that onset during or before pregnancy (Watson *et al*, 1984; Gotlib *et al*, 1989).

The rate of recurrence after a subsequent pregnancy having been depressed after the first is 27.3–48.9% with the onset of recurrent episodes clustering close to delivery (Garfield *et al*, 2004; Wisner *et al*, 2004).

Predictors of postnatal depression

Four meta-analyses of predictors have been conducted (Beck, 1996; 2001; O'Hara & Swain, 1996; Robertson *et al*, 2004). The last of these combined data from the previous three with other large-scale studies and calculated overall effect sizes. Strong to moderate and small risk factors are listed in Box 2.1. However, it should be noted that women in the included studies were mainly White, 25–35 years old and of mid–high socio-economic status (Ross *et al*, 2006).

Factors that do not appear to have a relationship with postnatal depression in these meta-analyses are:

- parity or number of children
- level of education
- length of relationship with partner
- gender of the child in Western societies.

A recent large prospective study in a more diverse population found low income to be the single largest significant predictor of postnatal depression (Segre *et al*, 2007).

Age is not a risk factor in samples over the age of 18 years, but studies suggest that adolescent mothers are at increased risk (Coletta, 1983; Hudson *et al*, 2000; Rubertsson *et al*, 2003). Barnet *et al* (1996) observed

---

Box 2.1 Risk factors for postnatal depression

Strong to moderate risk factors

- Depression or anxiety during pregnancy
- Past history of mental disorder
- Life events
- Lack of or perceived lack of social support

Moderate risk factors

- Neuroticism
- A difficult martial relationship during pregnancy

Small risk factors

- Obstetric factors
- Socio-economic status

---

that stress and conflict with the infant's father were associated with depressive symptoms, whereas a supportive relationship with the infant's father was associated with fewer symptoms. Additionally, support from a case-worker or support group can be protective (Thompson & Peebles-Wilkins, 1992). Social isolation, maternal competence and weight/shape concerns have also been identified as predictors of depressive symptoms in teenage mothers (Birkeland et al, 2005).

Ross et al (2004) found that biological variables (progesterone and cortisol) did not have a direct effect on depressive symptoms during pregnancy but rather acted indirectly via psychosocial stressors and anxiety.

Halbreich (2005) has proposed a bio-psychosocial-cultural model of the processes that might lead to postpartum mental disorders (Fig. 2.1).

Past psychiatric history, mood during pregnancy and the early puerperium

A past history of depression is a clear risk factor for postnatal depression. Depressed or anxious mood during pregnancy (particularly in the last trimester) predicts depression postpartum and is also associated with increased reporting of somatic symptoms during pregnancy (Kelly et al, 2001). Anxiety disorder in the third trimester predicts high scores on the EPDS postpartum independently of the presence of major depressive disorder during pregnancy (Sutter-Dallay et al, 2004).

Boyce (2003) reported that those with a past history of psychopathology (particularly depression or anxiety) were at increased risk of developing depression after childbirth. A family history of mental illness, a history of postnatal depression in the participant's mother and alcoholism in the participant's brother were also predictors. Bloch et al (2005) identified premenstrual dysphoric disorder, mood symptoms on days 2–4 postpartum, a past history of depression and report of mood symptoms during past oral contraceptive use as being associated with major depression at 6–8 weeks postpartum.

Mood disturbance in the week after delivery is clearly related to the development of postnatal depression. Several retrospective and prospective studies have demonstrated links between postpartum 'blues' and postnatal depression (for a review see Henshaw, 2003). One prospective controlled study identified severe blues as an independent predictor of major and minor depression (Henshaw et al, 2004). Depression was almost three times more likely to occur in women with severe blues, their depressive episodes onset earlier in the puerperium, lasted longer and were more likely to be associated with major than minor depression. In Nigeria, a strong relationship between scores on the Yoruba translation of the Maternity Blues Scale on day 5 postpartum and major or minor depression at 4 and 8 weeks after delivery has been observed (Adewuya, 2006). It is also clear that women who are elated in the early puerperium are also more likely to become depressed at a later date (Hannah et al, 1993; Glover et al, 1994).

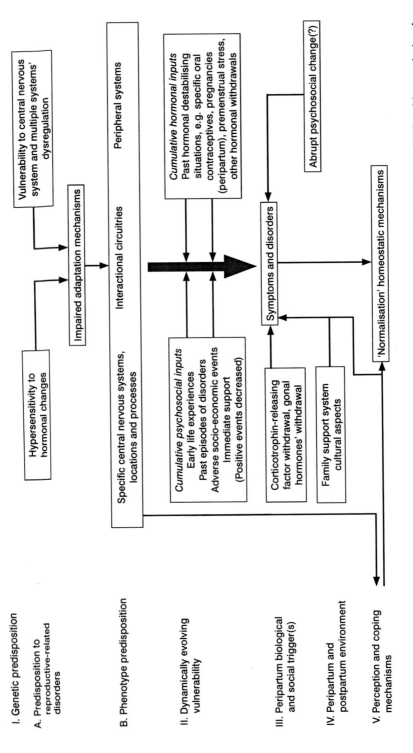

Fig. 2.1 A bio-psychosocial-cultural model of the process leading to postpartum disorders. From Halbreich, 2005, with permission from Elsevier.

Heron *et al* (2005) have reviewed the literature on early postnatal euphoria and pose the question as to whether it is an indicator of bipolarity.

Life events, adversity and social support

Stressful life events are known to trigger the onset of unipolar depression. Additional life events occurring during pregnancy were found to be strong predictors in O'Hara & Swain's meta-analysis (1996) and women who have depression after delivery experience more life events and more negative life events in the preceding 12 months than women who do not become depressed (Oretti *et al*, 2003). Those with a prior history of major depression are more likely to relapse within 6 months of delivery if they experience a stressful life event in the 12 months before illness onset (Marks *et al*, 1992).

However, O'Hara & Swain (1996) found no relationship with life events in Asian populations and a Brazilian study reports similar findings (Faisal-Cury *et al*, 2004). A Lebanese study found no relationship in a Beirut sample but one of borderline significance in a rural area (Chaaya *et al*, 2002).

Domestic violence has an association with high EPDS scores in pregnant and postpartum women (Leung *et al*, 2002; Bacchus *et al*, 2003) and three systematic reviews have identified a consistent negative relationship between poor social support and postnatal depression (Beck 1996, 2001; O'Hara & Swain, 1996; Robertson *et al*, 2004).

There is some evidence that poor parenting is a risk factor (Boyce *et al*, 1991a). The prevalence of women with a history of child sexual abuse ranges from 9 to 23%; women with histories of child sexual abuse are over-represented in psychiatric populations. Fifty per cent of women admitted to an Australian mother and baby unit (with major depression or adjustment disorders) had histories of child sexual abuse that was associated with higher scores on the Beck Depression Inventory (BDI), longer admissions and impaired mother–infant interactions (Buist, 1998). Follow-up 2.5–3.5 years later found that those with child sexual abuse histories had higher depression scores and more life stresses than controls (Buist & Janson, 2001). Battle *et al* (2006) reported 15% of perinatal psychiatric patients as having a history of physical abuse and 22% a history of child sexual abuse. A North American telephone survey of 200 postpartum women found childhood emotional abuse (but not physical or sexual abuse) predicted postnatal depression (Cohen *et al*, 2002).

Socio-demographic factors

Low family income, unemployment, lower social status and mother's occupation are associated with a significant increased risk of postnatal depression (Robertson *et al*, 2004; Segre *et al*, 2007).

Obstetric factors

Obstetric factors, including pregnancy and delivery complications, have a small but significant effect on the development of depression after delivery. However, some specific interventions may be important. Women who conceive via assisted reproductive technologies are more likely to experience depressive symptoms postpartum (relative risk (RR)=4; Fisher *et al*, 2005) and those delivered by Caesarean section have a more negative cognitive appraisal of delivery and higher level of post-traumatic stress disorder (PTSD) symptoms (Ryding *et al*, 1997, 1998). However, despite earlier studies suggesting a relationship between Caesarean section and postnatal depression, a recent meta-analysis concluded 'a link between Caesarean section and postpartum depression has not been established' (Carter *et al*, 2006).

Early discharge from hospital after birth is associated with higher levels of distress (Lane *et al*, 1999) and depression (Hickey *et al*, 1997).

Women whose previous pregnancy has ended in stillbirth experience higher levels of depressive and anxiety symptomatology in the third trimester of the next pregnancy and a trend towards more depressive symptoms at 1 year postpartum if they became pregnant less than 12 months after the stillbirth (Hughes *et al*, 1999).

Physical health problems associated with depressive symptoms 7–9 months after delivery include tiredness, urinary incontinence, back pain, sexual problems, increased coughs and colds, and bowel problems (Brown & Lumley, 2000), and there is an association between low haemoglobin levels on day 7 postpartum and depressive symptoms on day 28 (Corwin *et al*, 2003).

A large study examining outcomes in women who experienced severe obstetric morbidity (massive haemorrhage, pre-eclampsia, sepsis or uterine rupture) found those with high EPDS scores took longer to resume sexual activity and were more likely to cite fear of becoming pregnant again as a reason for this (Waterstone *et al*, 2003).

Personality

Premorbid personality is an important vulnerability factor. In addition to neuroticism, hostility, anxiety, a perception of being out of control during pregnancy and a negative cognitive attributional style have been found to be associated with postnatal depressive symptoms (Hayworth *et al*, 1980; O'Hara *et al*, 1982; Cutrona, 1983) as has interpersonal sensitivity (Boyce *et al*, 1991*b*). Women scoring high on the Vulnerable Personality Scale are at increased risk of depression (Boyce, 2003) as are those with 'immature defence styles' and attachment styles that are characterised by anxiety over relationships (McMahon *et al*, 2005). Insecure avoidant attachment styles are associated with antenatal depression, whereas insecure enmeshed styles are associated with postnatal depression (Bifulco *et al*, 2004). Church *et al* (2005) have suggested that dysfunctional cognitions mediate the relationship between risk factors and postpartum depressive symptoms.

Marital relationship

A poor marital relationship during pregnancy is a risk factor observed in many studies. Paykel *et al* (1980) found poor marital support to be a vulnerability factor leading to depression. Women who report that their partners are not easy to talk to, do not give emotional support, provide low levels of care, are over-controlling or who reported global dissatisfaction with the relationship are more likely to experience puerperal depression (Boyce *et al*, 1991a; Boyce, 2003).

Social support

Poor social support during pregnancy is predictive of postnatal depression with lack of support from the baby's father associated with high levels of symptoms. Lack of perceived support from a woman's primary support group and lack of support in relation to becoming pregnant are risk factors in first-time mothers (Brugha *et al*, 1998) but the size of a woman's primary social network does not seem to be important. Women reporting that they were unable to access satisfactory support in a crisis or were dissatisfied with the psychological support received after a crisis were at increased risk (Boyce, 2003). In India, where a woman often lives with her husband's family after marriage, a poor relationship with her mother-in-law has been identified as a risk factor for the development of postnatal depression (Chandran *et al*, 2002).

Sleep deprivation and fatigue

Two studies have demonstrated that fatigue is a predictor of depressed mood postpartum (Bozoky & Corwin 2002; Corwin *et al*, 2005). Ross *et al* (2005) reviewed the relationship between sleep and perinatal mood disorders, concluding that there is a significant relationship but that the evidence base is limited. The links between sleep deprivation and puerperal psychosis are discussed in Chapter 3.

Infant factors

It is clear that infant factors are independent risk factors for postnatal depression. Neonatal irritability and poor motor function have been shown to predict depression in first-time mothers (Murray *et al*, 1996) and infant sleep problems are associated with high EPDS scores (Hiscock & Wake, 2001). There is randomised controlled trial (RCT) evidence of a behavioural intervention which improves both infant sleep and maternal depressive symptoms (Hiscock & Wake, 2002).

Culture-specific factors, for example the preference for a son over a daughter, may be important in some communities (see Chapter 11).

Biological factors

The close temporal relationship between the rapid post-delivery decline in gonadal steroid hormones, cortisol, corticotrophin-releasing hormone and the onset of early puerperal mood change has led to the assumption that there must be a causal relationship with postnatal depression. Early studies of the role of biological risk factors which focused on hormone levels, correlating these with various measures of postnatal mood, have largely been unfruitful (Bloch *et al*, 2003).

17

However, a higher cortisol response to a psychosocial stress test in women who scored >9 on the EPDS within 13 days of delivery has been reported (Nierop et al, 2006), as has dysregulation of the hypothalamic–pituitary–adrenal (HPA) axis in women with depressive symptoms (Jolley et al, 2007) and higher day 3 oestradiol levels in women with major depressive disorder (Klier et al, 2007). Kammerer et al (2006) have reviewed the possible role of the HPA axis in perinatal affective disorders.

Challenge tests looking at functional neurotransmitter systems may be more likely to yield positive findings. Replicating the rapid post-delivery fall in gonadal steroids by administering a gonadotrophin-releasing hormone agonist to women who did and did not have histories of postnatal depression and then administering supraphysiological doses of oestradiol and progesterone and withdrawing under double-blind conditions led to 62.5% of the women with a history of depression developing mood symptoms during the withdrawal period, providing indirect evidence that women with past postnatal depression are sensitive to mood-destabilising effects of gonadal steroids (Bloch et al, 2000).

The growth hormone response to apomorphine is a measure of the functional state of D_2 receptors. This was measured in 14 postpartum women currently well but with a history of major depression. Five women who went on to relapse had enhanced growth hormone responses (suggesting increased sensitivity of D_2 receptors) that were particularly marked in those who had anxiety disorders (McIvor et al, 1996).

Newport et al (2004) identified alterations in serotonin transporter binding in women with postnatal depression (compared with healthy women and pregnant women with depression, and healthy postpartum women).

Lowering serum cholesterol is associated with violent death and suicide. Scrum cholesterol rises during pregnancy and falls rapidly after delivery. This fall is associated with depressed mood in the first 4 days postpartum (Ploeckinger et al, 1996). Lower cholesterol levels are associated with fatigue and depressed mood (Nasta et al, 2002), anxiety, anger and irritability (Troisi et al, 2002). The latter group also found lower high-density lipoprotein concentrations associated with anxiety. However, van Dam et al (1999) followed 266 women from 32 weeks gestation until 34 weeks postpartum and found little to support the hypothesis that the rapidity of cholesterol decline is associated with postnatal depression.

Alterations in serum fatty acid composition have been observed in major depression. One study found lower serum n-3 polyunsaturated fatty acid levels in women who went on to develop a postpartum major depressive episode compared with those who remained euthymic (de Vriese et al, 2003) and another demonstrated lower docosahexaenoic acid levels at 32 weeks postpartum in women with EPDS scores >10 (Otto et al, 2003).

Clara cell protein is a natural immunosuppressor and anti-inflammatory protein thought to have a role in inflammatory response system activation in mental disorders. Serum concentrations appear to be lower in women with postpartum major or minor depression (Maes *et al*, 1999). Recently delivered women with a history of major depression have been shown to have greater activation of the inflammatory response system in the first 3 days postpartum than women without such a history (Maes *et al*, 2001).

Thyroid dysfunction is well known to be associated with mood disturbance and follows around 10% of deliveries. Pop *et al* (1991) and Harris *et al* (1989) both found an association between thyroid dysfunction (measured by T3, T4 and thyroid stimulating hormone) and depression after childbirth, but a later study (Lucas *et al*, 2001) failed to replicate this.

Around 10% of women of childbearing age are thyroid antibody positive. Those who are positive during pregnancy are more likely to develop clinical thyroid disease and depression after delivery (Harris *et al*, 1992; Kuijpens *et al*, 2001) but giving thyroxine daily to such women after delivery does not prevent the onset of depression (Harris *et al*, 2002). Pregnant women with total and free thyroxine concentrations in the lower euthyroid range may be more likely to develop depression postpartum (Pedersen *et al*, 2007).

Genetics

Genetic factors are estimated to explain 38% of the variance in depressive symptoms postpartum and 25% of DSM–IV postpartum major depression (Treloar *et al*, 1999). Having a postpartum depressive episode predicts a sibling's depression after delivery (odds ratio (OR) = 3.97; Murphy-Ebernez *et al*, 2006). Significant associations between tryptophan hydroxylase gene polymorphisms and depression, anxiety and comorbid depression and anxiety in postpartum women have been demonstrated (Sun *et al*, 2004) and familial factors appear to be important in the vulnerability to triggering narrowly defined postpartum episodes (onset within 6–8 weeks of delivery) in women with recurrent depressive disorder (Forty *et al*, 2006).

Depression during pregnancy

Depressive symptoms are more prevalent during pregnancy than in the postpartum period (Green & Murray 1994: Evans *et al*, 2001; Josefsson *et al*, 2001) and in non-childbearing women (O'Hara *et al*, 1990). However, rates of depressive disorder diagnosed by standardised interview appear to be similar in the months before and after delivery (e.g. O'Hara, 1986; Cooper *et al*, 1988; O'Hara, *et al*, 1990) and similar to those in non-childbearing populations.

A systematic review and meta-analysis of prevalence studies (Bennett *et al*, 2004) confirmed rates of 7.4%, 12.8% and 12.0% in the first, second and third trimesters respectively. A large Swedish study which screened 1734 consecutive attendees of routine ultrasound screening found 3.3% of women had major depression, 6.9% minor depression and 6.6% anxiety disorders. Only 5.5% of those diagnosed had had any treatment (Andersson *et al*, 2003).

Depressive symptoms in women attending inner city antenatal clinics are associated with low educational status, being unmarried, unemployed, being in a second or subsequent pregnancy, having poor social and partner support, and chronic stressors (such as housing and financial problems) (Séguin et al, 1995; Bolton et al, 1998). A Swedish study reported more than two life events in the year before pregnancy and a native language other than Swedish as risk factors. Risk factors for primiparous women were unfortunate timing of pregnancy, previous miscarriage and age <25, whereas for multiparous women, lack of support from her partner when returning home with a newborn, single status, negative experience in a previous birth and unemployment were important.

A US study of women from Black and minority ethnic groups found that perceived social support and an avoidant coping style were associated with depressed mood in pregnancy, accounting for 34% of the variance (Rudnicki et al, 2001). Women reporting less social support tend to use avoidant coping strategies such as denial and experience higher levels of depressed mood. Loss of a parent or separation for over a year before the age of 16 has also been found to be associated with depressive disorder in pregnancy (Kitamura et al, 1994). Black pregnant women in the eastern USA have higher levels of depressive symptoms than White women (Orr et al, 2006).

Women reporting a history of child sexual abuse are more likely to experience depressive symptoms during pregnancy (Benedict et al, 1999) and those with a history of physical or sexual abuse or both are more likely to experience suicidal ideation (Farber et al, 1996).

In Kuwait, 16.9% of pregnant women had experienced assault or victimisation, with 9% suffering physical assault in the past month (Nayak & Al-Yattama, 1999). Assault history, with marital conflict, family stress and stressful life events were all associated with depressive symptoms; assault history remained a significant predictor even when the other variables were controlled for. A study in London found 23.5% of women had a lifetime history of domestic violence, 3% reporting this during the current pregnancy. Those with a history of domestic violence were more likely to have depressive symptoms, to have smoked during and/or in the year prior to pregnancy and to be single, separated or living alone (Mezey et al, 2005). Depressive, somatic and PTSD symptoms are higher in pregnant women who report intimate partner abuse or sexual coercion (Varma et al, 2007). These are often associated with alcohol misuse in the partner.

Depression in the year before delivery is an independent risk factor for sudden infant death syndrome along with smoking and having a male infant (Howard et al, 2007). Depressive symptoms are associated with substance misuse, smoking and psychosocial difficulties (Pritchard, 1994; Pajulo et al, 2001). Women with depression find it harder to stop smoking when they become pregnant (Ludman et al, 2000). Substance misuse, depression and a history of physical or sexual abuse are closely related in pregnancy (Horrigan et al, 2000).

High-risk pregnancy does not appear to lead to increased psychological distress (Dulude *et al*, 2002).

Anxiety, stress and adjustment

Anxiety symptoms are as common as depression after delivery and possibly more prevalent during pregnancy (Ross & McLean, 2006). Anxiety during pregnancy has been identified as an independent predictor of childhood behavioural and emotional problems (O'Connor *et al*, 2002).

Rates of between 5 and 57% have been reported in postpartum populations (Stuart *et al*, 1998; Brockington *et al*, 2006) and between 4 and 16% of new mothers meet DSM–IV criteria for generalised anxiety disorder, panic or phobia (Wenzel *et al*, 2003). A US study found postpartum prevalence rates of 8.2% for generalised anxiety disorder (higher than in the general population of women), 1.4% for panic disorder and 4.1% for social phobia (Wenzel *et al*, 2005). Anxiety symptoms frequently coexist with depressive symptoms and comorbid generalised anxiety disorder, and major depression is also common (Beeghly *et al*, 2002).

Common themes of severe anxiety during pregnancy are fear of foetal loss (particularly if there is a history of reproductive loss or fertility problems) or abnormality, whereas after delivery the fear of cot death or of mothering skills being criticised are most common. A comprehensive review is found in Brockington *et al* (2006).

In non-puerperal depression, the presence of anxiety symptoms renders episodes more severe and long lasting than episodes without anxiety symptoms. One small study suggests that this might also be the case for postnatal depression (Hendrick *et al*, 2000).

A large US community study of postpartum women with depressive symptoms found 11% experiencing panic attacks, 8% obsessional thoughts and 9% compulsions (Wenzel *et al*, 2001). Overall, 2.3% had both subsyndromal panic and obsessive–compulsive disorder symptoms, while 1.5% met DSM–IV criteria for panic disorder and 3.9% for obsessive–compulsive disorder; 1% had comorbid major depressive disorder and panic disorder, 2.4% had major depression comorbid with obsessive–compulsive disorder. Ross & McLean (2006) have systematically reviewed the relationship between panic disorder, generalised anxiety disorder, PTSD and obsessive–compulsive disorder and pregnancy and the postpartum period.

Around half of postnatal mothers with depression experience intrusive obsessional thoughts that are frequently aggressive in nature and directed towards their infant (Wisner *et al*, 1999a). Obsessions of infanticide have been reported in the literature since the late 1950s (Button & Reivich, 1972). Careful history taking is essential in order to distinguish between obsessions of infanticide and thoughts of harming an infant that a mother may be at risk of carrying out.

21

Obsessional symptoms are commonly centred on cleaning or hand washing, and concerns that the infant might ingest something dirty or be contaminated with germs. Checking compulsions tend to focus on the infant's health and in particular whether they are still breathing during the night and have not died from sudden infant death syndrome (Weightman *et al*, 1998). The relationship between obsessive–compulsive symptoms, pregnancy and the puerperium has been reviewed by Abramowitz *et al* (2003).

Distress, measured by self-report scales, was found to occur in 37% of new mothers and 13% of new fathers, but only 9% of mothers and 2% of fathers reported severe intrusive stress (Skari *et al*, 2002). Rates had fallen to similar levels to those in the general population by 6 weeks and to 6 months after delivery. Being a single parent, multiparity and previous trauma in childbirth were predictors of severe distress.

Post-traumatic stress disorder in relation to childbirth has been described in the literature since the late 1970s. Rates in the postpartum population are estimated at between 1 and 5.6% (Creedy *et al*, 2000; Czarnocka & Slade 2000; Ayers & Pickering, 2001; Söderquist *et al*, 2006). They are higher (7.7%) in disadvantaged pregnant women (Loveland Cook *et al*, 2004). One small study based on self-report measures has found a prevalence of 28% after preterm delivery and 17% after pre-eclampsia (Engelhard *et al*, 2002) but the relationship between PTSD and specific obstetric interventions or mode of delivery is inconsistent.

Predictors of PTSD symptoms include perceptions of low levels of support from staff and partner, pain in the first stage, low perceived control and feelings of powerlessness in labour, increased medical intervention, trait anxiety, past history of mental health problems, and a history of sexual trauma and social support (Czarnocka & Slade, 2000; Soet *et al*, 2003). Mothers who have a very low-birth-weight infant report more distress at 1 month postpartum and continue to do so at 1 year if their infant remains at high risk. At 3 years, mothers report more parenting stress (Singer *et al*, 1999). Women who had previously delivered a stillborn infant had rates of PTSD of 21% in the third trimester of a subsequent pregnancy which had dropped to 4% after 1 year postpartum. The likelihood of PTSD was increased with a shorter interval between the stillbirth and the current pregnancy (Turton *et al*, 2001). However, the sample followed by Söderquist *et al* (2006) had no reduction in symptoms over the course of a year.

Querulant (or complaining) disorder has also been described in relation to stressful deliveries where women are so dissatisfied that they develop a morbid preoccupation with it and their mental health and functioning is substantially impaired. It is associated with PTSD (Brockington *et al*, 2006).

Phobic anxiety

Sved-Williams (1992) reports that 13.6% of 66 mothers admitted to a mother and baby unit experienced phobic avoidance of their infant sufficiently severe to warrant management in its own right. A behavioural programme involving exposure is the recommended treatment.

Tokophobia is an intense dread of childbirth that can lead to women avoiding pregnancy, terminating the pregnancy of a very much wanted baby or demanding a Caesarean section in subsequent pregnancies (Hofberg & Brockington, 2000). It can be classified as:

- primary in a nulliparous woman
- secondary if she has had previous traumatic deliveries
- secondary to a depressive illness or PTSD during pregnancy.

Heimstad *et al* (2006) report the prevalence of serious fear as 5.5% and associated with elective Caesarean section delivery. The aetiology is multifactoral and may involve:

- transmission of fear of childbirth over generations
- a woman's appraisal of her last delivery and associated anxiety
- a history of sexual abuse or assault, or traumatic gynaecological examination.

Women with a history of sexual abuse are less likely to have an uncomplicated vaginal delivery at term.

Panic disorder

De Armond (1954) described a case series in which 'sudden panic-like fear without precipitating cause' onset shortly after leaving hospital. Panic disorder occurs for the first time in the postpartum period more often than is expected in the general population, with 10.9% of women with panic disorder reporting postpartum onset (age-corrected estimate=0.92%; Sholomskas *et al*, 1993) but this was a retrospective study. A qualitative study of mothers with postpartum-onset panic disorder described how it became a great struggle to manage their attacks, leading to negative changes in their lifestyles and lowered self-esteem (Beck, 1998). The impact of pregnancy and the postpartum period on pre-existing panic disorder is described in Chapter 4.

Obsessive–compulsive disorder

Obsessive–compulsive disorder may onset for the first time during pregnancy or postpartum (e.g. Sichel *et al*, 1993*a*; Arnold 1999; Labad *et al*, 2005). The incidence is estimated at 4% at 6 weeks postpartum (Uguz *et al*, 2007). More than a third of parous women with obsessive–compulsive disorder report their first onset as occurring during pregnancy (Neziroglu *et al*, 1992) and there is a report of a woman who experienced first-onset obsessive–compulsive disorder after the birth of her first baby going into remission after treatment. Three years later she had a recurrence after her second child (Hertzberg *et al*, 1997). There are two case reports of the onset of obsessive–compulsive disorder in the fourth month of pregnancy that resolved spontaneously after delivery (Iancu *et al*, 1995; Kalra *et al*, 2005).

A case series of 15 women with new-onset puerperal obsessive–compulsive disorder found all were experiencing intrusive thoughts of harming their infants and had developed some degree of avoidance of their babies (Sichel *et al*, 1993*b*). None went on to harm their infants. Nine went on to develop a secondary depressive illness and ten were admitted during the acute phase of their illness. A year later, most were still taking medication (selective serotonin reuptake inhibitors (SSRIs) or clomipramine) and continued with some intrusive thoughts. None had developed checking or other compulsions. A case–control study of women with postpartum-onset obsessive–compulsive disorder found the onset was within 4 weeks of delivery and they reported significantly more aggressive obsessions (about harming the baby) than did controls who had not had postpartum onset (Maina *et al*, 1999).

Postpartum-onset obsessive–compulsive disorder can recur after later pregnancies and therefore a woman with a previous history should be monitored closely and if symptoms recur, rapid intervention offered. There is at present no evidence base to support the use of prophylactic medication but this is recommended (Brandes *et al*, 2004). Fathers have also been reported as experiencing first-onset obsessive–compulsive disorder coinciding with pregnancy or the birth of a child (Abramowitz *et al*, 2001). Pregnancy and the postpartum period in women with pre-existing obsessive–compulsive disorder is described in Chapter 4.

Adjustment and transition

Becoming a new mother or the mother of an additional child requires adjustment to a new set of personal and social circumstances. Cultural expectations that this is an inevitably easy and pleasurable experience may lead to idealised views of what motherhood should be like and render women vulnerable to depression when there is conflict between expectation and experience (Mauthner, 1998). Lack of comfort with the maternal role and low measures of maternal role attainment have been associated with postnatal depressive symptoms (Fowles, 1998).

The loss of ritual and traditional practices around birth and new motherhood has also been hypothesised as a causative factor (Seel, 1986; Cox, 1994). Psychologists writing from a feminist perspective argue that depression is a rational response to the loss and isolation resulting from childbirth and should not be medicalised. Nicolson (1998) argues that 'postnatal depression needs to be reconceptualised as part of the normal experience of motherhood'.

Cheryl Beck has undertaken a metasynthesis of 18 qualitative studies of postnatal depression from the 1960s to the 1990s. She identified common themes that brought together illustrate four different perspectives on postnatal depression (Beck, 2002):

- incongruity between expectations and the reality of motherhood
- spiralling downward
- pervasive loss
- making gains.

Pregnancy loss

Pregnancy loss is common, occurring after 15–20% of confirmed pregnancies and usually during the first trimester (Frost & Condon, 1996; Lee & Slade, 1996). Stillbirths after 24 weeks gestation account for 0.5% of births in England and Wales (MacFarlane *et al*, 2000). Mental disorder, particularly affective illness and substance misuse increase the risk of pregnancy loss (OR=1.8; Gold *et al*, 2007).

Studies have shown that women who miscarry have higher levels of depressive and anxiety symptoms (Neugebauer *et al*, 1992; Thapar & Thapar, 1992; Janssen *et al*, 1996; Brier, 2005), with those who are childless at highest risk (Neugebauer *et al*, 1992).

They are also at increased risk of minor (Klier *et al*, 2000) and major depression (Neugebauer *et al*, 1997) and a recurrent episode of obsessive–compulsive disorder (Geller *et al*, 2001). In the last study, over half of the women with a past history of depression had a recurrence after miscarrying.

Symptoms in mothers who experience stillbirth or neonatal death can persist for up to 30 months after the loss (Boyle *et al*, 1996). A comparison of attachment in infants born to mothers who had lost their child after 18 weeks gestation and controls found that those born subsequent to pregnancy loss had increased disorganised attachment to their mothers. This was predicted by maternal unresolved status with respect to loss (Hughes *et al*, 2001). Fathers also report anxiety and depression after stillbirth or neonatal death but at a lower level than mothers (Badenhorst *et al*, 2006; Cumming *et al*, 2007).

There is a non-significant trend towards having PTSD in pregnancy after a stillbirth if the mother has been encouraged to see or to hold the dead infant (Turton *et al*, 2001). Therefore this practice is not advised. Community follow-up should be arranged for women who experience stillbirth or neonatal death.

A large study of pregnant women reported that 121 out of 1370 women miscarried, most before 20 weeks. One month later, the prevalence of DSM–IV PTSD was 25%. These women were more likely to report depression and 4 months later 7% still met PTSD criteria. Length of gestation at the time of loss was associated with higher levels of PTSD symptoms (Engelhard *et al*, 2001). Of the women who miscarried, 70% reported peri-traumatic dissociation. This was predicted by prior low control of emotions, a tendency to dissociate and a lower educational level. It was not related to neuroticism or prior life events (Engelhard *et al*, 2003).

A recent UK study explored symptomatic women's experiences of miscarriage, the care they received and the views of primary healthcare professionals (Wong *et al*, 2003). The women felt a need for formal follow-up (there is currently no systematic follow-up for women who miscarry; they are expected to seek help if they need it). They felt unable to absorb information during their hospital stay and felt confused, wanted more specific information and answers to questions, and found the normalisation of miscarriage by healthcare professionals distressing. There was a tendency to feel guilty and have a sense of failure. The response to the care they received varied greatly and the health professionals interviewed identified skills deficits. The authors recommend that health visitors should be formally notified of a woman who has miscarried so that they can undertake a 6–8 week check of psychological and psychiatric morbidity, as they do with women who have delivered a live child.

How these risk factors might be incorporated into screening programmes and used during pregnancy to identify vulnerable women is discussed in Chapter 7.

Geller *et al* (2006) have reviewed a wide range of internet resources which health professionals and women might find helpful.

Termination of pregnancy

In 2007, 198 500 pregnancies were terminated on therapeutic grounds (National Statistics & Department of Health, 2007). A large number of studies have addressed the issue of abortion and subsequent mental health. Some appear to suggest that abortion increases the risk of depression, anxiety, suicidal behaviours and substance use disorders (e.g. Fergusson *et al*, 2006). However, this study has limitations (as do many others); for example, the comparison groups were women who had children and women who did not become pregnant. The authors are careful to say that their findings do not imply a causative link between abortion and mental health problems. Although the majority of women seeking termination may not be at risk in the same way that women identified and reviewed as being vulnerable to depression after miscarriage might be, those who are particularly vunerable at the time of undergoing termination of preganancy are also at risk. Those particularly at risk appear to be very young women, who are often multiply disadvantaged (Fergusson *et al*, 2006), those undergoing late termination for foetal anomaly (Davies *et al*, 2005; Korenromp *et al*, 2005; Kersting *et al*, 2007) and others listed in Box 2.2.

There are historical reports of psychosis following both termination and miscarriage (Brockington, 2005) and one study found that admission rates for bipolar disorder increased after abortion (Reardon *et al*, 2003). There appears to be no difference in depressive or anxiety symptoms whether women have a medical or surgical termination (Ashok *et al*, 2005).

Box 2.2 Risk factors for psychological disturbance after termination of pregnancy

- Negative religious or cultural attitudes
- Lack of support from social network
- Unstable relationship with partner
- Past psychiatric history
- Older multiparous women with children
- Therapeutic abortion for foetal anomaly

From Zolese & Blacker, 1992

Impact of anxiety and depression during pregnancy on obstetric outcomes

A variety of poor outcomes have been reported as being associated with either depression or anxiety during pregnancy including:

- pre-eclampsia
- increased nausea and vomiting, longer sick leave during pregnancy, and an increased number of visits to the obstetrician
- elective Caesarean delivery and epidural analgesia during labour
- admission of the infant to neonatal care
- spontaneous preterm labour
- preterm delivery
- low birth weight.

Field *et al* (2006), on reviewing the literature, concluded that increased foetal activity, delayed intrauterine growth, prematurity and low birth weight occur more frequently if there is maternal depression during pregnancy, while a systematic review of the literature published between 1990 and 2005 concluded that 'the majority of the reviewed studies did identify a negative influence of symptoms of anxiety and depression on obstetric, foetal and neonatal outcome measures' (Alder *et al*, 2007). However, a meta-analysis of the association between pregnancy anxiety and gestational age at birth and birth weight failed to demonstrate a link (Littleton *et al*, 2007).

There is a growing literature describing the impact of depression during pregnancy on the foetus and neonate. Van den Bergh *et al* (2005) identified 14 independent studies showing a link between maternal anxiety and stress and cognitive, behavioural and emotional problems in the child. The links between maternal depression and anxiety during and after pregnancy are further explored in Chapter 6.

Assessment and management

This chapter addresses the community assessment and management of women with non-psychotic disorder. The assessment and treatment of those with psychosis or who require in-patient admission will be addressed in Chapter 4.

Assessment

This is essentially the same as standard psychiatric history and examination but takes into consideration the context and the fact that there is a foetus or infant (and possibly other children) who must be accounted for in decisions relating to treatments and risk assessment. Hence, the social and psychological background of the pregnancy and the postpartum, the physical health in relation to pregnancy and delivery, and the relationship with the infant should all be systematically enquired about. In addition, screening for some symptoms requires adaptation when a women is pregnant or has a baby. For example, when screening for obsessional intrusive thoughts, Brandes et al (2004) suggest all postpartum women should be asked a simple screening question:

> It is not uncommon for new mothers to experience intrusive and unwanted thoughts that they might harm their baby. Have any thoughts like that happened to you?'

A positive answer should be followed up with probes for the frequency and intensity of thoughts and for any thoughts or reports of actually harming the infant. A woman who is suicidal should be considered as highly likely to involve her infant in any act of self-harm.

Questions relating to sleep, appetite, fatigue, activity levels and libido must take into consideration the norms for the stage of pregnancy or the postpartum.

As in any other situation, unusual symptoms should prompt consideration of alternative diagnoses. A 37-year-old woman presented with mood symptoms then progressive hyperphagia, hypersexuality, disinhibition and impaired judgement postpartum. She was treated for depression for months before a frontotemporal dementia was dignosed (Dell & Halford, 2002). Women with serious physical illness have died owing to their symptoms being wrongly attributed to mental disorder, for example tachycardia of 140–160 being attributed to panic attacks and anxiety when in fact the patient had sepsis and cardiac arrhythmia (Lewis & Drife, 2004).

Interventions for depression

There are several reviews of treatment studies of postnatal depression (e.g. Boath & Henshaw, 2001; Dennis, 2004; Dennis & Stewart, 2004; Boath et al, 2007; Morrell, 2008). Many studies have methodological limitations, and thus the number of studies that can be entered into systematic reviews is restricted. At the time of writing, five have been completed (Lawrie *et al*, 2000; Granger & Underwood, 2001; Hoffbrand *et al*, 2001; Bledsoe & Grote, 2006; Dennis & Hodnett, 2007), the last two including meta-analyses. Almost all studies have small sample sizes. Bledsoe & Grote (2006) found the largest effect sizes were for cognitive–behavioural therapy (CBT) or medication alone, followed by group therapies, individual therapies, counselling and education. Postpartum implementations provided larger effect sizes than interventions delivered during pregnancy. The RCTs of psychological and psychosocial interventions are outlined in Appendix I.

Psychological therapies

Rogerian non-directive counselling, offered by UK health visitors and Swedish child health nurses, has been shown to be superior to standard care for mild to moderate cases of postnatal depression (Holden *et al*, 1989; Wickberg & Hwang, 1996). Many health visitors now offer a limited number of such 'listening visits' (usually four to eight, each lasting around an hour) to women in their homes. However, training and supervision vary, as does the availability of specialist secondary services for women for whom this approach is unsuitable or who do not respond to the intervention.

A qualitative study of women who had received listening visits revealed that they felt positive about the intervention if they had a prior good relationship with their health visitor but were less positive if that relationship was poor. Women perceived the intervention as supportive rather than therapeutic and attributed their recovery to other factors (Shakespeare *et al*, 2006). Morse *et al* (2004) evaluated the effectiveness of training Australian maternal and child health nurses in the early detection and management of new mothers with mild distress. These nurses had access to a liaison psychiatric network that provided support and consultation. There was no difference in the rates or levels of distress or psychosocial functioning between the intervention group and those receiving routine care. However, satisfaction with the intervention was high. Nursing care (six weekly visits) was superior to problem-solving when administered to women with high EPDS scores in the first week postpartum (Tezel & Gozum, 2006).

Health visitors can also be trained in cognitive–behavioural counselling skills. This intervention comprised childcare advice, reassurance, encouraging participation in enjoyable activities, accessing support from others and setting targets. Both cognitive–behavioural counselling (Appleby *et al*, 1997) and CBT (Misri *et al*, 2004) have been shown to be as effective as antidepressant treatment for postnatal major depression, but cognitive–behavioural counselling or CBT in addition to drug treatment did not confer any additional benefit. However, the trials are small and may be underpowered to detect any difference. Training health visitors in cognitive–behavioural counselling not only improved their skills but also improved screening and treatment, and increased referral rates to mental health services (Appleby *et al*, 2003).

In their meta-analysis, Bledsoe & Grote (2006) found larger effect sizes (>0.95) when medication was combined with CBT, interpersonal psychotherapy and group therapy with cognitive–behavioural, educational or transactional analysis components, and smaller effect sizes (<0.75) or no effect when the interventions used counselling, educational or psychodynamic approaches. The largest effect size was for medication in combination with CBT, followed by medication alone, then group therapy with cognitive–behavioural, educational or transactional analysis components.

Non-directive counselling, CBT and dynamic psychotherapy have all been shown in a RCT to have an impact on depressive symptoms, but only dynamic therapy was superior to a control in reducing depressive disorder (Cooper et al, 2003).

Interpersonal psychotherapy is a time-limited, manualised therapy that focuses on four main problem areas: grief, interpersonal disputes, role transitions and interpersonal deficits. It consists of three phases. The initial phase covers assessment, psychoeducation, selection of a treatment focus and negotiation of a treatment agreement. The problems are then worked on in the intermediate phase and a discussion of the progress made and how the patient feels about termination is carried out at the end.

Interpersonal psychotherapy has been adapted to deal with issues facing women with postpartum depression such as the relationship with the baby and partner, and returning to work, and there is one small RCT demonstrating efficacy (O'Hara et al, 2000). Klier et al (2001) reported an open trial of 12 sessions of interpersonal psychotherapy in a group setting. The participants received two individual sessions prior to the group intervention in order to explain how the group would work and three women required additional individual crisis management during the group intervention.

Interpersonal psychotherapy has also been adapted for use in pregnant women with depression with a focus on role transition in relation to pregnancy, interpersonal disputes related to pregnancy and motherhood, and complicated pregnancies (Spinelli & Endicott, 2003). Interpersonal counselling, a shorter intervention delivered by telephone aimed at distress rather than clinical depression, has been shown to reduce depressive symptoms in women with sub-syndromal depression following a miscarriage (Neugebauer et al, 2007).

A modified form of Gruen therapy which encompasses relaxation techniques, problem-solving strategies and CBT delivered by telephone over a 10-week period by nurse therapists is reported in a small pilot study (Ugarriza & Schmidt, 2006). It resulted in reduced BDI scores and may be particularly suitable for house-bound mothers or those in remote rural areas.

Group interventions

Many interventions can be delivered in a group setting. Being part of a group can reduce the sense of isolation that many mothers with mental health problems feel and enable them to share experiences and coping strategies. It can also be a cost-effective way of delivering an intervention as several women can be treated at the same time. However, some mothers will have specific issues that may be better dealt with on a one-to-one basis and others may require some individual work before they feel able to cope with a group.

The majority of group treatments consist of several components, for example education, social support and CBT. They may involve partners in some or all sessions (Morgan *et al*, 1997; Misri *et al*, 2000; Ugarriza, 2004). Setting up, running and evaluating a group intervention has been described by Milgrom *et al* (1999). Their book includes material for all their group sessions.

Focused interventions can also be offered; for example, a psychoeducational group has been shown to be superior to routine primary care in reducing depressive symptoms (Honey *et al*, 2002). An uncontrolled study examining counselling in the voluntary sector reported success in treating women both individually and in groups with therapy based on Gestalt, person-centred and psychodynamic principles (Alder & Truman, 2002). Small studies suggest group interpersonal psychotherapy is effective in treating postnatal depression (Clark *et al*, 2003; Reay *et al*, 2006) but larger controlled studies are needed.

Mothers can be trained in baby massage one to one or in a group setting and this may improve mother–infant interaction (Onozawa *et al*, 2001). There is no evidence as yet that it has an impact on maternal mental disorder. Services may also offer groups (which are usually closed) targeted at mothers with specific problems, for example survivors of child sexual abuse, those who have been bereaved or adolescent mothers. Saisto *et al* (2006) describe a psychoeducational group approach to women with fear of childbirth which led to withdrawn requests for Caesarean section.

Social support is often the main focus or an important component of group treatment. Many health visitors have set up such groups, with some becoming self-help groups beyond the lifetime of the original group. Groups may be open or closed and consist of just mothers, or fathers may attend some or all of the sessions. There are, however, limited data relating to the efficacy of support groups and it is not clear whether they are superior to other interventions.

There is some evidence that exercise (group-based pram-walking programmes or individual support) can reduce postpartum depressive symptoms. These and the possible mechanisms by which exercise may have such an effect have been reviewed by Daley *et al* (2007). The feasibility of exercise as an intervention, however, might be limited by the difficulties in engaging women with postpartum depression in exercise programmes (Daley *et al*, 2008).

Information and education

Women with high EPDS scores 4 weeks after delivery were randomised to receive an information leaflet at 6 weeks postpartum or not. Those who received the leaflet had lower scores when reassessed at 3 months (Heh & Fu, 2003). Over 90% of those who had received the leaflet said that it was useful to them and their families. Many had not known about postnatal depression before reading it and because of this information those in the experimental group gained more practical help from their families. There are a number of organisations that provide information via literature, websites or telephone support lines. Some also offer befriending or practical help in the home (Appendix II).

Caution must be exercised with respect to websites as several have been found not to contain much useful information or their information does not accurately reflect the evidence base or state the science relating to postnatal depression (Summers & Logsdon, 2005).

Antidepressants

Compared with the large body of evidence supporting antidepressant treatment of major depressive disorder, there is relatively little evidence to guide the clinician treating postnatal depression. Efficacy is discussed here and issues related to drug and other physical treatments in pregnant and breastfeeding women are described in Chapters 8 and 9.

There are several open label studies. Eight women with DSM–IV major depressive disorder were treated for 8 weeks with bupropion sustained release using a flexible dosing schedule of between 150 and 400 mg/day. This resulted in a significant reduction of Hamilton Rating Scale for Depression (HRSD) scores but only three women achieved remission. The women were permitted to use zolpidem for insomnia and lorazepam for anxiety, and some were receiving psychotherapy, so the improvement cannot be attributed to the antidepressant alone (Nonacs et al, 2005). Two of the women were breastfeeding.

An open label study of nefazodone in doses up to 500 mg/day in four women (Suri et al, 2005) reported one dropping out due to lethargy and the others improving. Stowe et al (1995) treated 21 women with sertraline and 14 were reported to have achieved remission. Those with onsets less than 4 weeks postpartum appeared to respond more quickly and require less medication. Of 15 women who received venlafaxine in a mean dose of 162.5 mg/day (Cohen et al, 2001), 12 responded with an improvement in depressive and anxiety symptoms.

There is one double-blind RCT of sertraline v. nortriptyline. There were no differences between the two drugs with respect to time to response and remission, improvement in psychosocial functioning and in the total side-effect burden, although side-effect profiles differed (Wisner et al, 2006).

A chart review of women attending psychiatric out-patient services for treatment of postnatal depression noted that although they were as likely as non-postpartum women to respond to medication, their time to respond was longer and they were more likely to be taking more than one antidepressant at a time (Hendrick et al, 2000).

A small naturalistic study compared response to SSRIs and tricyclic antidepressants in women with postnatal depression: SSRIs appeared to be superior (Wisner *et al*, 1999*b*). Atypical augmentation of an SSRI when treating postpartum depression with intrusive obsessional thoughts resulted in resolution of resistant obsessional symptoms in a small case series (Corral *et al*, 2007).

Risks of discontinuing antidepressants during pregnancy

Women who discontinue antidepressants on discovering they are pregnant or who have taken them in the 2 years prior to conception and have stopped are more likely to report depressive symptoms during pregnancy (Marcus *et al*, 2005). They may even experience suicidal ideation or need admission (Einarson *et al*, 2001). Cohen *et al* (2004) followed up 32 women with a history of depression who were euthymic before discontinuing medication around the time of conception. Three-quarters relapsed during pregnancy, most in the first trimester, with 38% resuming their medication.

However, care must be taken when treating women with a family history of bipolar disorder with antidepressants as there are reports of this triggering psychosis, a mixed affective episode or hypomania (Sharma, 2006). The difficulties in treating pregnant women with depression are clearly articulated by Freeman (2007).

Hormones

The assumption that postnatal depression must have a hormonal aetiology led to attempts to treat the disorder with oestrogens, progesterone and progestogens.

Uncontrolled studies performed by Dalton (1985, 1989, 1995) claimed success with progesterone as a treatment and prevention, but the studies have serious methodological problems and, as yet, there are no controlled data to support this. A Cochrane review concludes:

> 'There is no place for synthetic progestogens in the prevention of treatment of postnatal depression. Long-acting norethisterone enanthate is associated with an increased risk of postnatal depression.' (Lawrie *et al*, 2000).

Two small studies (one uncontrolled, one RCT) support the use of oestradiol in the treatment of severe postnatal depression (Gregoire *et al*, 1996; Ahokas *et al*, 2001). It should be noted that most of the women had previous or concurrent antidepressant or psychological therapy, so oestradiol has not been tested as a monotherapy. There are also concerns about using high doses of oestradiol in the postnatal period, owing to the increased risk of deep-vein thrombosis, difficulties with breastfeeding and endometrial hyperplasia. The optimum dose and route of administration has not been established. Until more data are available, the use of oestradiol is best limited to use as adjunct therapy for severe depressive disorders in women with no additional risk factors for thromboembolic disease or hormone-dependent tumours. For a review see Gentile (2005).

Omega-3 fatty acids

There has been interest in exploring the role of omega-3 fatty acids in the treatment for postnatal depression. Supporting this is evidence that fish consumption and omega-3 status after childbirth are not associated with postnatal depression (Browne *et al*, 2006).

Chiu *et al* (2003) report a pregnant woman with depression being treated successfully at 24-weeks gestation with omega-3 fatty acids. Rees *et al* (2005) report an open trial in which 12 pregnant women with major depression achieved a 40% reduction in EPDS and HRSD scores, and Freeman *et al* (2006*a*) report 15 pregnant women with major depression achieving a 40% reduction in EPDS scores. A small RCT in which 16 women were randomised to 0.5, 1.4 or 2.8 g omega-3 fatty acids demonstrated significant improvement in EPDS and HRSD scores (Freeman *et al*, 2006*b*). There was no advantage in giving higher doses over 0.5 g. However, a later study by this group found no advantage over placebo in adding omega-3 fatty acids to supportive psychotherapy though the study may have been underpowered to detect any difference (Freeman *et al*, 2008).

Bright light therapy

There is an open trial of morning bright light therapy in pregnant women with major depression reporting improvement in depression scores and no adverse effects over 5 weeks (Oren *et al*, 2002). A small RCT with 10 pregnant women with major depression reported an effect size similar to that of antidepressants seen over 10 weeks (Epperson *et al*, 2004).

Sleep deprivation

Sleep deprivation may help pregnant and postpartum women with depression. Parry *et al* (2000) exposed nine women with major depressive disorder who were either pregnant or postpartum to late-night and early-night deprivation. More women responded to late-night deprivation and more responded after a night of recovery sleep. However, only pregnant women responded to early-night and not to late-night deprivation. Clearly further research with controlled conditions is needed.

Complementary therapies

Mantle (2002) reviewed herbalism, homeopathy, massage and hypnosis, supported by the House of Lords Select Committee on Science and Technology as having an evidence base, plus Ayurvedic and traditional Chinese medicine which are not. Her paper is intended to be a resource for health professionals (particularly health visitors) whose clients may reject conventional therapies and are looking for alternatives. Weier & Beal (2004) reviewed the role of complementary therapies on the treatment of postnatal depression and concluded that although these may be used as adjuncts to conventional treatment for moderately or severely ill women, there is almost no evidence base supporting their use in this condition and most health professionals would not know how to prescribe or provide many of the therapies.

Over a third of women use herbal medicine during pregnancy (Forster *et al*, 2006). Thirty per cent reported using complementary therapies. The most commonly used were massage, herbal medicine and acupuncture. A third were using more than one treatment. Schnyer *et al* (2003) have described the conceptual framework for the use of acupuncture to treat depression in pregnancy in two case studies and there is a case report of a woman successfully treated with hypnosis (Yexley, 2007).

Interventions for anxiety

Some of the psychological interventions described can be adapted to deal with anxiety symptoms, particularly CBT. In addition, some specific interventions have been developed for perinatal anxiety disorders, although the literature remains limited.

There are interventions for fear of delivery. One study gave women in the intervention group support from a psychosomatic gynaecologist (mean 3.4 sessions) and some received brief psychotherapy (mean 7.4 sessions) during pregnancy. Before the intervention, 68% had requested Caesarean section. Afterwards, this dropped to 38%. Obstetric outcomes in those who had vaginal deliveries were similar to controls but they were more likely to have had induced labour, epidural anaesthesia or a pudendal nerve block (Sjögren & Thomasson, 1997).

An RCT of an intervention comprising information, education and cognitive therapy delivered to pregnant women with fear of vaginal delivery produced a reduction in unnecessary Caesarean sections, pregnancy and birth-related concerns, and shorter labours when compared with a control group who received information only (Saisto *et al*, 2001).

Forty women randomised to video and verbal feedback during ultrasound examinations or usual care had reduced scores on the Spielberger State–Trait Anxiety Inventory (STAI), reduced foetal activity and fewer delivery complications (Field *et al*, 1985). Another study compared seven sessions of applied relaxation therapy with usual antenatal care in pregnant women with high scores on the STAI. The intervention group had significant reductions in anxiety symptoms and perceived stress (Bastani *et al*, 2005).

In Sweden, 'fear of childbirth teams' have been established to meet the needs of women with fears of delivery and/or who had previous traumatic labours. Midwives trained in counselling talked to the women and invited them to express their fears and devised individual birth plans. Although women were very satisfied with their care, those in the intervention group had more frightening experiences of delivery and higher rates of PTSD symptoms than those in the control group (Ryding *et al*, 2003).

Interventions for obsessive–compulsive disorder

There is no RCT evidence to guide the clinician in treating postpartum onset obsessive–compulsive disorder but management is likely to include CBT with exposure and response-prevention and/or thought-stopping. This might also be the treatment of choice in pregnant women to avoid foetal exposure to drugs. Support for the patient, her partner and family are essential. Women with obsessive–compulsive disorder may be afraid of being left alone with the infant in case they harm the baby. This can lead to pressures on the extended family and there are reports of fathers giving up work to be with their partner (Jennings *et al*, 1999).

Selective serotonin reuptake inhibitors venlafaxine and clomipramine have a substantial evidence base behind their use in obsessive–compulsive disorder and there are small open trials postpartum onset. Sichel *et al* (1993*a*) treated the women in her study with fluoxetine, clomipramine, desipramine or a combination of these and reported significant improvement in symptoms. Buttolph & Holland (1990) describe four women successfully treated with fluoxetine and Arnold (1999) reported a case series of seven women of whom three entered into an open-label trial of fluvoxamine 50–300 mg daily. Two of the three had more than 30% improvement in their score on the Yale–Brown Obsessive Compulsive Scale (YBOCS). A small, uncontrolled study of women with obsessive–compulsive disorder (most of whom had new onsets postpartum) who had not responded to 8 weeks of antidepressant therapy (SSRIs and serotonin noradrenaline reuptake inhibitors (SNRIs)) found that adding quetiapine produced a full response (assessed by YBOCS and Clinical Global Impression scale) in 11 out of 17 patients (Misri & Milis, 2004).

What do women think about treatments?

There is a small but growing literature exploring women's views on treatments for perinatal depression. Concerns about treatment may stem from a reluctance to be labelled as suffering from depression. Over 90% of mothers interviewed by Whitton *et al* (1996) recognised there was something wrong, but only a third believed they had postnatal depression. Primiparous women and those from social classes I (professional), II (semi-professional, e.g. teachers) and III (skilled manual, clerical) were less likely to recognise themselves as having depression. Over 80% had not reported their symptoms to any health professional and 81% said they would not consider antidepressants. A more recent study from Wales found that mothers had little knowledge of postnatal depression before pregnancy, felt that it happened to 'other people' and tended to shield their emotions from their family (Hanley & Long, 2006).

In a German study, only 18% of those offered a variety of interventions took up the offer. Thirty-nine per cent refused for what were described as 'factual reasons,' for example thinking that psychiatric or psychotherapeutic treatments would not help (Ballestrem *et al*, 2005). There may also be stigma attached to accessing mental healthcare. One study found 50% of women with depressive symptoms who were offered a psychiatric assessment by the clinic staff refused it. The staff reported spending up to an hour with women after they had been told there was a strong suggestion that they had depression. They suggested that important factors in the women's decisions were stigma, differing expectations of well-being and the inconvenience of attending appointments. Women also preferred not to see a psychologist (Robinson & Young, 1982).

However, a US study reports that although only 5% of pregnant women with anxiety or depressive symptoms had discussed this with their obstetrician, 82.4% said they would be willing to and would accept a referral to a mental health professional (Birndoff *et al*, 2001). The study did not follow-up the women to see if this actually happened. Women with PTSD may also not want treatment. A variety of factors inform their decision including avoidance of reminders of the trauma, expensive and difficult to access services, childcare difficulties, and the stigma of mental health treatments (Loveland Cook *et al*, 2004).

Women with postnatal depression have worries about antidepressants. Of 35 who had been prescribed antidepressants, a third refused to take them because they were breastfeeding, 20 found them helpful but 11 did not. Four women did take them as prescribed but others missed doses or did not increase the dose when requested to do so, suggesting some degree of self-regulation. Most did not take them beyond remission (Boath *et al*, 2004a). Being provided with more information about treatments does not appear to increase acceptability (Chabrol *et al* 2001, 2004). Office-based therapies were more acceptable than those delivered at home but very few women found antidepressants acceptable. Being provided with more information about the interventions made little difference to the acceptability rating of psychotherapy and reduced that of antidepressants further.

However, Pearlstein *et al* (2006) found most women chose interpersonal psychotherapy with or without sertraline and observed a trend towards those with a history of depression being more likely to opt for the antidepressant.

A study comparing the satisfaction of women with postnatal depression with treatment in primary care with that in a specialist multidisciplinary parent and baby day-unit offering individualised programmes of care found overall levels of satisfaction greater in women who had attended the unit. They particularly valued the peer support received (Boath *et al*, 2004b). More of these mothers would like the same treatment again, would recommend it to a friend and felt better informed about postnatal depression. There were a few negative comments about the unit, but there were many more made by the women who had been treated in primary care. These most often related to the short length of time they had in consultations with their general practitioner (GP). A third were dissatisfied with the treatment they received from their GP and a fifth with the treatment they received from their health visitor. These women were less likely to recommend the care they had received to a friend. An Australian study found women scoring high on the EPDS were more likely to visit a GP and other professionals than low scorers but were less satisfied with the care they received from their GP. This mostly related to lack of information and not feeling listened to (Webster *et al*, 2001). These findings raise concern, as specialist services are limited and not uniformly accessible across the UK. Primary care professionals will treat most women with perinatal depression and it appears that a significant minority of those women will not be satisfied with that care.

Women with postnatal depression may also have practical reasons for not taking up treatment offers. They may have multiple roles: 26% of those offered self-help, out-patient treatment, out-patient psychotherapy or in-patient therapy, did not take up any of these interventions, saying they did not have time (Ballestrem *et al*, 2005). There may be difficulty accessing services owing to public transport or attending appointments that take place outside school hours or in services that do not provide childcare.

References

Abramowitz, J., Moore, K., Carmin, C., *et al* (2001) Acute onset of obsessive–compulsive disorder in males following childbirth. *Psychosomatics*, **42**, 429–431.

Abramowitz, J. S., Schwartz, S. A., Moore, K. M., *et al* (2003) Obsessive–compulsive symptoms in pregnancy and the puerperium: a review of the literature. *Anxiety Disorders*, **17**, 461–478.

Adewuya, A. O. (2006) Early postpartum mood as a risk factor for postnatal depression in Nigerian women. *American Journal of Psychiatry*, **163**, 1435–1437.

Ahokas, A., Kaukoranta, J., Wahlbeck, K., *et al* (2001) Estrogen deficiency in severe postpartum depression: successful treatment with sublingual physiologic 17beta-estradiol: a preliminary study. *Journal of Clinical Psychiatry*, **62**, 332–336.

Alder, E. & Truman, J. (2002) Counselling for postnatal depression in the voluntary sector. *Psychology and Psychotherapy: Theory, Research and Practice*, **75**, 207–220.

Alder, J., Fink, N., Bitzer, J., *et al* (2007) Depression and anxiety during pregnancy: a risk factor for obstetric, fetal and neonatal outcome? A critical review of the literature. *Journal of Maternal–Fetal & Neonatal Medicine*, **20**, 189–209.

Andersson, L., Sundstrom-Poromaa, I., Bixo. M., *et al* (2003) Point prevalence of psychiatric disorders during the second trimester of pregnancy: a population-based study. *American Journal of Obstetrics & Gynecology*, **189**, 148–154.

Appleby, L., Warner, R., Whitton, A., *et al* (1997) A controlled study of fluoxetine and cognitive–behavioural counselling in the treatment of postnatal depression. *BMJ*, **314**, 932.

Appleby, L., Hirst, E., Marshall, S., *et al* (2003) The treatment of postnatal depression by health visitors: impact of brief training on skills and clinical practice. *Journal of Affective Disorders*, **77**, 261–266.

Arnold, L. M. (1999) A case-series of women with postpartum onset obsessive–compulsive disorder. *Primary Care Companion to the Journal of Clinical Psychiatry*, **1**, 103–108.

Ashok, P. W., Hamoda, H., Flett, G. M., *et al* (2005) Psychological sequelae of medical and surgical abortion at 10–13 weeks gestation. *Acta Obstetricia Gynecologica Scandinavica*, **84**, 761–766.

Ayers, S. & Pickering, A. D. (2001) Do women get posttraumatic stress disorder as a result of childbirth? A prospective study of incidence. *Birth*, **28**, 111–118.

Badenhorst, W., Riches, S., Turton, P., et al (2006) The psychological effects of stillbirth and neonatal death on fathers: systematic review. *Journal of Psychosomatic Obstetrics and Gynaecology*, **27**, 245–256.

Ballestrem, C. L., Strauss, M. & Kaechele, H. (2005) Contribution to the epidemiology of postnatal depression in Germany – implications for the utilization of treatment. *Archives of Women's Mental Health*, **8**, 29–35.

Barnet, B., Joffe, A., Duggan, A. K., et al (1996) Depressive symptoms, stress, and social support in pregnant and postpartum adolescents. *Archives of Pediatrics & Adolescent Medicine*, **150**, 64–69.

Bastani, F., Hidarnia, A., Kazemnejad, A., et al (2005) A randomized controlled trial of the effects of applied relaxation training on reducing anxiety and perceived stress in pregnant women. *Journal of Midwifery and Women's Health*, **50**, 36–40.

Battle, C. L., Zlotnick, C., Miller, I. W., et al (2006) Clinical characteristics of perinatal patients: a chart review study. *Journal of Nervous and Mental Disease*, **194**, 369–377.

Beck, C. T. (1996) A meta-analysis of predictors of postpartum depression. *Nursing Research*, **45**, 297–303.

Beck, C. T. (1998) Postpartum onset of panic disorder. *Journal of Nursing Scholarship*, **30**, 131–135.

Beck, C. T. (2001) Predictors of postpartum depression. *Nursing Research*, **50**, 275–285.

Beck, C. T. (2002) Postpartum depression: a meta-synthesis. *Qualitative Health Research*, **12**, 453–472.

Beeghly, M., Weinberg, M. K., Olsen, K. A., et al (2002) Stability and change in level of maternal depressive symptomatology during the first postpartum year. *Journal of Affective Disorders*, **71**, 169–180.

Benedict, M. I., Paine, L. L., Paine, L. A., et al (1999) The association of childhood sexual abuse with depressive symptoms during pregnancy, and selected pregnancy outcomes. *Child Abuse and Neglect*, **23**, 659–670.

Bennett, H. A., Einarson, A., Taddio, A., et al (2004) Prevalence of depression during pregnancy: systematic review. *Obstetrics and Gynecology*, **103**, 698–709.

Bifulco, A., Figueiredo, B., Guedeney, N., et al (2004) Maternal attachment style and depression associated with childbirth: preliminary results from a European and US cross-cultural study. *British Journal of Psychiatry*, **184(Suppl. 46)**, s31–s37.

Birkeland, R., Thompson, J. K. & Phares, V. (2005) Adolescent motherhood and postpartum depression. *Journal of Clinical Child and Adolescent Psychology*, **34**, 292–300.

Birndorf, C. A., Madden, A., Portera, L., et al (2001) Psychiatric symptoms, functional impairment and receptivity towards mental health treatment among obstetrical patients. *International Journal of Psychiatry in Medicine*, **31**, 355–365.

Bledsoe, S. E. & Grote, N. K. (2006) Treating depression during pregnancy and the postpartum: a preliminary meta-analysis. *Research in Social Work Practice*, **16**, 109–120.

Bloch, M., Daly, R. C. & Rubinow, D. R. (2003) Endocrine factors in the etiology of postpartum depression. *Comprehensive Psychiatry*, **44**, 234–236.

Bloch, M., Schmidt, P. J., Danaceau, M., et al (2000) Effects of gonadal steroids in women with a history of postpartum depression. *American Journal of Psychiatry*, **157**, 924–930.

Bloch, M., Rotenberg, N., Koren, D., et al (2005) Risk factors associated with the development of postpartum mood disorders. *Journal of Affective Disorders*, **88**, 9–18.

Boath, E. & Henshaw, C. (2001) The treatment of postnatal depression: a comprehensive literature review. *Journal of Reproductive and Infant Psychology*, **19**, 215–248.

Boath, E., Bradley, E. & Henshaw, C. (2004a) Women's views of antidepressants in the treatment of postnatal depression. *Journal of Psychosomatic Obstetrics and Gynaecology*, **25**, 221–236.

Boath, E., Bradley, E. & Anthony, P. (2004b) Users' views of two alternative approaches to the treatment of postnatal depression. *Journal of Reproductive and Infant Psychology*, **22**, 13–24.

39

Boath, E., Henshaw, C. & Dennis, C.-L. (2007) The treatment of postnatal depression: an update and critical review. *Archives of Women's Mental Health*, **10**, XII.

Bolton, H. L., Hughes, P. M., Turton, P., *et al* (1998) Incidence and demographic correlates of depressive symptoms during pregnancy in an inner London population. *Journal of Psychosomatic Obstetrics and Gynaecology*, **19**, 202–209.

Boyce, P. (2003) Risk factors for postnatal depression: a review and risk factors in Australian populations. *Archives of Women's Mental Health*, **6**, S43–S50.

Boyce, P., Hickie, I. & Parker, G. (1991a) Parents, partners or personality? Risk factors for post-natal depression. *Journal of Affective Disorders*, **21**, 245–255.

Boyce, P., Parker, G., Barnett, B., *et al* (1991b) Personality as a vulnerability factor to depression. *British Journal of Psychiatry*, **159**, 106–114.

Boyce, P., Johnstone, S. A., Hickey, A. R., *et al* (2000) Functioning and well-being at 24 weeks postpartum of women with postnatal depression. *Archives of Women's Mental Health*, **3**, 91–97.

Boyle, F. M., Vance, J. C., Najman, J. M., *et al* (1996) The mental health impact of stillbirth, neonatal death or SIDS: prevalence and patterns of distress among mothers. *Social Science and Medicine*, **43**, 1273–1282.

Bozoky, I. E. & Corwin, J. (2002) Fatigue as a predictor of postpartum depression. *Journal of Obstetric Gynecologic and Neonatal Nursing*, **31**, 436–443.

Brandes, M., Soares, C. N. & Cohen, L. S. (2004) Postpartum onset obsessive–compulsive disorder: diagnosis and management. *Archives of Women's Mental Health*, **7**, 99–110.

Brier, N. (2005) Anxiety after miscarriage: a review of the empirical literature and implications for clinical practice. *Birth*, **31**, 138–142.

Brockington, I. F. (2005) Post-abortion psychosis. *Archives of Women's Mental Health*, **8**, 53–54.

Brockington, I. F., Macdonald, E. & Wainscott, G. (2006) Anxiety, obsessions and morbid preoccupations in pregnancy. *Archives of Women's Mental Health*, **8**, 253–263.

Brown, S. & Lumley, J. (2000) Physical health problems after childbirth and maternal depression at six to seven months postpartum. *British Journal of Obstetrics and Gynaecology*, **107**, 1194–201.

Browne, J. C., Scott. K. M. & Silvers, M. (2006) Fish consumption in pregnancy and omega-3 status after birth are not associated with postnatal depression. *Journal of Affective Disorders*, **90**, 131–139.

Brugha, T. S., Sharp, H. M., Cooper, S. A., *et al* (1998) The Leicester 500 project: social support and the development of postnatal depressive symptoms, a prospective cohort study. *Psychological Medicine*, **28**, 63–79.

Buist, A. (1998) Childhood abuse, parenting and postpartum depression. *Australian and New Zealand Journal of Psychiatry*, **32**, 479–487.

Buist, A. & Janson, H. (2001) Childhood sexual abuse, parenting and postpartum depression – a 3-year follow-up study. *Child Abuse and Neglect*, **25**, 909–921.

Buttolph, L. M. & Holland, A. D. (1990) Obsessive compulsive disorders in pregnancy and childbirth. In *Obsessive Compulsive Disorders: Theory and Management* (eds M. Jenike, L. Baer & W. Minichiello), pp. 89–97. Year Book Medical.

Button, J. H. & Reivich, R. S. (1972) Obsessions of infanticide. *Archives of General Psychiatry*, **27**, 235–240.

Carter, F. A., Frampton, C. M. A. & Mulder, R. T. (2006) Caesarean section and postpartum depression: a review of the evidence examining the link. *Psychosomatic Medicine*, **68**, 321–330.

Chaaya, M., Campbell, O. M., El Kak, F., *et al* (2002) Postpartum depression: prevalence and determinants in Lebanon. *Archives of Women's Mental Health*, **5**, 65–72.

Chabrol, H., Teissedre, F., Santrisse, K., *et al* (2001) Acceptabilité des antidépresseurs et des psychotherapies dans les depressions du post-partum: enquête chez 198 accouchées. *Encéphale*, **27**, 380–382.

Chabrol, H., Teissedre, F., Armitage, J., *et al* (2004) Acceptability of psychotherapy and antidepressants for postnatal depression among newly delivered mothers. *Journal of Reproductive and Infant Psychology*, **22**, 5–12.

Chandran, M., Tharyan, P., Muliyil, J., *et al* (2002) Post-partum depression in a cohort of women from a rural area of Tamil Nadu, India: incidence and risk factors. *British Journal of Psychiatry*, **181**, 499–504.

Chiu, C-C., Huang, S-Y., Shen, W. W., *et al* (2003) Omega-3 fatty acids for depression in pregnancy. *American Journal of Psychiatry*, **160**, 385.

Church, N. F., Brechman-Toussaint, M. L. & Hine, D. W. (2005) Do dysfunctional cognitions mediate the relationship between risk factors and postnatal depression symptomatology? *Journal of Affective Disorders*, **87**, 65–72.

Clark, R., Tluczek, A. & Wenzel, A. (2003) Psychotherapy for postpartum depression: a preliminary report. *American Journal of Orthopsychiatry*, **73**, 441–454.

Cohen, L. S., Viguera, V. C., Bouffard, S. M., *et al* (2001) Venlafaxine in the treatment of postpartum depression. *Journal of Clinical Psychiatry*, **62**, 592–596.

Cohen, L. S., Nonacs, R. M., Bailey, J. W., *et al* (2004) Relapse of depression during pregnancy following antidepressant discontinuation: a preliminary prospective study. *Archives of Women's Mental Health*, **7**, 217–221.

Cohen, M. M., Schei, B., Ansara, D., *et al* (2002) A history of personal violence and postpartum depression: Is there a link? *Archives of Women's Mental Health*, **4**, 83–92.

Coletta, N. D. (1983) At risk for depression: a study of young mothers. *Journal of Genetic Psychology*, **142**, 301–310.

Cooper, P. J. & Murray, L. (1995) Course and recurrence of postnatal depression. Evidence for the specificity of the diagnostic concept. *British Journal of Psychiatry*, **166**, 191–195.

Cooper, P. J., Campbell, E. A. & Day, A., *et al* (1988) Non-psychotic psychiatric disorder after childbirth. A prospective study of prevalence, incidence, course and nature. *British Journal of Psychiatry*, **152**, 799–806.

Cooper, P. J., Tomlinson, M., Swartz, L., *et al* (1999) Post-partum depression and the mother–infant relationship in a South African peri-urban settlement. *British Journal of Psychiatry*, **175**, 554–558.

Cooper, P. J., Murray, L., Wilson, A., *et al* (2003). Controlled trial of the short- and long-term effect of psychological treatment of post-partum depression: 1. Impact on maternal mood. *British Journal of Psychiatry*, **182**, 412–419.

Corral, M., Misri, S. & Wardrop. (2007) Atypical augmentation of postpartum depression. *Archives of Women's Mental Health*, **9**, 161–171.

Corwin, E. J., Murray-Kolb, L. E. & Beard, J. L. (2003) Low hemoglobin level is a risk factor for postpartum depression. *Journal of Nutrition*, **133**, 4139–4142.

Corwin, E. J., Brownstead, J., Barton, N., *et al* (2005) The impact of fatigue on the development of postpartum depression. *Journal of Obstetric, Gynecologic and Neonatal Nursing*, 34, 577–586.

Cox, J. L. (1994) Prevention of postnatal mental illness: sociocultural facets. *Topics in Preventive Psychiatry*, **165**, 40–48.

Cox, J. L., Murray, D. & Chapman, G. (1993) A controlled study of the onset, duration and prevalence of postnatal depression. *British Journal of Psychiatry*, **163**, 27–31.

Creedy, D. K., Shochet, I. M. & Horsfall, J. (2000) Childbirth and the development of acute trauma symptoms: incidence and contributing factors. *Birth*, **27**, 104–1011.

Cumming, G., Klein, S., Bolsover, D., *et al* (2007) The emotional burden of miscarriage for women and their partners: trajectories of anxiety and depression over 13 months. *British Journal of Obstetrics and Gynaecology*, **114**, 1138–1145.

Cutrona, C. E. (1983) Causal attributions and perinatal depression. *Journal of Abnormal Psychology*, **92**, 161–172.

Czarnocka, J. & Slade, P. (2000) Prevalence and predictors of post-traumatic stress symptoms following childbirth. *British Journal of Clinical Psychology*, **39**, 35–51.

Dalton, K. (1985) Progesterone prophylaxis used successfully in postnatal depression. *Practitioner*, **229**, 507–508.

Dalton, K. (1989) Successful progesterone prophylaxis for idiopathic postnatal depression. *International Journal of Prenatal and Perinatal Studies*, **1**, 322–327.

Dalton, K. (1995) Progesterone prophylaxis for postnatal depression. *International Journal of Prenatal Perinatal and Psychology Medicine*, **7**, 447–450.

Daley, A. J., MacArthur, C. & Winter, H. (2007) The role of exercise in treating postpartum depression: a review of the literature. *Journal of Midwifery & Women's Health*, **52**, 56–62.

Daley, A., Winter, H., Grimmett, C., *et al* (2008) Feasibility of an exercise intervention for women with postnatal depression: a pilot randomised controlled trial. *British Journal of General Practice*, **58**, 178–183.

Davies, V., Gledhill, J. McFadyen, A., *et al* (2005) Psychological outcome in women undergoing termination of pregnancy for ultrasound-detected fetal anomaly in the first and second trimesters: a pilot study. *Ultrasound in Obstetrics and Gynecology*, **25**, 389–392.

de Armond, M. (1954) A type of postpartum anxiety reaction. *Diseases of the Nervous System*, **15**, 26–29.

de Vriese, S. R., Christophe, A. B., Maes, M., *et al* (2003) Lowered serum n-3 polyunsaturated fatty acid (PUFA) levels predict the occurrence of postpartum depression: Further evidence that lowered n-PUFA are related to major depression. *Life Sciences*, **73**, 3181–3187.

Dean, C., Dean, N. R., White, A., *et al* (1995) An adoption study comparing the prevalence of psychiatric illness in women who have adoptive and natural children and women who have adoptive children only. *Journal of Affective Disorders*, **34**, 55–60.

Dell, D. L. & Halford, J. J. (2002) Dementia presenting as postpartum depression. *Obstetrics and Gynecology*, **99**, 925–928.

Dennis, C. L. (2004) Treatment of postpartum depression, part 2: a critical review of nonbiological interventions. *Journal of Clinical Psychiatry*, **65**, 1252–1265.

Dennis, C. L. & Stewart, D. E. (2004) Treatment of postpartum depression, part 1: a critical review of biological interventions. *Journal of Clinical Psychiatry*, **65**, 1242–1251.

Dennis, C. & Hodnett, E. (2007) Psychosocial and psychological interventions for treating postpartum depression. *Cochrane Database of Systematic Reviews*, **4**, CD006116.

Dulude, D., Bélanger, C., Wright, J., *et al* (2002) High-risk pregnancies, psychological distress, and dyadic adjustment. *Journal of Reproductive & Infant Psychology*, **20**, 101–123.

Einarson, A., Selby, P. & Koren, G. (2001) Abrupt discontinuation of psychotropic drugs during pregnancy: fear of teratogenic risk and impact of counselling. *Journal of Psychiatry and Neuroscience*, **26**, 44–48.

Engelhard, I. M., van den Hout, M. A. & Amtz, A. (2001) Posttraumatic stress disorder after pregnancy loss. *General Hospital Psychiatry*, **23**, 62–66.

Engelhard, I. M., van Rij, M., Boullart, I., *et al* (2002) Posttraumatic stress disorder after pre-eclampsia: an exploratory study. *General Hospital Psychiatry*, **24**, 260–264.

Engelhard, I. M., van den Hout, M. A., Kindt, M., *et al* (2003) Peritraumatic dissociation and posttraumatic stress after pregnancy loss: a prospective study. *Behaviour Research and Therapy*, **41**, 67–78.

Epperson, C. N., Terman, M., Terman, J. S., *et al* (2004) Randomized clinical trial of bright light therapy for antepartum depression: preliminary findings. *Journal of Clinical Psychiatry*, **65**, 421–425.

Evans, J., Heron, J., Francomb, H., *et al* (2001) Cohort study of depressed mood during pregnancy and after childbirth. *BMJ*, **323**, 257–260.

Faisal-Cury, A., Tedesco, J. J. A., Kahhale, S., *et al* (2004) Postpartum depression in relation to life-events. *Archives of Women's Mental Health*, **7**, 123–131.

Farber, E. W., Herbert, S. E. & Reviere, S. L. (1996) Childhood sexual abuse and suicidality in obstetrics patients in a hospital-based urban prenatal clinic. *General Hospital Psychiatry*, **18**, 56–60.

Feggetter, G., Cooper, P. & Gath, D. (1981) Non-psychotic psychiatric disorders in women one year after childbirth. *Journal of Psychosomatic Research*, **25**, 369–372.

Felice, E., Saliba, J., Grech, V., *et al* (2004) Prevalence rates and psychosocial characteristics associated with depression in pregnancy and postpartum in Maltese women. *Journal of Affective Disorders*, **82**, 297–301.

Fergusson, D. M., Horwood, L. J. & Ridder, E. M. (2006) Abortion in young women and subsequent mental health. *Journal of Child Psychology and Psychiatry*, **47**, 16–24.

Field, T., Sandberg, D., Quetel, T. A., et al (1985) Effects of ultrasound feedback on pregnancy anxiety, fetal activity and neonatal outcome. Obstetrics and Gynaecology, **66**, 525–528.

Field, T., Diego, M. & Hernandez-Reif, M. (2006) Prenatal depression effects on the fetus and newborn: a review. Infant Behavior and Development, **29**, 445–455.

Fisher, J. R., Hammarberg, K. & Baker, H. W. (2005) Assisted conception is a risk factor for postnatal mood disturbance and early parenting difficulties. Fertility and Sterility, **84**, 426–430.

Forster, D. A., Denning, A., Wills, G., et al (2006) herbal medicine use during pregnancy in a group of Australian women. BMC Pregnancy and Childbirth, **6**, 21.

Forty, L., Jones, L., Macgregor, S., et al (2006) Familiality of postpartum depression in unipolar disorder: results from a family study. American Journal of Psychiatry, **163**, 1549–1553.

Fowles, E. R. (1998) The relationship between maternal role attainment and postpartum depression. Health Care for Women International, **19**, 83–94.

Freeman, M. P. (2007) Antenatal depression: navigating the treatment dilemmas. American Journal of Psychiatry, **164**, 1162–1165.

Freeman, M. P., Hibbeln, J. R., Wisner, K. L., et al (2006a) An open trial of omega-3 fatty acids for depression in pregnancy. Acta Neuropsychiatrica, **18**, 21–24.

Freeman, M. P., Hibbeln, J. R., Wisner, K. L., et al (2006b) Randomized dose-ranging pilot trial of omega-3 fatty acids for postpartum depression. Acta Psychiatrica Scandinavica, **113**, 31–35.

Freeman, M. P., Davis, M., Sinha, P., et al (2008) Omega-3 fatty acids and supportive psychotherapy for perinatal depression: a randomized placebo-controlled study. Journal of Affective Disorders, **110**, 142–148.

Frost, M. & Condon, J. T. (1996) The psychological sequelae of miscarriage: a critical review of the literature. Australian and New Zealand Journal of Psychiatry, **30**, 54–62.

Garfield, P., Kent, A., Paykel, E. S., et al (2004) Outcome of postpartum disorders: a 10 year follow-up of hospital admissions. Acta Psychiatrica Scandinavica, **109**, 434–439.

Geller, P. A., Klier, C. M. & Neugebauer, R. (2001) Anxiety disorders following miscarriage. Journal of Clinical Psychiatry, **62**, 432–438.

Geller, P. A., Psaros, C. & Kerns, D. (2006) Web-based resources for healthcare providers and women following pregnancy loss. Journal of Obstetric, Gynecological and Neonatal Nursing, **35**, 523–532.

Gentile, S. (2005) The role of estrogen therapy in postpartum psychiatric disorders. CNS Spectrums, **10**, 944–952.

Glover, V., Liddle, P., Taylor, A., et al (1994) Mild hypomania (the highs) can be a feature of the first postpartum week. Association with later depression. British Journal of Psychiatry, **164**, 517–521.

Gold, K. J., Dalton, V. K., Schwenk, T. L., et al (2007) What causes pregnancy loss? Preexisting mental illness as an independent risk factor. General Hospital Psychiatry, **29**, 207–213.

Gordon, R. E. G. & Gordon K. K. (1959) Social factors in the prediction and treatment of emotional disorders of pregnancy. American Journal of Obstetrics and Gynecology, **77**, 1074–1083.

Gotlib, I. H., Whiffen, V. E., Mount, J. H. et al (1989) Prevalence rates and demographic characteristics associated with depression in pregnancy and the postpartum. Journal of Consulting and Clinical Psychology, **57**, 269–274.

Granger, A. C. & Underwood, M. R. (2001) Review of the role of progesterone in the management of postnatal mood disorders. Journal of Psychosomatic Obstetrics and Gynecology, **22**, 49–55.

Green, J. M., Murray, D. (1994) The use of the Edinburgh Postnatal Depression Scale in research to explore the relationship between antenatal and postnatal dysphoria. In Perinatal Psychiatry: Use and Misuse of the Edinburgh Postnatal Depression Scale (eds J. Cox & J. Holden), pp. 180–189. Gaskell.

Gregoire, A. J. P., Kumar, R., Everitt, B., *et al* (1996) Transdermal oestrogen for treatment of severe postnatal depression. *Lancet*, **347**, 930–933.

Halbreich, U. (2005) Postpartum disorders: multiple interacting underlying mechanisms and risk factors. *Journal of Affective Disorders*, **88**, 1–7.

Halbreich, U. & S. Karkun (2006) Cross-cultural and social diversity of prevalence of postpartum depression and depressive symptoms. *Journal of Affective Disorders*, **91**, 97–111.

Hanley, J. & Long, B. (2006) A study of Welsh mothers' experience of postnatal depression. *Midwifery*, **22**, 147–157.

Hannah, P., Cody, D., Glover, V., *et al* (1993) The tyramine test is not a marker for postnatal depression: early postpartum euphoria may be. *Journal of Psychosomatic Obstetrics and Gynecology*, **14**, 295–304.

Harris, B., Fung, H., Johns, S., *et al* (1989) Transient postpartum thyroid dysfunction and postnatal depression. *Journal of Affective Disorders*, **17**, 243–249.

Harris, B., Othman, S., Davies, J. A., *et al* (1992) Association between postpartum thyroid dysfunction and thyroid antibodies and depression. *BMJ*, **305**, 152–156.

Harris, B., Oretti, R., Lazarus, J. *et al* (2002) Randomised trial of thyroxine to prevent postnatal depression in thyroid-antibody-positive women. *British Journal of Psychiatry*, **180**, 327–330.

Hayworth, J., Little, B., Bonham-Carter, S., *et al* (1980) A predictive study of post-partum depression: some predisposing characteristics. *British Journal of Medical Psychology*, **53**, 161–167.

Heh, S-S. & Fu, Y-Y. (2003) Effectiveness of informational support in reducing the severity of postnatal depression in Taiwan. *Journal of Advanced Nursing*, **42**, 30–36.

Heimstad, R., Dahloe, R., Laache, I., *et al* (2006) Fear of childbirth and history of abuse: implications for pregnancy and delivery. *Acta Obstetricia et Gynecologica Scandinavica*, **85**, 435–440.

Henderson, J. J., Evans, S. F., Straton, J. A., *et al* (2003) Impact of postnatal depression on breastfeeding duration. *Birth*, **30**, 175–180.

Hendrick, V., Altshuler, L., Strouse, T., *et al* (2000) Postpartum and nonpostpartum depression: differences in presentation and response to pharmacologic treatment. *Depression and Anxiety*, **11**, 66–72.

Henshaw, C. (2003) Mood disturbance in the early puerperium: a review. *Archives of Women's Mental Health*, **6**, S33–S42.

Henshaw, C., Foreman, D. & Cox, J. (2004) Postnatal blues: a risk factor for postpartum depression. *Journal of Psychosomatic Obstetrics and Gynaecology*, **25**, 267–272.

Heron, J., Craddock, N. & Jones, I. (2005) Postnatal euphoria – are 'the highs' an indicator of bipolarity? *Bipolar Disorders*, **7**, 103–110.

Hertzberg, T., Leo, R. J. & Kim, K. Y. (1997) Recurrent obsessive–compulsive disorder associated with pregnancy and childbirth. *Psychosomatics*, **38**, 386–388.

Hickey, A. R., Boyce, P. M., Ellwood, D., *et al* (1997) Early discharge a risk factor for postnatal depression. *Medical Journal of Australia*, **167**, 244–247.

Hiscock, H. & Wake, M. (2001) Infant sleep problems and postnatal depression: a community-based study. *Pediatrics*, **107**, 6.

Hiscock, H. & Wake, M. (2002) Randomised controlled trial of behavioural infant sleep intervention to improve infant sleep and maternal mood. *BMJ*, **324**, 1062–1065.

Hofberg, K. & Brockington, I. F. (2000) Tokophobia: an unreasoning dread of childbirth. A series of 26 cases. *British Journal of Psychiatry*, **176**, 83–85.

Hoffbrand, S., Howard, L., Crawley, H. (2001) Antidepressant treatment for post-natal depression. *Cochrane Database of Systematic Reviews*, **2**, CD002018.

Holden, J. M., Sagovsky, R. & Cox, J. L. (1989) Counselling in a general practice setting: controlled study of health visitor intervention in treatment of postnatal depression. *BMJ*, **298**, 223–226.

Honey, K. L., Bennett, P. & Morgan, M. (2002) A brief psycho-educational group intervention for postnatal depression. *British Journal of Clinical Psychology*, **41**, 405–409.

Horrigan, T. J., Schroeder, A. V. & Schaffer, R. M. (2000) The triad of substance abuse, violence, and depression are interrelated in pregnancy. *Journal of Substance Abuse Treatment*, **18**, 55–58.

Howard, L. M., Kirkwood, G. & Latinovic, R. (2007) Sudden infant death syndrome and maternal depression. *Journal of Clinical Psychiatry*, **68**, 1279–1283.

Hudson, D. B., Elek, S. M. & Campbell-Grossman, C. (2000) Depression, self-esteem, loneliness, and social support among adolescent mothers participating in the new parents project. *Adolescence*, **35**, 445–453.

Hughes, P. M., Turton, P. & Evans, C. D. (1999) Stillbirth as risk factor for depression and anxiety in the subsequent pregnancy: cohort study. *BMJ*, **318**, 1721–1724.

Hughes, P., Turton, P., Hopper, E., *et al* (2001) Disorganised attachment behaviour among infants born subsequent to stillbirth. *Journal of Child Psychology and Psychiatry and Allied Disciplines*, **42**, 791–801.

Iancu, I., Lepkifker, E., Dannon, P., *et al* (1995) Obsessive–compulsive disorder limited to pregnancy. *Psychotherapy and Psychosomatics*, **64**, 109–112.

Janssen, H. J., Cusinier, M. C. & Hoogduin, K. A. (1996) Controlled prospective study on the mental health of women following pregnancy loss. *American Journal of Psychiatry*, **153**, 226–230.

Jennings, K. D., Ross, S., Popper, S., *et al* (1999) Thoughts of harming infants in depressed and nondepressed mothers. *Journal of Affective Disorders*, **54**, 21–28.

Jolley, S. N., Elmore, S., Barnard, K. E., *et al* (2007) Dysregulation of the hypothalamic–pituitary–adrenal axis in postpartum depression. *Biological Research for Nursing*, **8**, 210–222.

Josefsson, A, Berg, G., Nordin, C., *et al* (2001) Prevalence of depressive symptoms in late pregnancy and postpartum. *Acta Obstetricia et Gynecologica Scandinavica*, **80**, 251–255.

Kalra, H., Tandon, R., Trivedi, J. K., *et al* (2005) Pregnancy-induced obsessive compulsive disorder: a case-report. *Annals of General Psychiatry*, **4**, 12.

Kammerer, M., Taylor, A. & Glover, V. (2006) The HPA axis and perinatal depression: a hypothesis. *Archives of Women's Mental Health*, **9**, 187–196.

Kelly, R. H., Russo, J. & Katon, W. (2001) Somatic complaints among pregnant women cared for in obstetrics: normal pregnancy or depressive and anxiety symptom amplification revisited? *General Hospital Psychiatry*, **23**, 107–113.

Kersting, A., Kroker, K., Steinhard, J., *et al* (2007) Complicated grief after traumatic loss: a 14 month follow up study. *European Archives of Psychiatry and Clinical Neuroscience*, **257**, 437–443.

Kitamura, T., Toda, M., Shima, S., *et al* (1994) Early loss of parents and early rearing experience among women with antenatal depression. *Journal of Psychosomatic Obstetrics and Gynaecology*, **15**, 133–139.

Klier, C. M., Geller, P. A. & Neugebauer, R. (2000) Minor depressive disorder in the context of miscarriage. *Journal of Affective Disorders*, **59**, 13–21.

Klier, C. M., Muzik, M., Rosenblum, K. L., *et al* (2001) Interpersonal psychotherapy adapted for the group setting in the treatment of postpartum depression. *Journal of Psychotherapy Practice and Research*, **10**, 124–131.

Klier, C. M., Muzik, M., Dervic, K., *et al* (2007) The role of estrogen and progesterone in depression after birth. *Journal of Psychiatric Research*, **41**, 273–279.

Korenromp, M. J., Christiaens, G. C., van den Bout, J., *et al* (2005) Long-term psychological consequences of pregnancy termination for fetal abnormality: a cross-sectional study. *Prenatal Diagnosis*, **25**, 253–260.

Kuijpens, J. L., Vader, H. L., Drexhage, H. A., *et al* (2001) Thyroid peroxidase antibodies during gestation are a marker for subsequent depression postpartum. *European Journal of Endocrinology*, **145**, 579–584.

Labad, J., Menchon, J. M., Alonso, P., *et al* (2005) Female reproductive cycle and obsessive-compulsive disorder. *Journal of Clinical Psychiatry*, **66**, 428–435.

Lane, D. A., Kauls, L. S., Ickovics, J. R., *et al* (1999) Early postpartum discharges. Impact on distress and outpatient problems. *Archives of Family Medicine*, **8**, 237–242.

Lawrie, T. A., Herxheimer, A. & Dalton, K. (2000) Oestrogens and progestogens for preventing and treating postnatal depression. *Cochrane Database of Systematic Reviews*, **2**, CD001690.

Lee, C. & Slade, P. (1996) Miscarriage as a traumatic event: a review of the literature and new implications for intervention. *Journal of Psychosomatic Research*, **40**, 235–244.

Leung, W. C., Kung, F., Lam, J., *et al* (2002) Domestic violence and postnatal depression in a Chinese community. *International Journal of Gynaecology and Obstetrics*, **79**, 159–166.

Lewis, G. & Drife, J. (2004) *Why Mothers Die 2000–2002. The Sixth Report of the Confidential Enquiries into Maternal Deaths in the United Kingdom*. RCOG Press.

Littleton, H. L., Breitkopf, C. R. & Berenson, A. B. (2007) Correlates of anxiety symptoms during pregnancy and association with perinatal outcomes: a meta-analysis. *American Journal of Obstetrics and Gynecology*, **196**, 424–432.

Loveland Cook, C. A., Flick, L. H., Homan, S. M., *et al* (2004) Posttraumatic stress disorder in pregnancy: prevalence, risk factors, and treatment. *Obstetrics and Gynecology*, **103**, 710–717.

Lucas, A., Pizarro, E., Granada, M. L., *et al* (2001) Postpartum thyroid dysfunction and postpartum depression: are they two linked disorders? *Clinical Endocrinology*, **55**, 809–14.

Ludman, E. J., McBride, C. M., Nelson, J. C. *et al* (2000) Stress, depressive symptoms, and smoking cessation among pregnant women. *Health Psychology*, **19**, 21–27.

MacFarlane, A., Mugford, M., Henderson, J., *et al* (2000) *Birth Counts: Statistics of Pregnancy and Childbirth (Volume 2)*, pp. 63–67. TSO (The Stationery Office).

Maes, M., Ombelet, W., Libbrecht, I., *et al* (1999) Effects of pregnancy and delivery on serum concentrations of Clara cell protein (CC16), an endogenous anticytokine: lower serum CC16 is related to postpartum depression. *Psychiatry Research*, **87**, 117–127.

Maes, M., Ombelet, W., De Jongh, R., *et al* (2001) The inflammatory response following delivery is amplified in women who previously suffered from major depression, suggesting that major depression is accompanied by a sensitization of the inflammatory response system. *Journal of Affective Disorders*, **63**, 85–92.

Maina, G., Albert, U., Bogetto, F., *et al* (1999) Recent life events and obsessive–compulsive disorder (OCD): the role of pregnancy/delivery. *Psychiatry Research*, **89**, 49–58.

Mandl, K. D., Tronick, E. Z., Brennan, T. A., *et al* (1999) Infant health care use and maternal depression. *Archives of Pediatrics and Adolescent Medicine*, **153**, 808–813.

Mantle, F. (2002) The role of alternative medicine in treating postnatal depression. *Complementary Therapies in Nursing and Midwifery*, **8**, 197–203.

Marcus, S. M., Flynn, H. A., Blow, F., *et al* (2005) A screening study of antidepressant treatment rates and mood symptoms in pregnancy. *Archives of Women's Mental Health*, **8**, 25–27.

Marks, M., Wieck, A., Checkley, S. A., *et al* (1992) Contribution of psychological and social factors to psychotic and non-psychotic relapse after childbirth in women with previous histories of affective disorder. *Journal of Affective Disorder*, **29**, 253–264.

Mauthner, N. S. (1998) 'It's a woman's cry for help': a relational perspective on postnatal depression. *Feminism and Psychology*, **8**, 325–355.

McIvor, R, Davies, R., Wieck, A., *et al* (1996) The growth hormone response to apomorphine at 4 days postpartum in women with a history of major depression. *Journal of Affective Disorders*, **40**, 131–136.

McMahon, C., Barnett, B., Kowalenko, N., *et al* (2005) Psychological factors associated with persistent postnatal depression: past and current relationships, defence styles and the mediating role of insecure attachment style. *Journal of Affective Disorders*, **84**, 15–24.

Mezey, G., Bacchus, L., Bewley, S., *et al* (2005) Domestic violence, lifetime trauma and psychological health of childbearing women. *British Journal of Obstetrics and Gynaecology*, **112**, 197–204.

Milgrom, J., Martin, P. R. & Negri, L. M. (1999). *Treating Postnatal Depression. A Psychological Approach for Health Care Practitioners*. Wiley.

Misri, S. & Milis, L. (2004) Obsessive–compulsive disorder in the postpartum: open-label trial of quetiapine augmentation. *Journal of Clinical Psychopharmacology,* **24,** 624–627.

Misri, S., Kostaras, X., Fox, D., *et al* (2000) The impact of partner support in the treatment of postpartum depression. *Canadian Journal of Psychiatry,* **45,** 554–558.

Misri, S., Reebye, P., Corral, M., *et al* (2004) The use of paroxetine and cognitive–behavioral therapy in postpartum depression and anxiety: a randomized controlled trial. *Journal of Clinical Psychiatry,* **65,** 1236–1241.

Morgan, M., Matthey, S., Barnett, B., *et al* (1997) A group programme for postnatally distressed women and their partners. *Journal of Advanced Nursing,* **26,** 913–920.

Morse, C., Durkin, S., Buist, A., *et al* (2004) Improving the postnatal outcomes of new mothers. *Journal of Advanced Nursing,* **45,** 465–474.

Murphy-Eberenz, K., Zandi, P. P., March, D., *et al* (2006) Is perinatal depression familial? *Journal of Affective Disorders,* **90,** 49–55.

Murray, L., Stanley, C., Hooper, R., *et al* (1996) The role of infant factors in postnatal depression and mother–infant interactions. *Developmental Medicine and Child Neurology,* **38,** 109–119.

Nasta, M. T., Grussu, P., Quatraro, R. M., *et al* (2002) Cholesterol and mood states at 3 days after delivery. *Journal of Psychosomatic Research,* **52,** 61–63.

National Statistics & Department of Health (2007) *Statistical Bulletin. Abortion Statistics, England and Wales: 2007.* Department of Health.

Nayak, M. B. & Al-Yattama, M. (1999) Assault victim history as a factor in depression during pregnancy. *Obstetrics and Gynecology,* **94,** 204–208.

Neugebauer, R., Kline, J., O'Connor, P., *et al* (1992) Depressive symptoms in women in the six months after miscarriage. *American Journal of Obstetrics and Gynecology,* **166,** 104–109.

Neugebauer, R., Kline, J., Shrout, P., *et al* (1997) Major depressive disorder in the 6 months after miscarriage. *JAMA,* **277,** 383–388.

Neugebauer, R., Kline, J., Bleiberg, K., *et al* (2007). Preliminary open trial of interpersonal counseling for subsyndromal depression following miscarriage. *Depression and Anxiety,* **24,** 219–222.

Newport, D. J., Owens, M. J., Knight, D. L., *et al* (2004) Alterations in platelet serotonin transporter binding in women with postpartum onset major depression. *Journal of Psychosomatic Research,* **38,** 467–473.

Neziroglu, F., Anemone, R., & Yaryura-Tobias, J.A. (1992) Onset of obsessive–compulsive disorder in pregnancy. *American Journal of Psychiatry,* **149,** 947–950.

Nicolson, P. (1998) *Post-Natal Depression: Psychology, Science and the Transition to Motherhood.* Routledge.

Nierop, A., Bratiskas, A., Zimmerman, R. *et al* (2006) Are stress induced cortisol changes during pregnancy associated with postpartum depressive symptoms? *Psychosomatic Medicine,* **68,** 931–937.

Nonacs, R. M., Soares, C. N., Viguera, A. C., *et al* (2005) Bupropion SR for the treatment of postpartum depression: a pilot study. *International Journal of Psychopharmacology,* **8,** 445–449.

O'Connor, T. G., Heron, J., Glover, V., *et al* (2002) Antenatal anxiety predicts child behavioral/emotional problems independently of postnatal depression. *Journal of the American Academy of Child & Adolescent Psychiatry,* **41,** 1470–1477.

O'Hara, M. (1986) Social support, life events, and depression during pregnancy and the puerperium. *Archives of General Psychiatry,* **43,** 569–573.

O'Hara, M. W. & Swain, A. M. (1996) Rates and risks of postpartum depression: a meta analysis. *International Review of Psychiatry,* **8,** 37–54.

O'Hara, M., Rehm, L. P. & Campbell, S. (1982) Predicting depressive symptomatology cognitive–behavioral models and postpartum depression. *Journal of Abnormal Psychology,* **91,** 457–461.

O'Hara, M., Neunaber, D. J. & Zekowski, E. M. (1984) Prospective study of postpartum depression: prevalence, course and predictive factors. *Journal of Abnormal Psychology,* **93,** 158–171.

47

O'Hara, M. W., Zekowski, E. M., Phipps, L. H., *et al* (1990) Controlled prospective study of postpartum mood disorders: comparison of childbearing and nonchildbearing women. *Journal of Abnormal Psychology*, **99**, 3–15.

O'Hara, M. W., Stuart, S., Gorman, L. L., *et al* (2000) Efficacy of interpersonal psychotherapy for postpartum depression. *Archives of General Psychiatry*, **57**, 1039–45.

Onozawa, K., Glover, V., Adams, D., *et al* (2001) Infant massage improves mother–infant interaction for mothers with postnatal depression. *Journal of Affective Disorders*, **63**, 201–207.

Onozawa, K., Kumar, R., Adams, D., et al (2003) High EPDS scores in women from ethnic minorities living in London. *Archives of Women's Mental Health*, **6**, s51–s55.

Oren, D. A., Wisner, K. L., Spinelli, M., *et al* (2002) An open trial of morning light therapy for treatment of antepartum depression. *American Journal of Psychiatry*, **159**, 666–669.

Oretti, R. G., Harris, B., Lazarus, I. H., *et al* (2003) Is there an association between life events, postnatal depression and thyroid dysfunction in thyroid antibody positive women? *International Journal of Social Psychiatry*, **49**, 70–76.

Orr, S. T., Blazer, D. G. & James, S. A. (2006) Racial disparities in elevated prenatal depressive symptoms among Black and White women in eastern North Carolina. *Annals of Epidemiology*, **16**, 463–468.

Otto, S. J., de Groot, R. H. & Hornstra, G. (2003) Increased risk of postpartum depressive symptoms is associated with slower normalization after pregnancy of the functional docosahexaenoic acid status. *Prostaglandins, Leukotrines and Essential Fatty Acids*, **69**, 237–243.

Pajulo, M., Savonlahti, E., Sourander, A., *et al* (2001) Antenatal depression, substance dependency and social support. *Journal of Affective Disorders*, **65**, 9–17.

Parry, B. L., Curran, M. L., Stuenkel, C. A., *et al* (2000) Can critically timed sleep deprivation be useful in pregnancy and postpartum depressions? *Journal of Affective Disorders*, **60**, 201–212.

Paykel, E. S., Emms, E. M., Fletcher, J., *et al* (1980) Life events and social support in puerperal depression. *British Journal of Psychiatry*, **136**, 339–346.

Pearlstein, T. B., Zlotnick, C., Battle, C. L., *et al* (2006) Patient choice of treatment for postpartum depression. *Archives of Women's Mental Health*, **9**, 303–308.

Pedersen, C. A., Johnson, J. L., Silva, S., *et al* (2007) Antenatal thyroid correlates of postpartum depression. *Psychoneuroendocrinology*, **32**, 235–245.

Peindl, K. S., Wisner, K. L, Zolnik, E. J., *et al* (1995) Effects of postpartum psychiatric illness on family planning. *International Journal of Psychiatry in Medicine*, **25**, 291–300.

Petrou, S., Cooper, P., Murray, L., *et al* (2002) Economic costs of post-natal depression in a high–risk British cohort. *British Journal of Psychiatry*, **181**, 505–512.

Pitt, B. (1968) 'Atypical' depression following childbirth. *British Journal of Psychiatry*, **114**, 1325–1335.

Ploeckinger, B., Dantendorfer, K., Ulm, M., *et al* (1996) Rapid decrease of serum cholesterol concentration and postpartum depression. *BMJ*, **313**, 664.

Pop, V. J., de Rooy, H. A. & Vader, H. L. (1991) Postpartum thyroid dysfunction and depression in an unselected population. *New England Journal of Medicine*, **324**, 1815–1816.

Pritchard, C. W. (1994) Depression and smoking in pregnancy in Scotland. *Journal of Epidemiology and Community Health*, **48**, 377–382.

Rahman, A. & Creed, F. (2007) Outcome of prenatal depression and risk factors associated with persistence in the first postnatal year: Prospective study from Rawalpindi, Pakistan. *Journal of Affective Disorders*, **100**, 115–121.

Reardon, D. C., Cougle, J. R. Rue, V. M., *et al* (2003) Psychiatric admission of low–income women following abortion and childbirth. *Canadian Medical Association Journal*, **168**, 1253–1256.

Reay, R., Fisher, Y., Robertson, M., *et al* (2006) Group interpersonal psychotherapy for postnatal depression: a pilot study. *Archives of Women's Mental Health*, **9**, 31–39.

Rees, A–M., Austin, M–P., Parker, G. (2005) Role of omega-3 fatty acids as a treatment for depression in the perinatal period. *Australian and New Zealand Journal of Psychiatry*, **39**, 274–280.

Roberts, J., Sword, W., Watt, S., *et al* (2001) Costs of postpartum care: examining associations from the Ontario mother and infant survey. *Canadian Journal of Nursing Research*, **33**, 19–34.

Robertson, E., Grace, S., Wallington, T., *et al* (2004) Antenatal risk factors for postpartum depression: a synthesis of recent literature. *General Hospital Psychiatry*, **26**, 289–295.

Robinson, R. & Young, J. (1982) Screening for depression and anxiety in the postnatal period: acceptance or rejection of a subsequent treatment offer. *Australian and New Zealand Journal of Psychiatry*, **16**, 47–51.

Ross, L. E. & McLean, L. M. (2006) Anxiety disorders during pregnancy and the postpartum period: a systematic review. *Journal of Clinical Psychiatry*, **67**, 1285–1298.

Ross, L. E., Murray, B. J. & Steiner, M. (2005) Sleep and perinatal mood disorders: a critical review. *Journal of Psychiatry and Neuroscience*, **30**, 247–256.

Ross, L. E., Sellers, E. M., Gilbert Evans, S. E., *et al* (2004) Mood changes during pregnancy and the postpartum period: development of a biopsychosocial model. *Acta Psychiatrica Scandinavica*, **109**, 457–466.

Ross, L. E., Campbell, V. L., Dennis, C–L., *et al* (2006) Demographic characteristics of participants in studies of risk factors, prevention and treatment of postpartum depression. *Canadian Journal of Psychiatry*, **51**, 704–710.

Rubertsson, C., Waldenström, U. & Wickberg, B. (2003) Depressive mood in early pregnancy: prevalence and women at risk in a national Swedish sample. *Journal of Reproductive and Infant Psychology*, **21**, 113–123.

Rudnicki, S. R, Graham, J. L., Habboushe, D. F., *et al* (2001) Social support and avoidant coping: correlates of depressed mood during pregnancy in minority women. *Women and Health*, **34**, 19–34.

Ryding, E. L., Wijma, B. & Wijma, K. (1997) Posttraumatic stress reactions after emergency Cesarean section. *Acta Obstetricia et Gynecologica Scandinavica*, **76**, 856–861.

Ryding, E. L., Wijma, K. & Wijma, B. (1998) Psychological impact of emergency Cesarean section in comparison with elective Cesarean section, instrumental and normal vaginal delivery. *Journal of Psychosomatic Obstetrics and Gynecology*, **19**, 135–144.

Ryding, E. L., Persson, A., Onell, C., *et al* (2003) An evaluation of midwives' counseling of pregnant women in fear of childbirth. *Acta Obstetricia et Gynecologica Scandinavica*, **82**, 10–17.

Saisto, T., Salmela Aro, K., Nurmi, J–E., *et al* (2001) A randomized controlled trial of intervention in fear of childbirth. *Obstetrics and Gynecology*, **98**, 820–826.

Saisto, T., Toivanen, R., Samela–Arp, K., *et al* (2006) Therapeutic group psychoeducation and relaxation in treating fear of childbirth. *Acta Obstetricia et Gynecologica Scandinavica*, **85**, 1315–1319.

Schnyer, R. N., Manber, R. & Fitzcharles, A. J. (2003) Acupuncture treatment for depression during pregnancy: conceptual framework and two case reports. *Complementary Health Practice Review*, **8**, 40–53.

Seel, R. M. (1986) Birth rite. *Health Visitor*, **59**, 182–184.

Segre, L. S., O'Hara, M. W., Arndt, S., *et al* (2007) The prevalence of postpartum depression: the relative significance of three social indices. *Social Psychiatry and Psychiatric Epidemiology*, **42**, 316–321.

Séguin, L., Potvin, L., Denis, M. S., *et al* (1995) Chronic stressors, social support and depression during pregnancy. *Obstetrics and Gynecology*, **85**, 583–589.

Shakespeare, J., Blake, F. & Garcia, J. (2006) How do women with postnatal depression experience listening visits in primary care? A qualitative interview study. *Journal of Reproductive and Infant Psychology*, **24**, 149–162.

Sharma, V. (2006) A cautionary note on the use of antidepressants in postpartum depression. *Bipolar Disorders*, **8**, 411–414.

Sholomskas, D. E., Wickamaratne, P. J., Dogolo, L., *et al* (1993) Postpartum onset of panic disorder: a coincidental event? *Journal of Clinical Psychiatry*, **54**, 476–480.

Sichel, D. A, Cohen, L. S., Rosenbaum, J. F., *et al* (1993a) Postpartum onset of obsessive–compulsive disorder. *Psychosomatics*, **34**, 277–279.

Sichel, D. A, Cohen, L. S., Dimmock, J. A., *et al* (1993b) Postpartum obsessive compulsive disorder: a case series. *Journal of Clinical Psychiatry*, **54**, 156–159.

Singer, L. T., Salvator, A., Guo, S., *et al* (1999) Maternal psychological distress and parenting stress after the birth of a very low-birth-weight infant. *Journal of the American Medical Association*, **281**, 799–805.

Sjögren, B. & Thomasson, P. (1997) Obstetric outcome in 100 women with severe anxiety over childbirth. *Acta Obstetricia et Gynecologica Scandinavica*, **76**, 948–952.

Skari, H., Skreden, M., Malt, U. F., *et al* (2002) Comparative levels of psychological distress, stress symptoms, depression and anxiety after childbirth – a prospective population-based study of mothers and fathers. *British Journal of Obstetrics and Gynaecology*, **109**, 1154–1163.

Söderquist, J., Wijma, B. & Wijma, K. (2006) The longitudinal course of post-traumatic stress after childbirth. *Journal of Psychosomatic Obstetrics and Gynecology*, **27**, 113–119.

Soet, J. E., Brack, G. A. & Dilorio, C. (2003) Prevalence and predictors of women's experience of psychological trauma during childbirth. *Birth*, **30**, 36–46.

Spinelli, M. G. & Endicott, J. (2003) Controlled clinical trial of interpersonal psychotherapy versus parenting education program for depressed pregnant women. *American Journal of Psychiatry*, **160**, 555–562.

Stowe, Z. N., Casarella, J., Landry, J., *et al* (1995) Use of Lustral™ (sertraline) in post-natal depression. *Depression*, **3**, 49–55.

Stuart, S., Couser, G., Schilder, K., *et al* (1998) Postpartum anxiety and depression: onset and comorbidity in a community sample. *Journal of Nervous and Mental Disease*, **186**, 420–424.

Summers, A. L. & Logsdon, M. C. (2005) Web sites for postpartum depression: convenient, frustrating, incomplete, and misleading. *American Journal of Maternal Child Nursing*, **30**, 88–94.

Sun, H. S., Tsai, H-W., Ko, H-C., *et al* (2004) Association of tryptophan hydroxylase polymorphisms with depression, anxiety and comorbid depression and anxiety in a population-based sample of postpartum Taiwanese women. *Genes, Brain and Behavior*, **3**, 328–336.

Suri, R., Burt, V. K. & Altshuler, L. L. (2005) Nefazodone for the treatment of postpartum depression. *Archives of Women's Mental Health*, **8**, 55–56.

Sutter-Dallay, A. L., Giaconne-Marchese, V., Glatigny-Dallay, E., *et al* (2004) Women with anxiety disorders during pregnancy are at increased risk of intense postnatal depressive symptoms: a prospective survey of the MATQUID cohort. *European Psychiatry*, **19**, 459–463.

Sved-Williams, A. E. (1992) Phobic reactions of mothers to their own babies. *Australian and New Zealand Journal of Psychiatry*, **26**, 631–638.

Tezel, A. & Gozum, S. (2006) Comparison of effects of nursing care to problem solving training on levels of depressive symptoms in post partum women. *Patient Education and Counseling*, **63**, 64–73.

Thapar, A. K. & Thapar, A. (1992) Psychological sequelae of miscarriage: a controlled study using the general health questionnaire and the hospital anxiety and depression scale. *British Journal of General Practice*, **42**, 94–96.

Thompson, M. S. & Peebles-Wilkins, W. (1992) The impact of formal, informal and societal support networks on the psychological well-being of black adolescent mothers. *Social Work*, **37**, 322–328.

Treloar, S. A., Martin, N. G., Bucholz, K. K., *et al* (1999) Genetic influences on post-natal depressive symptoms: findings from an Australian twin sample. *Psychological Medicine*, **29**, 645–654.

Troisi, A., Moles, A., Panepuccia, L., *et al* (2002) Serum cholesterol levels and mood symptoms in the postpartum period. *Psychiatry Research*, **109**, 213–219.

Turton, P., Hughes, P., Evans, C. D. H., *et al* (2001) Incidence, correlates and predictors of post-traumatic stress disorder in the pregnancy after stillbirth. *British Journal of Psychiatry*, **178**, 556–560.

Ugarriza, D. N. (2004) Group therapy and its barriers for women suffering from postpartum depression. *Archives of Psychiatric Nursing*, **18**, 39–48.

Ugarriza, D. N. & Schmidt, L. (2006) Telecare for women with postpartum depression. *Journal of Psychosocial Nursing and Mental Health Services*, **44**, 37–45.

Uguz, F., Akamn, C. Kaya, N., *et al* (2007) Post-partum onset obsessive–compulsive disorder: incidence, clinical features and related factors. *Journal of Clinical Psychiatry*, **68**, 132–138.

van Dam, R. M., Schuit, A. J., Schouten, G., *et al* (1999) Serum cholesterol decline and depression in the postpartum period. *Journal of Psychosomatic Research*, **46**, 385–390.

Van den Bergh, B. R., Mulder, E. J., Mennes, M., *et al* (2005) Antenatal maternal anxiety and stress and the neurobehavioural development of the fetus and child: links and possible mechanisms. A review. *Neuroscience and Biobehavioral Reviews*, **29**, 237–258.

Varma, D., Chandra, P. S., Thomas, T., *et al* (2007) Intimate partner violence and sexual coercion among pregnant women in India: relationship with depression and post-traumatic stress disorder. *Journal of Affective Disorders*, **102**, 227–235.

Waterstone, M., Wolfe, C., Hooper, R., *et al* (2003) Postnatal morbidity after childbirth and severe obstetric morbidity. *British Journal of Obstetrics and Gynaecology*, **110**, 128–133.

Watson, J. P., Elliott, S. A., Rugg, A. J., *et al* (1984) Psychiatric disorder in pregnancy and the first postnatal year. *British Journal of Psychiatry*, **144**, 453–462.

Webster, J., Pritchard, M. A., Linnane, J. W. J., *et al* (2001) Postnatal depression: Use of health services and satisfaction with health-care providers. *Journal of Quality in Clinical Practice*, **21**, 144–148.

Weier, K. M. & Beal, M. W. (2004) Complementary therapies as adjuncts in the treatment of postpartum depression. *Journal of Midwifery and Women's Health*, **49**, 96–104.

Weightman, H., Dalal, B. M. & Brockington, I. F. (1998) Pathological fear of cot death. *Psychopathology*, **31**, 246–249.

Wenzel, A., Gorman, L., O'Hara, M., *et al* (2001) The occurrence of panic and obsessive compulsive symptoms in women with postpartum dysphoria: a prospective study. *Archives of Women's Mental Health*, **4**, 5–12.

Wenzel, A., Haugen, E., Jackson, L. C., *et al* (2003) Prevalence of generalised anxiety at eight weeks postpartum. *Archives of Women's Mental Health*, **6**, 43–49.

Wenzel, A., Haugen, E., Jackson, L. C., *et al* (2005) Anxiety symptoms and disorders at eight weeks postpartum. *Anxiety Disorders*, **19**, 295–311.

Whitton, A., Warner, R. & Appleby, L. (1996) The pathway to care in post-natal depression: women's attitudes to post-natal depression and its treatment. *British Journal of General Practice*, **46**, 427–428.

Wickberg, B. & Hwang, C. P. (1996) Counselling of postnatal depression: a controlled study on a population based Swedish sample. *Journal of Affective Disorders*, **39**, 209–216.

Wisner, K. L., Peindl, K. S., Gigliotti, T. V., *et al* (1999a) Obsessions and compulsions in women with postpartum depression. *Journal of Clinical Psychiatry*, **60**, 176–180.

Wisner, K. L., Peindl, K. S., Gigliotti, T. V., *et al* (1999b) Tricyclics vs SSRIs for postpartum depression. *Archives of Women's Mental Health*, **1**, 189–191.

Wisner, K. L., Perel, J. M., Peindl, K. S., *et al* (2004) Timing of depression recurrence in the first year after birth. *Journal of Affective Disorders*, **78**, 249–252.

Wisner, K. L., Hanusa, B. H., Perel, J. M., *et al* (2006) Postpartum depression: a randomized trial of sertraline versus nortriptyline. *Journal of Clinical Psychopharmacology*, **26**, 353–360.

Wong, M. K. Y., Crawford, T., Gask, L., *et al* (2003) A qualitative investigation into women's experiences after a miscarriage: implications for the primary healthcare team. *British Journal of General Practice*, **53**, 697–702.

Yexley, M. (2007) Treating postpartum depression with hypnosis: addressing specific symptoms presented by the client. *American Journal of Clinical Hypnosis*, **49**, 219.

Zolese, G. & Blacker, C. V. (1992) The psychological complications of therapeutic abortion. *British Journal of Psychiatry*, **160**, 742–749.

Further reading

Alder, J., Fink, N., Bitzer, J., *et al* (2007) Depression and anxiety during pregnancy: a risk factor for obstetric, fetal and neonatal outcome? A critical review of the literature. *Journal of Maternal-Fetal and Neonatal Medicine*, **20**, 189–209.

Halbriech, U. (2006) The association between pregnancy processes, preterm delivery, low birth weight, and postpartum depressions – the need for interdisciplinary integrations. *American Journal of Obstetrics and Gynecology*, **193**, 1312–1322.

Raphael-Leff, J. (1991) *Psychological Processes of Childbearing*. Chapman and Hall.

Stowe, Z. N., McCreary, P., Hostetter, A., *et al* (2001) Management of treatment-resistant depression during pregnancy and the postpartum period. In *Treatment-Resistant Mood Disorders* (eds J.D. Amsterdam, M. Hornig & A.A. Nierenberg), pp. 321–349. Cambridge University Press.

The Royal College of Psychiatrists

Information leaflets on postnatal depression for patients, carers and professionals, and on mental illness after childbirth (www.rcpsych.ac.uk/mentalhealthinformation/mentalhealthproblems/postnatalmentalhealth.aspx).

www.mededppd.org/

A website supported by the US National Institute of Mental Health, providing information to help screen, diagnose and treat women with postnatal depression. There are sections for professionals (which include continuing professional development material), women with postnatal depression and their families.

CHAPTER 3

Puerperal psychosis

Studies have suggested that the few weeks after delivery are when a woman is at highest risk of a psychotic illness. Kendell *et al* (1976) demonstrated that in the 3 months following childbirth, women are more than 20 times as likely to be admitted with a diagnosis of a psychotic disorder. However, Terp & Mortensen (1998), using women from the general population as controls, found that the relative risk of all admissions was only increased slightly (RR=1.09) but that for a first admission with functional psychosis between days 2 and 28 after delivery the relative risk was 3.21. Harlow *et al* (2007) found a similar incidence of hospitalisation in first-time mothers (0.01%), noting that this was largely confined to women who had previously had a psychotic or bipolar illness and that most of the postpartum episodes occurred within 4 weeks of delivery. More recently, using women who had delivered in the 11–12 months previously as controls, a Danish group (Munk-Olsen *et al*, 2006) found the risk raised in the first 3 months and highest for first-time mothers 10–19 days postpartum (RR=7.31). Similarly, the risk of psychiatric out-patient contact was increased in the first 3 months and highest 10–19 days after delivery (RR=2.67). The prevalence for the first 3 months was 1.03 per 1000 births. Women with schizophrenia-like disorders were more likely to be admitted within the first month after delivery and women with bipolar illness within the first 2 months of delivery. Kendell *et al* (1976) identified a later peak of admissions from the 10–24th month after delivery.

Puerperal psychoses are severe illnesses that onset within 2–4 weeks of delivery and will usually require admission. Affective illnesses predominate, most often fulfilling diagnostic criteria for major depression with psychotic features, mania or schizoaffective psychosis (Dean & Kendell, 1981; Meltzer & Kumar, 1985; Pfuhlmann *et al*, 1998). A proportion can only be classified as 'unspecified functional psychosis' and around half meet Leonhard's criteria for cycloid psychosis (Pfuhlmann *et al*, 1998).

Organic psychoses occurring in relation to childbirth have been recognised and documented since the time of Hippocrates and include idiopathic confusional states, stupor, post-eclamptic psychosis, infective delirium,

delirium associated with anaemia and alcohol withdrawal (Brockington, 1996), subdural haematoma (e.g. Campbell & Varma, 1993) and, more recently, meningioma (Khong *et al*, 2007) as presenting with psychotic symptoms postpartum. Organic psychoses, particularly infective delirium, may still be a common cause of puerperal psychosis in some low- and middle-income countries (Ndosi & Mtawali, 2002).

Phenomena

The early signs of illness are often non-specific, for example insomnia, agitation, perplexity and odd behaviour. Such symptoms can easily be overlooked or attributed to postpartum blues and their significance not recognised. However, the patient may be floridly psychotic within a few hours as onset is frequently very rapid and often occurs only a few days after delivery.

When the symptomatology of 58 women with puerperal psychosis and 52 women with non-puerperal psychotic illnesses (including schizophrenia) was compared, the puerperal group were found to be less likely to have persecutory or systematised delusions, auditory hallucinations, odd affect and social withdrawal than the non-puerperal controls. However, they were more likely to have manic features such as elation, lability of mood, rambling speech and distractibility as well as more confusion and increased need to be supervised during tasks (Brockington *et al*, 1981). Conversely, a South African study comparing 20 puerperal women with psychosis and 20 age-matched controls with mania (Oosthuizen *et al*, 1995) observed the puerperal group to be more likely to have delusions of control, auditory hallucinations, blunted affect and emotional turmoil. However, their findings are limited by the following: many puerperal women with psychosis have a depressive illness but were excluded from the study; the patients were not randomly selected; a third of the puerperal group had a history of treatment for schizophrenia. Four women meeting criteria for delusional misidentification as in the Fregoli syndrome have been described (O'Sullivan & Dean, 1991).

Apparent cognitive deficits are not unusual. A US study compared 21 women who had childbearing-related affective psychoses with 96 women whose psychosis was not related to delivery. They found that the recently delivered group had 'more prominent symptoms relating to cognitive impairment and bizarre behaviour' and more homicidal ideas than the control group (Wisner *et al*, 1994). Mood-incongruent delusions are not infrequent, for example delusions of reference or persecution, and there may be visual, tactile or olfactory hallucinations which again suggest an organic syndrome.

Catatonic symptoms such as waxy flexibility, stupor, mutism, immobility and negativism have been reported in the literature (e.g. Hanson & Brown, 1973; Lai & Huang, 2004) and observed in clinical practice, but their true prevalence in the postpartum population is not known. One case of catatonic stupor reported in the literature was found to have an atypical posterior reversible encephalopathy syndrome (Kitabayashi *et al*, 2007).

Epidemiology

The last few decades have seen a fall in mortality and morbidity from childbirth but this has not been paralleled by a fall in the incidence of puerperal psychosis, which has remained remarkably stable at 0.5–1.0 per 1000 deliveries (Meltzer & Kumar, 1985; Terp & Moretensen, 1998; Munk-Olsen *et al*, 2006; Harlow *et al*, 2007). However, if a woman has had a past episode, the risk rises to one in seven (Kendell *et al*, 1987).

Risk factors for admission in the puerperium identified in early studies include being primiparous, single and having had a Caesarean section (Kendell *et al*, 1976, 1981, 1987; Meltzer & Kumar, 1985). Kendall *et al* (1987) found an association with a history of perinatal death not found in the other studies. Paffenbarger (1964) also identified being older, having longer intervals between pregnancies and fertility problems as being risk factors. A large study of first-time mothers in Sweden over a 12-year period ($n=502\,767$), identified older age and being single as risk factors (Nager *et al*, 2005). Analysis on the same data-set also found that those living in the poorest neighbourhoods had a significantly higher risk of admission (Nager *et al*, 2006). In a within-participant comparative study of 129 women with bipolar affective puerperal psychosis, Blackmore *et al* (2006) identified primiparity (OR=3.76) and delivery complications (OR=2.68) as independent risk factors.

There are differences in the sleep patterns of women in late pregnancy and the postpartum period that are more marked in first-time mothers. Women with puerperal psychosis may have a longer labour and be more likely to deliver at night than controls (Sharma *et al*, 2004), and sleep loss has been suggested as a final common pathway for various causal factors in the development of psychosis in vulnerable women (Sharma & Mazmanian, 2003).

In low- and middle-income countries there is high comorbidity with physical health problems including anaemia, infection and oedema proteinuria hypertension gestosis (Agarwal *et al*, 1990; Ndosi & Mtawali, 2002) but some authors have noted the close match between the incidence, pattern of illness and associated findings in a Black African population and those described in the literature in populations in the Western world (Allwood *et al*, 2000).

Onset, course and prognosis

Paffenbarger (1964) reported that there was usually a 'lucid interval' after delivery before the development of symptoms. A third of his sample developed symptoms within the first week, 68% within the first months and 80% inside 6 weeks. In a study of women admitted to hospital in Japan, half had an onset of illness in the first week postpartum and 56% in the second week; 80% became ill within the first month (Okano *et al*, 1998). However, a recent study refutes the notion of a latent period, with 50% of women with bipolar experiencing puerperal psychotic symptoms on days 1–3 with 22% of onsets on day 1 (Heron *et al*, 2007). Early symptoms include feeling excited, elated or high, not sleeping, feeling energetic or active and talking more (Heron *et al*, 2008).

There is often a time lag between onset of illness and admission but several studies indicate that women with manic episodes are admitted more quickly than those with depressive psychoses (Dean & Kendell, 1981; Meltzer & Kumar, 1985; Okano *et al*, 1998) and that psychotic depressions onset earlier than non-psychotic illnesses (Meltzer & Kumar, 1985).

The course of illness can be fluctuating and involve very severe disturbance but the prognosis of the acute episode is good, with most women making a good recovery and returning to premorbid functioning. In the longer term, however, there is a risk of further episodes both after subsequent pregnancies and at other times.

Brockington *et al* (1982) summed the findings of six studies published between 1956 and 1972 and estimated the combined risk of recurrence to be about one in five for each subsequent pregnancy. Others estimate it at 25–50%. For example, Pfuhlmann *et al* (2000) followed up women 6–26 years after a first-episode puerperal psychosis and observed a 47% recurrence rate after later deliveries. Puerperal recurrence after subsequent pregnancies in a recent 10-year follow-up was 75–80% for women whose index illness was a psychosis and 27.3% for those in whom it was depression (Garfield *et al*, 2004). The risk of non-puerperal episodes appears to be higher.

Da Silva & Johnstone (1981) found 50% of a hospitalised sample remaining well after 1–6 years follow-up. Of the remainder, 2 had died by suicide, 3 were long-term in-patients, 14 were in out-patient care, 1 was on lithium but well, and 3 were not in treatment and unwell. They noted a poorer outcome in women with an index schizophrenia illness. Dean *et al* (1989) observed a 36% recurrence rate if the index episode was puerperal but 50% if it was not. Similar findings were reported by Schöpf & Rust (1994), but others found a higher recurrence rate in those with index puerperal episodes (40% *v*. 31%), though this was a smaller sample (Hunt & Silverstone 1995). Videbech & Gouliaev (1995) followed up 50 women 7–14 years after their first psychotic episode which was puerperal. Forty per cent of the women were not working to full capacity owing to mental disorder, 60% had had recurrences and schizophreniform symptoms in the index episode predicted incapacity to work. Only 4% of women had exclusively puerperal episodes.

Garfield *et al* (2004) followed up 66 women 10 years after hospitalisation with a puerperal illness. The recurrence rate was 87.2% and the readmission rate 63.3%. The strongest predictor of recurrence was a past psychiatric history. Women with no previous psychiatric history or who had only experienced previous puerperal episodes do better at follow-up (only 38.9% relapsed) than those who had a prior history of non-puerperal illness (70.9%). Most of the women in this study had a diagnosis of major depression. Of 61 women reviewed after 25 years since a puerperal psychotic episode (various diagnoses), 63.9% had had further episodes, with the average number of episodes being 4.8 (Rohde & Marneros, 1993). A 9-year follow-up of women with clearly defined bipolar affective puerperal psychosis found 57% experiencing additional puerperal illnesses and 62% non-puerperal episodes (Robertson *et al*, 2005).

Psychosis in pregnancy

There are case-reports of psychosis occurring (Brockington *et al*, 1990) and recurring during pregnancy (Glaze *et al*, 1991). Howe & Srinavasan (1999) report a case of Cotard's syndrome occurring around the 33rd week of pregnancy. The woman jumped out of the upstairs window of the obstetric unit sustaining multiple fractures. Her baby was delivered by Caesarean section and she was treated with electroconvulsive therapy (ECT). In 2003, Friedman & Rosenthal reported a case of delusional disorder and borderline personality disorder in the third trimester. The patient was treated successfully with olanzapine and psychotherapy. Another report describes a woman presenting at 28 weeks gestation with symptoms initially like eclampsia but who within 48 h of Caesarean delivery of her infant became floridly psychotic. It was then assumed that her initial presentation had in fact been catatonic stupor (Ranzini *et al*, 1996). Mbassa Mencik (2005) reports 12.5% of women with psychotic disorders relating to childbirth presenting to a hospital in Cameroon becoming acutely ill while pregnant.

There are also case-reports of psychosis occurring after termination of pregnancy or miscarriage (e.g. da Silva & Johnstone, 1981; Davidson & Clare, 1998; Brockington, 2005), hydatidiform mole (Hopker & Brockington, 1991) and male-to-female gender reassignment (Mallett *et al*, 1989).

Many of these women have gone on to suffer from puerperal psychoses after subsequent pregnancies which went to term, suggesting a link between late pregnancy, post-abortion and postpartum triggers.

Relationship to bipolar disorder

Chaudron & Pies (2003) reviewed the evidence base from 1966 to 2002, which includes the follow-up studies cited above, and concluded that it 'supported a link between postpartum psychosis and bipolar disorder' with many but not all puerperal psychotic episodes falling within the bipolar spectrum. The evidence base to support this is growing. The high risk of recurrence of bipolar disorder after delivery and management of this is discussed in Chapter 4.

Aetiology

Genetics

In the early 19th century, Esquirol noted that puerperal psychosis tended to run in families (Esquirol, 1838). Dean *et al* (1989) observed a significant and substantial increase in affective morbidity in first-degree relatives of women who had experienced puerperal psychosis compared with women with bipolar who had not had a puerperal episode. Puerperal psychosis has a close relationship with bipolar disorder and there is compelling evidence from family, twin and adoption studies that genes influence susceptibility to bipolar disorder, although the mode of inheritance appears complex and it is likely that interaction of several susceptibility genes is required. There are case reports of monozygotic twin pairs concordant for puerperal psychosis (e.g. Kane, 1968) and a familial clustering where there was consanguinity (Craddock *et al*, 1994). Jones & Craddock (2001) have demonstrated that women with bipolar whose first-degree relative has had an episode of puerperal psychosis are more likely to experience a puerperal episode following subsequent pregnancies than those who have no first-degree relatives with puerperal psychosis. In addition, women with bipolar who have had a puerperal episode are more likely to have a first-degree relative with an affective disorder than women without a history of puerperal episodes (Jones & Craddock, 2001).

Variation at the serotonin transporter gene is influenced by oestradiol. The presence of one allele (Stin2.12) was associated with an almost four times risk of puerperal psychosis (OR=3.9), an effect that increased when the phenotype was restricted to women who had experienced multiple episodes (Coyle *et al*, 2000); recent work has shown linkage with chromosomes 16p13 and 8q24 (Jones *et al*, 2007).

Dopamine

Oestrogen modulates monoamine neurotransmitter systems including the dopaminergic system. The rapid fall of circulating gonadal steroid hormones after delivery paralleling the often acute onset of symptoms led to the hypothesis that women who become psychotic may have supersensitive dopamine receptors, particularly D_2 receptors. Two cases in which puerperal psychosis was accompanied by abnormal extrapyramidal movements support this idea (Vinogradov & Csernansky, 1990) and there are case reports of puerperal psychosis following treatment with bromocriptine (e.g. Canterbury *et al*, 1987; Reeves & Pinkofsky, 1997; Pinardo Zabala *et al*, 2003). The dopamine agonist apomorphine was used by Wieck *et al* (1991) to test this by giving apomorphine to postpartum women with a history of psychosis and to controls 4 days after delivery. The women who had recurrences of psychosis had greater growth hormone responses than the controls and those who remained well. However, a later study was unable to replicate these findings and found no difference between those at high risk of recurrence and controls (Meakin *et al*, 1995).

Wieck *et al* (2003) demonstrated that women predisposed to bipolar relapses in the puerperium had greater growth hormone responses than controls in the midluteal phase of the menstrual cycle but not in the follicular phase.

Thyroid

The relationship between non-psychotic puerperal depression and thyroid function has been described in Chapter 2. The literature relating to psychotic puerperal illnesses and thyroid abnormalities is limited to a case-report of a woman who developed psychotic depression at 3 months postpartum and who also had thyroiditis. Her symptoms resolved when she became biochemically euthyroid (Bokhari *et al*, 1998).

Women's experiences

Women who have suffered from postnatal depression feel very strongly that it is different from other mental illnesses, precipitated by childbirth and with a biological aetiology. As such, they feel that it requires specialised treatment. Those who had been treated in general psychiatric services felt frustrated and angry that their specific needs were not met and that they had been treated like everyone else. Other important themes were loss of aspects of motherhood, control, future pregnancies, and disruption of social roles and relationships (Robertson & Lyons, 2003). Hanzak (2005) has written a vivid account of her illness, hospitalisation and recovery.

Suicide

'Why Mothers Die 2000–2002' (Lewis & Drife, 2004), highlighted suicide as a major cause of maternal death, and, like the 1997–1999 CEMD report (Lewis & Drife, 2001), found suicide to be the leading cause of indirect or late-indirect deaths for the year following delivery. The majority of these deaths appeared to be of women suffering from psychosis or a very severe depressive illness. Oates (2003) has estimated the suicide rate for puerperal psychosis to be 2 per 1000 women. Lindahl *et al* (2005) estimate that suicide accounts for 20% of maternal deaths even though the rate for all delivered women in the year after birth is lower than that of the general population. 'Saving Mothers' Lives' (Lewis, 2007) found a decrease in the numbers of maternal suicide, which if it persists in the next triennium, will suggest that some of the strategies recommended are being implemented.

The most common profile of a woman who is at risk of suicide in late pregnancy or after delivery is a White, older woman in her second or subsequent pregnancy, married and living in comfortable circumstances. She is likely to have had contact with psychiatric services and a history of mental illness, and may be in current treatment. She is likely to die violently (e.g. by hanging, drowning, jumping from a height or in front of a train, by causing an intentional road traffic accident, self-immolation or throat cutting).

Self-harm

A review in 1968 estimated that between 5 and 12% of women attempting suicide were pregnant (Whitlock & Edwards, 1968). In 1984, 0.07% of calls to a US metropolitan poison control centre were from or about pregnant women (Rayburn *et al*, 1984) and the attempt reported was usually her first. Half of the overdoses reported were taken during the first trimester, most commonly using an over-the-counter analgesic, iron or a vitamin.

Studies in Sweden and the USA have found that issues relating to pregnancy and interpersonal difficulties are often cited as the main provoking factors for self-harm in pregnant women. These may include prior loss of children (through death, termination or adoption), desire for a termination or the potential loss of a partner as reasons for their act.

One review assessed 27 studies that reported rates of suicidal ideation, intention, attempts and completed suicide in pregnant and postpartum women (Lindahl *et al*, 2005). Suicidal thoughts (assessed by endorsement of item 10 on the EPDS, 'the thought of harming myself has occurred to me') occurred in up to 14% of pregnant women. The authors observed lower rates of suicide during pregnancy than that in the general population, but that when suicide did occur, violent methods were used. Particular groups at risk are teenagers and women from cultures where being unmarried and pregnant is stigmatised. Women with past histories of abuse are also more likely to die by suicide. A US study of over 2000 women who attempted suicide found that those more likely to harm themselves were young, single, multiparous, less well-educated and more likely to be African-American. Of these, 26% misused substances (Gandhi *et al*, 2006). Follow-up found that those who self-harmed were more likely than controls to have a preterm labour, a Caesarean delivery and require a blood transfusion. Their infants showed an increased risk of respiratory distress syndrome and low birth weight.

Infanticide

Although the majority of women who die by suicide do not also kill their infant, the 2000–2002 CEMD report (Lewis & Drife, 2004) identified three cases where the infant was also killed at the time of the suicide. In two cases, an older child was also killed at the same time and four suicides occurring in pregnancy near term also resulted in the death of a viable infant. Infanticidal ideas are common in populations with severe postpartum mental illness. Chandra *et al* (2002) report 43% having suicidal ideas, 36% reporting infanticidal behaviour and 34% reporting both. Depression and psychotic ideas predicted infanticidal ideas, while the presence of psychotic ideas towards the infant predicted infanticidal behaviour.

Infanticide is a legal term used in the UK to refer to the killing of a child under the age of 12 months. Neonaticide is not a legal term but refers to the killing of a child within 24h of birth. Craig (2004) has reviewed the associated factors and Friedman *et al* (2005*a*) included infanticide and neonaticide in a wider review of child murder. Women who commit neonaticide are usually young, poorly educated and primiparous. They are often living at home with their parents and often have concealed their pregnancy. Most do not have a mental illness at the time of killing their child. Very few of them have a psychotic disorder and where a psychiatric diagnosis is found, this is more likely to be a personality disorder or a mild or borderline learning disability.

Mothers who commit infanticide are more likely to be older and married or living with a partner. There is more likely to be a mental illness present and the infant death is often part of an extended suicide or occasionally an altruistic act based upon a delusional idea that some terrible fate was about to befall the infant. Mothers with schizophrenia who relapse in relation to pregnancy or childbirth may incorporate the infant into their delusional system or be acutely disturbed and carry out the act with no rational reason.

Substance misuse is a factor often associated with infanticide and only very rarely is it the consequence of factitious disorder by proxy.

Friedman *et al* (2005*b*) examined a case series of mothers who had killed their children and were adjudicated as 'not guilty by reason of insanity' (n=9). Their children's ages ranged from birth to 16 years (mean=3.7; a third were infants). Over 80% of the mothers had a psychotic disorder or mood disorder with psychotic features and many had had recent contact with psychiatric services. Almost half had made previous suicide attempts and 56% had planned suicide along with the death of their child. Half of these women had depression and the majority were experiencing auditory hallucinations including command hallucinations to kill their children. Three-quarters were delusional at the time of the killing and two-thirds of these had delusions that involved their children. These delusions frequently involved a belief that the child was possessed by the devil or demons, that the mother herself was a god or religious figure and that some terrible thing would happen to the child. Over a third were pregnant or within the first postpartum year. The most common method used was suffocation.

In England and Wales, women who kill a child under the age of 12 months are usually disposed of by the judiciary by means of Chapter 36 of the Infanticide Act 1938 (Office of Public Sector Information, 1938). This allows for the occasion when a mother:

> '...causes death of her child under the age of 12 months by wilful act or omission, but at the time of the act or omission the balance of her mind was disturbed by reason of her having not fully recovered from the effect of having

61

given birth to the child or by reasons of the effect of lactation consequent on the birth of the child...'.

In Northern Ireland, the relevant legislation is the Infanticide Act (Northern Ireland) 1939. In Scotland, there is no specific legislation and general homicide laws are imposed instead.

Disposal is usually non-custodial and can be tied in with ongoing treatment in a community rehabilitation order with conditions of treatment or a hospital order. However, this somewhat outdated law gives rise to anomalies. For example, a women who kills her infant who is a day over a year old, despite clear evidence of her illness being consequent upon childbirth, will be charged with murder and despite a plea of diminished responsibility, will be much more likely to receive a custodial sentence. In 2006, the Homicide Act was revised and recommendations made (Law Commission, 2006; Box 3.1). However, at the time of writing these changes are still under discussion.

Management

Assessment

The assessment of any acutely ill puerperal woman is essentially the standard psychiatric examination (history, mental state examination and physical examination) with the addition of the bio-psychosocial context of recent childbirth and the infant's well-being to consider as well as the mother's, that of her partner, other children and family members.

Box 3.1 Homicide Act 2006 revisions and recommendations

Infanticide

9.27 We recommend that the offence/defence of infanticide be retained without amendment (subject to 'murder' being replaced with 'first degree murder or second degree murder'). (Paragraph 8.23)

9.28 We recommend that in circumstances where infanticide is not raised as an issue at trial and the defendant (biological mother of a child aged 12 months or less) is convicted by the jury of murder [first degree murder or second degree murder], the trial judge should have the power to order a medical examination of the defendant with a view to establishing whether or not there is evidence that at the time of the killing the requisite elements of a charge of infanticide were present. If such evidence is produced and the defendant wishes to appeal, the judge should be able to refer the application to the Court of Appeal and to postpone sentence pending the determination of the application. (Paragraphs 8.46 and 8.58)

Reproduced with permission from Law Commission, 2006

It is essential in all women with psychosis or depression to assess suicidality and infanticidal ideas. Delusions should be clearly defined and the content examined carefully for reference to harming herself and/or her infant and/or older children. A mother who believes that her child has changed in some way, looks strange, is not hers or is, for example, evil, is at risk of harming that child.

Chandra *et al* (2006) found that 53% of women with a severe postpartum illness and 78% of those with psychotic postpartum disorders had delusional beliefs about their infant. The mothers whose delusions involved believing that the baby was a devil, ill-fated or was someone else's baby were more likely to shout at or hit the infant or to have attempted to smother it. Caregivers of those women who believed their baby was God were more likely to consider her unsafe with her baby and other delusions (more elaborate or bizarre) were associated with being unable to manage chores related to the baby and with talking negatively about it.

A number of rating scales have been devised to assess disturbances of the mother–infant relationship. The Bethlem Mother–Infant Interaction Scale has seven sub-scales and was designed to be used on a weekly basis by nursing staff on an in-patient unit (Kumar & Hipwell, 1996). It can be repeated to monitor progress. There are also scales that assess mother–infant bonding (Brockington *et al*, 2001; Taylor *et al*, 2005). The two latter scales have been compared (Wittkowski *et al*, 2007).

Beware the patient who superficially appears to have an acute mental disorder but if an adequate history and examination are performed is found to have an acute medical or surgical problem. There are case reports of chronic subdural haematoma presenting as puerperal psychosis in which the patient's complaint of persistent headache after epidural anaesthesia was ignored (Campbell & Varma, 1993), and a woman appearing confused and complaining of auditory hallucinations and *déja vu* the day after a Caesarean delivery, who was found to have a meningioma (Khong *et al*, 2007). The misattribution of physical symptoms to functional psychiatric disorder can cause a delay in making the correct diagnosis or lead to the admission of acutely medically ill women to psychiatric hospitals. Such mistakes led to the deaths of several women reported to the last two CEMD reports (Lewis & Drife, 2004; Lewis, 2007).

In-patient care

Most women with acute psychosis will require admission, as will some of those with a severe depressive illness and other diagnosis. Women who require acute admission for a severe mental illness in the postpartum should be admitted to a specialist mother and baby unit unless there are compelling child protection issues which preclude this. In Scotland this is now enshrined within the Mental Health (Care and Treatment) Act 2003 (Office of Public Sector Information, 2003).

Drug treatment

Most women with psychotic illnesses will require antipsychotic medication in addition to antidepressants and/or mood stabilisers, depending on the precise nature of the episode. Care should be taken not to over sedate a woman caring for an infant, particularly if she is breastfeeding and needs to do night feeds. However, in the early days of an admission many women will require their baby to be looked after in the nursery at night to allow them to sleep. At other times even women with severe psychosis can, with the support of nursery nurses and psychiatric nurses skilled in the care of mothers, undertake a good deal of infant care and maintain a close bond with their baby.

There are case reports of neuroleptic malignant syndrome occurring in women with puerperal psychosis (e.g. Price *et al*, 1989; Alexander *et al*, 1998) and some authors have postulated that women with puerperal psychosis might be more likely to experience it. It can be difficult to distinguish clinically from the 'organic' features of the illness or acute sepsis and other physical complications of the postpartum period. However, it should be considered if a patient appears to deteriorate after medication with psychotropics and the serum creatinine phosphokinase level checked Prescribing for breastfeeding mothers is discussed in Chapter 9.

Women with depression in a retarded or stuperose state may need anticoagulating if they have recently delivered and are inactive. As such, women may well need ECT; an anaesthetic opinion should be sought well in advance.

Oestradiol

There are three small case series examining the role that oestradiol might have as an effective treatment for puerperal psychosis. The first two describe women with low oestradiol levels and refractory to antipsychotics being given sublingual 17B oestradiol. The rise in serum concentrations is reported as paralleling the improvement in symptoms (Ahokas & Aiko, 1999; Ahokas *et al*, 2000*a*). In the third study, 10 women with puerperal psychosis and low oestradiol levels after delivery were given sublingual 17B oestradiol three to six times daily until the serum concentration was 400 pmol/l (Ahokas *et al*, 2000*b*). Symptoms measured by the Brief Psychiatric Rating Scale improved by the end of the first week, but it should be noted that two-thirds of the women had had treatment before starting oestradiol (psychotherapy and antipsychotics), though this was reported as being ineffective. None of these studies report any safety data, which is important given the potential risks of thromboembolic events and endometrial hyperplasia. Clearly there is a need for larger, controlled, methodologically sound studies before oestradiol can be declared an effective and safe treatment for puerperal psychosis.

There is a published report of progesterone used as a treatment for puerperal mania (Meakin & Brockington, 1990) but the improvement in the two cases reported in this paper could be attributed to the antipsychotics that were also prescribed. There are no controlled data to support the use of progesterone as a treatment for puerperal psychosis.

Electroconvulsive therapy

There has long been a belief that puerperal psychosis is particularly responsive to ECT and this has been confirmed by one study (Reed *et al*, 1999) in which women with puerperal illnesses showed greater clinical improvement than those with non-puerperal disorder. The use of ECT in pregnant women is described in Chapter 8.

Psychological treatment

Although no specific intervention has been trialled in women with puerperal psychotic illnesses, it is clear that many would benefit from psychotherapeutic work, particularly when the acute phase of the disorder is settling. There may be specific issues that need addressing such as bereavement or coping with stressful life events and marital problems, in addition to coming to terms with having been acutely ill and what that means for the future. A woman with her first psychotic episode and her partner will benefit from education about the disorder, the risk of recurrence after later pregnancies or at other times and what can be done to prevent it recurring (the prevention of puerperal psychosis is described in Chapter 7).

Contraception

Contraceptive needs must be addressed and in place before a woman begins periods of home leave. Do not assume the primary care team will deal with this on discharge. Depot norethisterone enanthate given within 48 h of delivery has been associated with depressive symptoms (Dennis *et al*, 2008) so long-acting progestogens are unlikely to be the best option for women with mood disorders. If in doubt, seek advice from the midwife with a responsibility for contraceptive advice or the local family planning clinic. Mother and baby units should keep a stock of condoms to give to patients who have not made any contraceptive plans before going on leave.

References

Agrawal, P., Bhatia, M. S. & Malik, S. C. (1990) Postpartum psychosis: a study of indoor cases in a general hospital clinic. *Acta Psychiatrica Scandinavica*, **81**, 571–575.

Ahokas, A. & Aito, M. (1999) Role of estradiol in puerperal psychosis. *Psychopharmacology*, **147**, 108–110.

Ahokas, A., Aito, M. & Turiainen, S. (2000a) Association between oestradiol and puerperal psychosis. *Acta Psychiatrica Scandinavica*, **101**, 167–169.

Ahokas, A., Aito, M. & Rimon, R. (2000b) Positive treatment effect of estradiol in postpartum psychosis: a pilot study. *Journal of Clinical Psychiatry*, **61**, 166–169.

Alexander, P. J., Thomas, R. M. & Das, A. (1998) Is risk of neuroleptic malignant syndrome increased in the postpartum period? *Journal of Clinical Psychiatry*, **59**, 254–255.

Allwood, C. W., Berk, M. & Bodemer, W. (2000) An investigation into puerperal psychoses in black women admitted to Baragwanath Hospital. *South African Medical Journal*, **90**, 518–520.

Blackmore E. R., Jones, I., Doshi, M., *et al* (2006) Obstetric variables associated with bipolar affective puerperal psychosis. *British Journal of Psychiatry*, **188**, 32–36.

Bokhari, R., Bhatara, V. S., Bandettini, F., *et al* (1998) Postpartum psychosis and postpartum thyroiditis. *Psychoneuroendocrinology*, **23**, 643–650.

Brockington, I. (1996). *Motherhood and Mental Health*. Oxford University Press.

Brockington, I. F. (2005) Post-abortion psychosis. *Archives of Women's Mental Health*, **8**, 53–54.

Brockington, I. F., Winokur, G. & Dean, C. (1982) Puerperal psychosis. In *Motherhood and Mental Illness* (eds I. F. Brockington & R. Kumar), pp. 37–59. Academic Press.

Brockington, I. F., Oates, M. & Rose, G. (1990) Prepartum psychosis. *Journal of Affective Disorders*, **19**, 31–35.

Brockington, I. F., Czernik, K. F., Schofield, E. M., *et al* (1981) Puerperal psychosis: phenomena and diagnosis. *Archives of General Psychiatry*, **38**, 829–833.

Brockington, I. F., Oates, J., George, S., *et al* (2001) A screening questionnaire for mother–infant bonding disorders. *Archives of Women's Mental Health*, **3**, 133–140.

Campbell, D. A. & Varma, T. R. (1993) Chronic subdural haematoma following epidural anaesthesia, presenting as puerperal psychosis. *British Journal of Obstetrics and Gynaecology*, **100**, 782–784.

Canterbury, R. J., Haskins, B., Khan, N., *et al* (1987) Postpartum psychosis induced by bromocriptine. *Southern Medical Journal*, **80**, 1463–1464.

Chandra, P. S., Venkatasubramanian, G. & Thomas, T. (2002) Infanticidal ideas and infanticidal behavior in Indian women with severe postpartum psychiatric disorders. *Journal of Nervous and Mental Disease*, **190**, 457–461.

Chandra, P. S., Bhargavarman, R. P., Raghunandan, V. N. G. P., *et al* (2006) Delusions related to infant and their association with mother–infant interactions in postpartum psychotic disorders. *Archives of Women's Mental Health*, **9**, 285–288.

Chaudron, L. H. & Pies, R. W. (2003) The relationship between postpartum psychosis and bipolar disorder: a review. *Journal of Clinical Psychiatry*, **64**, 1284–1292.

Coyle, N., Jones, I., Robertson, E., *et al* (2000) Variation at the serotonin transporter gene influences susceptibility to bipolar affective puerperal psychosis. *Lancet*, **356**, 1490–1491.

Craddock, N., Brockington, I., Mant, R., *et al* (1994) Bipolar affective puerperal psychosis associated with consanguinity. *British Journal of Psychiatry*, **164**, 359–364.

Craig, M. (2004) Perinatal risk factors for neonaticide and infanticide: can we identify those at risk? *Journal of the Royal Society of Medicine*, **97**, 57–61.

da Silva, L. & Johnstone, E. C. (1981) A follow-up study of severe puerperal psychiatric illness. *British Journal of Psychiatry*, **139**, 346–354.

Davidson, K. & Clare, A. W. (1989) Psychotic illness following termination of pregnancy. *British Journal of Psychiatry*, **154**, 559–560.

Dean, C. & Kendell, R. E. (1981) The symptomatology of puerperal illnesses. *British Journal of Psychiatry*, **139**, 128–133.

Dean, C., Williams, R. J. & Brockington, I. F. (1989) Is puerperal psychosis the same as bipolar manic-depressive disorder? A family study. *Psychological Medicine*, **19**, 637–647.

Dennis, C. L., Ross, L. E. & Herxheimer, A. (2008) Oestrogens and progestins for preventing and treating postpartum depression. *Cochrane Database of Systematic Reviews*, **4**, CD001690.

Esquirol, E. (1838) *Des Maladies Mentales Considérées sous les Rapports Medical, Hygénique et Medico Legal*. Baillière.

Friedman, S. H. & Rosenthal, M. B. (2003) Treatment of perinatal delusional disorder: a case report. *International Journal of Psychiatry in Medicine*, **33**, 391.

Friedman, S. H., Horwitz, S. M. & Resnick, P. J. (2005a) Child murder by mothers: a critical analysis of the current state of knowledge and a research agenda. *American Journal of Psychiatry*, **162**, 1578–1587.

Friedman, S. H., Hrouda, D. R. & Holden, C. E. (2005b) Child murder committed by severely mentally ill mothers: an examination of mothers found not guilty by reason of insanity. *Journal of Forensic Science*, **50**, 1–6.

Gandhi, S. G., Gilbert, W. M., McElvy, S. S., *et al* (2006) Maternal and neonatal outcomes after attempted suicide. *Obstetrics and Gynecology*, **107**, 984–990.

Garfield, P., Kent, A., Paykel, E. S., *et al* (2004) Outcome of postpartum disorders: a 10 year follow-up of hospital admissions. *Acta Psychiatrica Scandinavica*, **109**, 434–439.

Glaze, R., Chapman, G. & Murray, D. (1991) Recurrence of puerperal psychosis during late pregnancy. *British Journal of Psychiatry*, **159**, 567–569.

Hanson, G. D. & Brown, M. J. (1973) Waxy flexibility in a postpartum woman: a case report and review of the catatonic syndrome. *Psychiatric Quarterly*, **47**, 95–103.

Hanzak, E. A. (2005) *Eyes Without Sparkle: A Journey Through Postnatal Illness*. Radcliffe Publishing.

Harlow, B. L., Vitonis, A. F., Sparen, P., *et al* (2007) Incidence of hospitalization for postpartum psychotic and bipolar episodes in women with and without prior prepregnancy or prenatal psychiatric hospitalizations. *Archives of General Psychiatry*, **64**, 42–48.

Heron, J., Robertson Blackmore, E., McGuinness, M., *et al* (2007) No 'latent period' in the onset of bipolar affective puerperal psychosis. *Archives of Women's Mental Health*, **10**, 79–81.

Heron, J., McGuinness, M., Blackmore, E. R., *et al* (2008) Early postpartum symptoms in puerperal psychosis. *British Journal of Obstetrics and Gynaecology*, **115**, 348–353.

Hopker, S. W. & Brockington, I. F. (1991) Psychosis following hydatidiform mole in a patient with recurrent puerperal psychosis. *British Journal of Psychiatry*, **158**, 122–123.

Howe, G. B. & Srinavasan, M. (1999) A case study on the successful management of Cotard's syndrome in pregnancy. *International Journal of Psychiatry in Clinical Practice*, **3**, 293–295.

Hunt, N. & Silverstone, T. (1995) Does puerperal illness distinguish a subgroup of bipolar patients? *Journal of Affective Disorders*, **34**, 101–107.

Jones, I. & Craddock, N. (2001) Familiality of the puerperal trigger in bipolar disorder: results of a family study. *American Journal of Psychiatry*, **158**, 913–917.

Jones, I., Hamshere, M., Nangle, J-M., *et al* (2007) Bipolar affective puerperal psychosis: genome-wide significant evidence for linkage to chromosome 16. *American Journal of Psychiatry*, **164**, 1099–1104.

Kane Jr., J. F. (1968) Postpartum psychosis in identical twins. *Psychosomatics*, **9**, 278–281.

Kendell, R. E., Chalmers, J. C. & Platz, C. (1987) Epidemiology of puerperal psychoses. *British Journal of Psychiatry*, **150**, 662–673.

Kendell, R. E., Wainwright, S., Hailey, A., *et al* (1976) The influence of childbirth on psychiatric morbidity. *Psychological Medicine*, **6**, 297–302.

Kendell, R. E., Maguire, R. J., Connor, Y., *et al* (1981) Mood changes in the first three weeks after childbirth. *Journal of Affective Disorders*, **3**, 317–326.

Khong, S-Y., Leach, J. & Greenwood, C. (2007) Meningioma mimicking puerperal psychosis. *Obstetrics and Gynecology*, **109**, 515–516.

Kitabayashi, Y., Hamamoto, Y., Hirosawa, R., *et al* (2007) Postpartum catatonia associated with atypical posterior reversible encephalopathy syndrome. *Journal of Neuropsychiatry and Clinical Neuroscience*, **19**, 91–92.

Kumar, R. & Hipwell, A. E. (1996) Development of a clinical rating scale to assess mother–infant interaction in a psychiatric mother and baby unit. *British Journal of Psychiatry*, **169**, 18–26.

Lai, J-Y. & Huang, T-I. (2004) Catatonic features noted in patients with post-partum mental illness. *Psychiatry and Clinical Neuroscience*, **58**, 157–162.

Law Commission (2006) *Murder, Manslaughter and Infanticide. Project 6 of the Ninth Programme of Law Reform: Homicide*. TSO (The Stationery Office).

Lewis, G. (2007) *Saving Mothers' Lives. Reviewing Maternal Deaths to Make Motherhood Safer – 2003–2005. The Seventh Report on Confidential Enquiries into Maternal Deaths in the United Kingdom.* Confidential Enquiry into Maternal and Child Health.

Lewis, G. & Drife, J. (2001) *Why Mothers Die 1997–1999. The Fifth Report of the Confidential Enquiries into Maternal Deaths in the United Kingdom.* RCOG Press.

Lewis, G. & Drife, J. (2004) *Why Mothers Die 2000–2002. The Sixth Report of the Confidential Enquiries into Maternal Death in the United Kingdom.* RCOG Press.

Lindahl, V., Pearson J. L. & Colpe, L. (2005) Prevalence of suicidality during pregnancy and the postpartum. *Archives of Womens' Mental Health,* **8,** 77–87.

Mallett, P., Marshall, E. J. & Blacker, C. V. (1989) 'Puerperal psychosis' following male-to-female sex reassignment? *British Journal of Psychiatry,* **155,** 257–259.

Mbassa Menick, D. M. (2005) Accidents psychiatriques et manifestations psychopathalogiques de la gravido-puerpéralité au Cameroun. *Médecine Tropicale,* **65,** 563–569.

Meakin, C. & Brockington, I. F. (1990) Failure of progesterone treatment in puerperal mania. *British Journal of Psychiatry,* **156,** 910.

Meakin, C. J., Brockington, I. F., Lynch, S., et al (1995) Dopamine supersensitivity and hormonal status in puerperal psychosis. *British Journal of Psychiatry,* **166,** 73–79.

Meltzer, E. S. & Kumar, R. (1985) Puerperal mental illness, clinical features and classification: a study of 142 mother-and-baby admissions. *British Journal of Psychiatry,* **147,** 647–654.

Munk-Olsen, T., Laursen, T. M., Pedersen, C. B., et al (2006) New parents and mental disorders: a population-based register study. *JAMA,* **296,** 2582–2589.

Nager, A., Johansson, L-M. & Sundquist, K. (2005) Are sociodemographic factors and year of delivery associated with hospital admission for postpartum psychosis? A study of 500, 000 first-time mothers. *Acta Psychiatrica Scandinavica,* **112,** 47–53.

Nager, A., Johansson, L-M. & Sundquist, K. (2006) Neighbourhood socioeconomic environment and risk of postpartum psychosis. *Archives of Women's Mental Health,* **9,** 81–86.

Ndosi, N. K. & Mtawali, M. L. (2002) The nature of puerperal psychosis at Muhimbili National Hospital: its physical co-morbidity associated main obstetric and social factors. *African Journal of Reproductive Health,* **6,** 41–49.

Oates, M. (2003) Perinatal psychiatric disorders: a leading cause of maternal morbidity and mortality. *British Medical Bulletin,* **67,** 219–229.

Office of Public Sector Information (1938) *Revised Statute from the UK Statute Law Database. Infanticide Act 1938.* TSO (The Stationery Office) .

Office of Public Sector Information (2003) *Mental Health (Care and Treatment) (Scotland) Act 2003.* TSO (The Stationery Office).

Okano, T., Nomura, J., Kumar, R., et al (1998) An epidemiological and clinical investigation of postpartum psychiatric illness in Japanese mothers. *Journal of Affective Disorders,* **48,** 233–240.

Oosthuizen, P., Russouw, H. & Roberts, M. (1995) Is puerperal psychosis bipolar mood disorder? A phenomenological comparison. *Comprehensive Psychiatry,* **36,** 77–81.

O'Sullivan, D. & Dean, C. (1991) The Fregoli syndrome and puerperal psychosis. *British Journal of Psychiatry,* **159,** 274–277.

Paffenbarger, R. S. (1964) Epidemiological aspects of parapartum mental illness. *British Journal of Preventive and Social Medicine,* **18,** 189–195.

Pfuhlmann, B., Stober, G., Franzek, E., et al (1998) Cycloid psychoses predominate in severe postpartum psychiatric disorders. *Journal of Affective Disorders,* **50,** 125–134.

Pfuhlmann, B., Stober, G., Franzek, E., et al (2000) Differential diagnosis, course and outcome of postpartum psychoses. A catamnestic investigation. *Nervenarzt,* **71,** 386–392.

Pinardo Zabala, A., Alberca Munoz, M. L. & Gimenez Garcia, J. M. (2003) Postpartum psychosis associated with bromocriptine. *Anales de Medicina Interna,* **20,** 50–51.

Price, D. K., Turnbull, G. J., Gregory, R. P., et al (1989) Neuroleptic malignant syndrome in a case of post-partum psychosis. *British Journal of Psychiatry,* **155,** 849–852.

Ranzini, A. C., Vinekar, A. S., Houlihan, C., et al (1996) Puerperal psychosis mimicking eclampsia. *Journal of Maternal–Fetal Medicine,* **5,** 36–38.

Rayburn, W., Aronow, R., DeLancey, B., *et al* (1984) Drug overdose during pregnancy: an overview from a metropolitan poison control center. *Obstetrics and Gynecology*, **64**, 611–614.

Reed, P., Sermin, N., Appleby, L., *et al* (1999) A comparison of clinical response to electroconvulsive therapy in puerperal and non-puerperal psychoses. *Journal of Affective Disorders*, **54**, 255–260.

Reeves, R. R. & Pinkofsky, H. B. (1997) Postpartum psychosis induced by bromocriptine and pseudoephedrine. *Journal of Family Practice*, **45**, 164–166.

Robertson, E. & Lyons, A. (2003) Living with puerperal psychosis: a qualitative analysis. *Psychology & Psychotherapy: Theory, Research and Practice*, **76**, 411–431.

Robertson, E., Jones, I., Haque, S., *et al*, (2005) Risk of puerperal and non-puerperal recurrence of illness following bipolar affective puerperal (post-partum) psychosis. *British Journal of Psychiatry*, **186**, 258–259.

Rohde A. & Marneros, A. (1993) Zur Prognose der Wochenbettpsychosen: Verlauf und Ausgand nach durchschnittlich 26 Jahren. *Nervenarzt*, **64**, 175–180.

Schöpf, J. & Rust, B. (1994) Follow-up and family study of postpartum psychoses. *Part I: Overview. European Archives of Psychiatry and Clinical Neuroscience*, **244**, 101–111.

Sharma, V., & Mazmanian, D. (2003) Sleep loss and puerperal psychosis. *Bipolar Disorders*, **5**, 98–105.

Sharma, V., Smith, A. & Khan, M. (2004) The relationship between duration of labour, time of delivery and puerperal psychosis. *Journal of Affective Disorders*, **83**, 215–220.

Taylor, A., Atkins, R., Kumar, R., *et al* (2005) A new Mother-to-Infant Bonding Scale: links with early maternal mood. *Archives of Women's Mental Health*, **8**, 45–51.

Terp, I. M., & Mortensen, P. B. (1998) Post-partum psychosis. Clinical diagnosis and relative risk of admission after parturition. *British Journal of Psychiatry*, **172**, 521–526.

Videbech, P. & Gouliaev, G. (1995) First admission with puerperal psychosis: 7–14 years of follow-up. *Acta Psychiatrica Scandinavica*, **91**, 167–173.

Vinogradov, S. & Csernansky, J. G. (1990) Postpartum psychosis with abnormal movements: dopamine supersensitivity unmasked by withdrawal of endogenous estrogens? *Journal of Clinical Psychiatry*, **51**, 365–366.

Whitlock, F. A. & Edwards, J. E. (1968) Pregnancy and attempted suicide. *Comprehensive Psychiatry*, **9**, 1–12

Wieck, A., Kumar, R., Hirst, A. D., *et al* (1991) Increased sensitivity of dopamine receptors and recurrence of affective psychosis after childbirth. *BMJ*, **303**, 613–616.

Wieck, A., Davies, R. A., Hirst, A. D., *et al* (2003) Menstrual cycle effects on hypothalamic dopamine receptor function in women with a history of puerperal bipolar disorder. *Journal of Psychopharmacology*, **17**, 204–209.

Wisner, K. L., Peindl, K. and Hanusa, B. H. (1994) Symptomatology of affective and psychotic illnesses related to childbearing. *Journal of Affective Disorders*, **30**, 77–87.

Wittkowski, A., Wieck, A. & Mann, S. (2007) An evaluation of two bonding questionnaires: a comparison of the Mother-to-Infant Bonding Scale with the Postpartum Bonding Questionnaire in a sample of primiparous mothers. *Archives of Women's Mental Health*, **10**, 171–175.

Further reading

Brockington, I. (1996) *Motherhood and Mental Health*. Oxford University Press.

Gentile, S. (2005) The role of oestrogen therapy in postpartum psychiatric disorders: an update. *CNS Spectrums*, **10**, 944–952.

Mahé, V. & Dumaine, A. (2001) Oestrogen withdrawal associated psychoses. *Acta Psychiatrica Scandinavica*, **104**, 323–331.

Sit, D., Rothschild, A. J. & Wisner, K. L. (2006) A review of postpartum psychosis. *Journal of Women's Health*, **15**, 352–368.

Spinelli, M. G. (2003) *Infanticide: Psychosocial and Legal Perspectives on Mothers who Kill*. American Psychiatric Publishing.

CHAPTER 4

Childbearing in women with existing mental disorders

It has long been observed that patients with serious mental disorders, particularly schizophrenia, have fewer children than the general population and to a certain extent this is true, especially of men. Several studies have shown reduced fertility rates in women with schizophrenia, particularly those over the age of 25 (Howard *et al*, 2002) and in White British rather than Caribbean or Asian women (Hutchinson *et al*, 1999). The lower rate is less marked or absent in women with affective psychosis (McGrath *et al*, 1999; Howard *et al*, 2002).

Estimates of the number of women with a psychotic illness who are mothers range from 56 to 63% (McGrath *et al*, 1999; Howard *et al*, 2001). Women with bipolar and unipolar affective disorders are more likely to be multiparous than women with schizophrenia (Jablensky *et al*, 2005). For a comprehensive review of fertility and pregnancy in women with psychotic disorders, see Howard (2005).

Unfortunately, many general medical and psychiatric services in primary and secondary care appear to be ignorant of the fact that their female patients with serious mental illness are current or potential parents. For example, women with psychotic disorders are less likely than matched controls drawn from the General Practice Research Database to have received contraceptive advice (Howard *et al*, 2004). Despite mental health workers estimating that 49% of their female patients were sexually active and 22% were using contraception, they had only discussed this with the patient in a third of cases (McLennan & Ganguli, 1999). They were more confident in knowing their patients' sexual activity status (93.5% of cases), than whether they were using contraception (69% of cases). There was no clinician gender bias. Half of the women were reported as having children, 46% living alone with the children. Clinicians had childcare concerns about 72% of cases where their patient was the sole carer; however, the majority of these families were not receiving support from childcare services and in those that were this did not appear to be directly related to the clinician's concern. A small study of mothers with severe mental illness observed that only 28.9% had full custody of their children, with the majority being cared for by partners or relatives and 26% fostered or in residential care settings (Sands *et al*, 2004).

Clearly, reduced fertility rates in psychosis are likely to be multifactoral in aetiology but it appears that some women may be advised by others not to become pregnant. A study of women with bipolar disorder attending a specialist perinatal psychiatry service for advice revealed that 45% had previously been advised not to become pregnant: 69% by a psychiatrist or other mental health professional and 14% by an obstetrician or GP (Viguera *et al*, 2002a). Family members including spouses, parents or siblings had also advised against pregnancy in 29% of cases. After consultation and a full risk–benefit analysis, 63% of women attempted to conceive and of these 69% were successful within 12 months. The 37% who chose not to pursue a pregnancy most frequently cited reasons of fear of the impact of medication on foetal development and the possibility of recurrence of illness if maintenance medication was stopped.

Many women with mental disorders also engage in other risk behaviours when pregnant or planning to conceive. They are significantly more likely to smoke (Shah & Howard, 2006) and are at increased risk of pregnancy loss (Gold *et al*, 2007). Attempts should be made to reduce or stop smoking in addition to limiting the intake of alcohol and drugs, tackling obesity and minimising caffeine intake. Some women will require support in attending antenatal care visits. As diet is often poor and medication may increase the risk of neural tube defects, vitamins and folic acid should be considered for women of reproductive age, especially those intending to conceive. The suggested dose of folic acid is 5 mg/day, although there is no clear evidence that this prevents neural tube defects though it may reduce the risk (Kjaer *et al*, 2008). *Saving Mothers' Lives* (Lewis, 2007) recommends that:

> 'Pre-conception counselling and support, both opportunistic and planned, should be provided for women of child-bearing age with pre-existing serious medical or mental health conditions which may be aggravated by pregnancy. This includes obesity. This recommendation especially applies to women prior to having assisted reproduction and other fertility treatments.'

Schizophrenia

Although women with tightly defined schizophrenia who remain on medication are less likely to relapse after delivery than women with affective illnesses or more broadly defined schizophrenia (Davies *et al*, 1995), a substantial minority (21.72%) of those who have been admitted before pregnancy will relapse postpartum (Harlow *et al*, 2007). Many features of schizophrenia and the lifestyle of women who have it can lead to poor outcomes for them and their children. For example, they are more likely to have multiple partners, no current partner, unplanned pregnancies, coercive sex, to be indulging in risky sexual behaviour, and to be the victim of violence during pregnancy (Miller *et al*, 1992; Miller, 1997).

They are also more likely to be single mothers or to have partners who are unemployed or disabled, to be socially disadvantaged and lacking in social support and to be either very young (<20) or older (>35) mothers (Jablensky et al, 2005). Women with psychotic disorders are more likely than controls to use illicit drugs before pregnancy, to drink and/or use illicit drugs during pregnancy, and to experience a relapse within 3 months of delivery, most frequently of a non-psychotic depressive or anxiety disorder (Howard et al, 2004). They are less likely to attend antenatal clinics and often receive poorer quality antenatal care.

Even when smoking and other relevant factors such as maternal age, education and pregnancy-induced hypertension are controlled for, the odds of poor outcomes such as low-birth-weight or small-for-gestational-age infants, preterm delivery and stillbirth are higher in women with schizophrenia (Bennedsen et al, 1999; Nilsson et al, 2002). An increased risk of sudden infant death syndrome has also been reported (Bennedsen et al, 2001). Being overweight and folate deficient when pregnant (which may relate to poor diet, weight gain on atypical antipsychotics or be a direct metabolic consequence of schizophrenia), increases the risk of neural tube defects (Freeman et al, 2002a; Koren et al, 2002), as does Vitamin B12 deficiency.

A large, well-controlled birth cohort study identified a higher rate of obstetric complications in women with schizophrenia, especially placental abruption and antepartum haemorrhages, a significantly increased OR (1.40) for the percentage of offspring with expected birth weight below the 10th centile and an excess of cardiovascular malformations (especially patent ductus arteriosus) whether diagnosed at birth or later (Jablensky et al, 2005). A meta-analysis of studies focused on this issue revealed a twofold increase in the relative risk for foetal death or stillbirth in the offspring of parents with psychosis, a magnitude similar to that of smoking (Webb et al, 2005). The aetiology and the relative contribution of maternal and paternal influences is uncertain but it is likely to be multifactorial. In addition, parental mental disorder involving past admissions doubles the risk of sudden infant death syndrome (King-Hele et al, 2007) and raises the risk of child homicide by five to ten times (Webb et al, 2007). Delayed walking, visual dysfunction, language disorders, enuresis and disturbed behaviour are significantly increased in the offspring of mothers with schizophrenia (Henriksson & McNeil, 2004).

Women with schizophrenia are also more likely to be separated from their children at birth or during childhood and to have reduced contact with them after their children go into care. This leaves many women very traumatised, a fact some health professionals do not always appear to recognise (Dipple et al, 2002). Health professionals are poor at recording information regarding the children of their patients; Dipple et al (2002) found a lack of information in the case notes of women who had experienced the trauma of being separated from children or even the death of a child. The Victoria Climbié Inquiry report (Laming, 2003) has highlighted the potentially disastrous consequences of failing to recognise and communicate information about children who may be at risk. 'Working Together to Safeguard Children' (HM Government, 2006a) was issued in 2006 and all health professionals should be able to understand the risk factors relevant to safeguarding issues, including the needs of parents for support and the risks to unborn children, and know where to refer for help. They should be prepared to share appropriate information with other agencies. 'What to do if you're Worried a Child is being Abused' (HM Government, 2006b) provides guidance on action where there are concerns about a child's welfare.

Psychotic denial of pregnancy may occur in a chronically unwell woman, particularly if she has previously had children removed and fears the removal of the current baby (Miller, 1990). There is also a case report of a pregnant woman with schizophrenia (unmedicated at the time) who performed her own Caesarean section at 37 weeks gestation (Yoldas et al, 1996). Childless women may have delusions of maternity, i.e. believing that they have children (Hrdlička, 1998).

There are numerous case reports of delusion of pregnancy since Esquirol first reported one in the 19th century (Vie & Bobe, 1932). It can occur in both male and female patients, in organic or functional psychoses, depression and dementia, and advances in reproductive technology has influenced the content of the delusions. For example, a case is described where a woman believed herself to have a 'test-tube pregnancy' (Manoj et al, 2004). There are also cases occurring in the context of antipsychotic-induced hyperprolactinaemia (Ahuja et al, 2008a, 2008b).

Kornischka & Schneider (2003) have stressed that delusions of pregnancy must be distinguished from:

- pseudocyesis: where a woman believes herself to be pregnant and develops signs and symptoms of pregnancy
- simulated pregnancy: the person is aware that she is not pregnant
- organic pseudo-pregnancy: where the symptoms may result from an endocrine tumour
- the Couvade syndrome: a father developing symptoms as if he were pregnant and about to or be giving birth.

Brockington (1996) provides a comprehensive review of the literature up to the 1990s.

Management

The aim of treating a woman with schizophrenia who becomes pregnant is to maximise functioning so that she can cope with pregnancy, the delivery and with parenting. Ideally, she should be jointly managed by her usual treating team with advice and support from a specialist perinatal service. Midwifery staff should be invited to care plan reviews, which will need to take place more frequently during pregnancy and postpartum. Pre-birth planning meetings should also involve child protection staff where there are concerns regarding parenting ability and child safety.

By 28 weeks a care plan for the remainder of the pregnancy, the perinatal period and the postpartum period should have been devised, agreed by all, copied to all parties concerned, including the obstetrician and GP, and a copy placed in the hand-held record. If there are significant concerns about the well-being of the child, a social services assessment must be sought.

Although there are interventions aimed at increasing mother–child sensitivity and attachment, the most efficacious being sensitivity-focused behavioural techniques and toddler–parent psychotherapy, none of the published studies have involved mothers with schizophrenia (Wan *et al*, 2008).

Medication

If possible, medication should be switched to low-dose haloperidol or other typical antipsychotics (chlorpromazine or trifluoperazine) unless the existing medication is the only one that is tolerated or which has been effective. Olanzapine carries risks of precipitating gestational diabetes and weight gain, so must be used very cautiously and a patient on clozapine should ideally be switched to an alternative if possible (however, most women on clozapine will be on it as they have failed to respond to or tolerate alternatives). Initiation of clozapine should be avoided during pregnancy but considered postpartum if the mother is not breastfeeding. Women on depot medication should not stop this but be made aware of possible extrapyramidal side-effects in the neonate. Initiating depot medication during pregnancy is not advised because of this.

See Chapter 8 for an outline of the issues regarding rapid tranquilisation of a pregnant or perinatal woman and detail regarding medication and physical treatments during pregnancy.

Bipolar disorder

Women with bipolar disorder have a high risk of recurrence related to childbirth, with up to 67% experiencing an episode in the immediate postpartum period (Kendell *et al*, 1987; Terp & Mortensen, 1998; Freeman *et al*, 2002*b*; Robertson *et al*, 2005). Those with a family history of puerperal relapse are particularly likely to relapse postpartum (Jones *et al*, 2001) and the risk of recurrence appears to be the same in patients with either bipolar I or II disorder but more likely if they have had more than four episodes (Viguera *et al*, 2000).

Symptoms tend to onset rapidly, within 48–72 h of delivery if it is a manic relapse; days or weeks after delivery, if a depressive relapse. Mixed affective states may be more common at this time (Wisner *et al*, 2004).

Relapse postpartum is particularly likely if maintenance medication has been discontinued (Viguera *et al*, 2000). The risk is greater with a rapid discontinuation; if a mood stabiliser must be discontinued, this should be tapered slowly rather than stopped abruptly to reduce the risk of recurrence.

Initially it was thought that women with bipolar were less likely to experience an episode of illness during pregnancy and this was supported by two studies (Sharma & Persad, 1995; Grof *et al*, 2000). However, it now seems clear that this is not the case. Blehar *et al* (1998) reported that almost a third of women experienced worsening of symptoms; Akdeniz *et al* (2003) reported 32% of women having pregnancy or postpartum episodes and Freeman *et al* (2002b) found 50% experienced symptoms while pregnant. Those who did were more likely to have a postpartum episode and such episodes were almost exclusively depressive. The women who had a postpartum episode after the birth of their first child all had a mood episode after subsequent pregnancies; those who did not have an episode after the birth of their first child were still at high risk of having one after subsequent pregnancies. Viguera & Cohen (1998) also identified that pregnancy episodes were more likely to be depressive or dysphoric mixed states.

Whether or not mood stabilisers are continued throughout pregnancy seems to be important. If they are discontinued, pregnant women relapse as frequently as non-pregnant women: 57% *v.* 52% (Viguera *et al*, 2000). The time to relapse is shortened with a rapid (within 2 weeks) rather than a slower (over 2–4 weeks) discontinuation. Cohen *et al* (1995) estimated the relative risk of recurrence for women who did not receive maintenance medication as 8.6 times that of women who did. Sodium valproate should be avoided during pregnancy if at all possible, owing to the increased risk of neural tube defects (see Chapter 8 for more details).

Prevention of postpartum recurrence

A non-randomised, single-blind study found that divalproex semisodium is no better than monitoring for preventing recurrent episodes (Wisner *et al*, 2004; for details, see Chapter 7) but there are more promising data for olanzapine (Sharma *et al*, 2006). Current best advice therefore is to provide prophylaxis with the drug a woman has responded to in the past and increase the dose rapidly if symptoms occur. If she intends to breastfeed then the medication must be compatible with this (see Chapter 9).

If medication is refused, then close monitoring is essential and all professionals involved in maternity (primary and secondary) care in the postpartum period should be aware of the risks. A clear management plan to follow if relapse occurs should be in the woman's hand-held record and in all her hospital and GP records (paper and electronic).

Management

Women with bipolar who are considering conceiving must have the opportunity to discuss how their care might be managed before and during pregnancy and postpartum in order to minimise the risk of recurrence (Fig. 4.1). Factors to consider are: how severe the illness is; response to previous medications; previous recurrences and their triggers; what effect previous

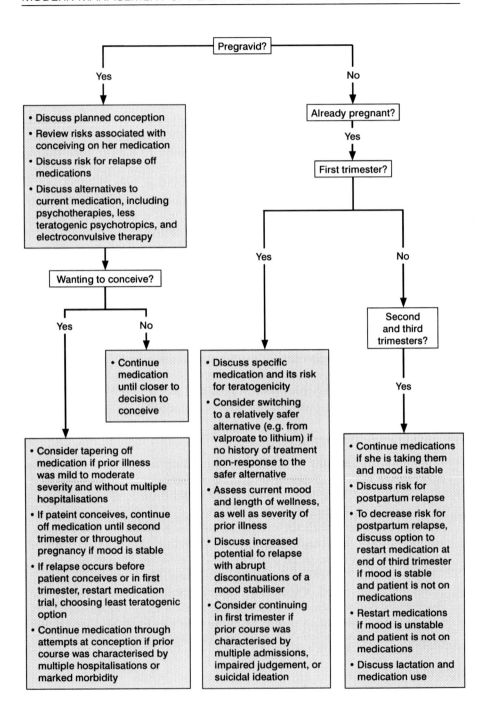

Fig. 4.1 Suggested approach for women with bipolar disorder who wish to conceive or are pregnant. Reproduced with permission from Altshuler *et al*, 2003.

reductions and discontinuations of medication have had, including the time to recurrence after discontinuation and time to recovery on re-introduction. Length of time the patient has been euthymic or stable and the reproductive risks of the medication being considered should be taken into account (see Chapter 8).

In reality, 50% of pregnancies in the UK are unplanned, so having to deal with a pregnant woman on medication when the period of greatest risk (first trimester) is underway is not unusual. In many cases the woman may have stopped maintenance medication on discovering her pregnancy or may have been advised to do so by someone else (often a health professional).

There should be a comprehensive risk–benefit assessment for each woman based on her history and current mental state, other risk factors for poor obstetric outcome such as smoking, alcohol and drug consumption, and how these might change should she relapse.

Detailed discussion of particular medications and their use in pregnancy is to be found in Chapter 8.

There should always be a discussion regarding the very high risk of recurrence after subsequent pregnancies which is estimated to be 50–90% (Reich & Winokur, 1970; Parry, 1989; Hunt & Silverstone, 1995; Viguera et al, 2002b). Although there is some evidence that women whose first bipolar episode is puerperal have significantly fewer episodes of mood disorder over a 5–10-year follow-up (Serretti et al, 2006), the fact that there are also likely to be non-puerperal episodes must be raised.

Anticonvulsants are increasingly being used as mood stabilisers and anitmanic medication. Clinicians should be aware that they might reduce the efficacy of oral contraceptives via enzyme induction, increased clearance or by increasing sex hormone binding globulin levels and reducing the availability of the free hormones. Carbamazepine is the most likely drug to act in this way, followed by topiramate, and women on these drugs using oral contraceptives will require a preparation with at least 50 µg of ethinylestradiol in order to maintain efficacy or consider a second or alternative form of contraception. Lamotrigine levels can be reduced by oral contraceptives but there does not appear to be any interaction between valproate or gabapentin and oral contraceptives (Kaplan, 2004).

If a woman with bipolar develops a mild to moderate depressive episode while pregnant, the first choice is to offer a psychological treatment such as CBT. However, if her depression is more severe, an SSRI antidepressant (other than paroxetine) or quetiapine is advised.

A woman with bipolar who becomes manic should be prescribed a typical or atypical antipsychotic with lithium, ECT or valproate being reserved for severe and/or unresponsive cases.

Anxiety disorders

Mulder et al (2002) reviewed the literature relating to the impact of maternal stress on pregnancy and the unborn child in both humans and animals, and considered possible mechanisms for effects. They concluded that 'recent well-controlled human studies indicate that pregnant women with high stress and anxiety levels are at increased risk for spontaneous abortion and preterm labour and for having a malformed or growth-retarded baby'. They were more cautious about suggesting any long-term functional disorders arising from stress or anxiety during pregnancy. Littleton *et al* (2007) conducted a meta-analysis and found no significant associations between anxiety symptoms during pregnancy and several perinatal outcomes (length of labour, birth weight, use of analgesia during labour, gestational age and 5-min APGAR score).

Studies with small sample sizes and potential selection bias due to the inclusion of potentially higher-risk populations have reported contradictory findings when examining whether or not anxiety disorders during pregnancy predict poor outcomes. Some (e.g. Crandon, 1979; Smith & Reif, 1994) report lower APGAR scores in infants, while others (Grimm & Venet, 1996; McCool *et al*, 1994) contradict these findings. A larger study comparing outcomes in women with anxiety symptoms and those without, recruited from a general population study in Norway and controlling for confounders, confirmed that the presence of anxiety was associated with lower APGAR scores at 1 and 5 min after delivery (Berle *et al*, 2005). Panic disorder is associated with an increased risk of anaemia, shorter gestational age and increased preterm births (Bánhidy *et al*, 2006).

The mechanisms are still uncertain but anxiety symptoms in pregnancy are associated with increased uterine artery resistance (Teixeira *et al*, 1999) and this might lead to poor foetal growth. Other possibilities are changes in the HPA axis and cortisol secretion, increased use of medication during pregnancy or delivery or other health-related behaviours that might affect foetal well-being such as smoking, alcohol use or poor nutrition.

Panic disorder

There is conflicting evidence regarding the impact pregnancy and the postpartum period have on the course of illness in women with pre-existing panic disorder. Two studies suggest that most women experience no change in their level of symptomatology (Cohen *et al*, 1996; Wisner *et al*, 1996). In another, 43% improved, 33% worsened and 23% reported no change (Northcott & Stein, 1994). Even if symptoms improve during pregnancy, they may recur postpartum (Curran *et al*, 1995; Bandelow *et al*, 2006), particularly if the woman has not continued to take prophylactic medication (Cohen *et al*, 1994).

Hendrick & Altshuler (1997) report a woman maintained on nortriptyline and CBT with lorazepam as required during attacks who became pregnant. She chose to stop the lorazepam when she attempted to conceive, her symptoms increased and her antidepressant had to be increased, gaining better control of her attacks.

The authors of a review of studies up to 1999 concluded that of the 215 pregnancies reported in the studies, 41% showed improvement during pregnancy but 38% recurred or onset postpartum (Hertzberg & Wahlbeck, 1999). All but one of the studies reviewed (Cohen *et al*, 1996) were retrospective. Recent findings suggest that women whose first onset of panic disorder occurred while pregnant are more likely to experience a recurrence in relation to a later pregnancy than those whose first illness onset was not linked with pregnancy (Dannon *et al*, 2006), and a small prospective study observed that most women found their symptoms improved in the early postpartum period (Guler *et al*, 2008).

Post-traumatic stress disorder

A US study examined 744 pregnant women and found that 7.7% met diagnostic criteria for PTSD. In half, the precipitating event had occurred before the age of 15 and only 12% had had any treatment. Those with PTSD were five times more likely to have a major depressive disorder and three times more likely to have a generalised anxiety disorder (Loveland Cook *et al*, 2004).

Pregnancy complications have been examined in women identified from Michigan Medicaid records as having PTSD and those with no mental health records (Seng *et al*, 2001). Of those with PTSD, 22% also had a substance misuse diagnosis. Those with PTSD had higher ORs for:

- ectopic pregnancy (OR=1.7, 95% confidence interval (CI) 1.1–2.8)
- hospitalisation for miscarriage (OR=1.9, 95% CI 1.3–2.9)
- hyperemesis (OR=3.9, 95% CI 2.0–7.4)
- preterm contractions (OR=1.4, 95% CI 1.1–1.9)
- macrosomia (OR=1.5, 95% CI 1.0–2.2).

There were no differences in labour or other complications such as gestational diabetes and pre-eclampsia. It was, however, difficult to determine the chronology of the events in this study. A more recent study of pregnant women with PTSD observed a non-significant increase in preterm delivery but no association with low birth weight (Rogal *et al*, 2007). This study may have been underpowered and could not control for all possible confounders, so this relationship has yet to be confirmed.

Management

Although intuitively we feel that actively treating anxiety disorders in pregnant women should lead to better neonatal outcomes, this is not borne out by good evidence as yet. One study has shown that US women with a low income (of whom up to a quarter reported 'negative mood', a composite indicator of various symptoms including anxiety) receiving at least 45 min of psychosocial care were less likely to have a low-birth-weight infant (Zimmer-Gembeck & Helfand, 1996). Field *et al* (1985) gave mothers video and verbal feedback during ultrasound scans. The women enjoyed the sessions, anxiety symptoms were reduced and foetal movements reduced. Infants of primiparous mothers appeared to have better outcomes but there were no biological markers to support the hypothesis that reducing anxiety was causal and the women did not have anxiety disorders.

Obsessive–compulsive disorder

Women with pre-existing obsessive–compulsive disorder may find their symptoms worsen, as did 29% of a retrospective study of 57 women (Williams & Koren, 1997). Four women reported symptom improvement during pregnancy but two of these had postpartum relapses. Miscarriage can also precipitate recurrences (Geller *et al*, 2001). Uguz *et al* (2007) found a prevalence of 3.5% in the third trimester and only 2 of 434 women had onset during pregnancy. In 6 (46.1%) patients, pre-existing symtoms were reported to have worsened during pregnancy and in 3 (23.1%) patients to have decreased. The most common obsessions were contamination and symmetry/exactness, with cleaning/washing and checking the most common compulsions.

Eating disorders

The majority of women with eating disorders are of childbearing age. The point prevalence in a London population has been reported as 4% (King, 1989) and although the fertility rate of women with eating disorders is lower than that of the general population, a study screening 530 women in a London antenatal clinic found that 4.9% scored above threshold on the Eating Attitudes Test (Turton *et al*, 1999). This instrument was not validated for use in pregnant women and does not confirm the diagnosis of an eating disorder but it is estimated that 2.4–3.3% might suffer from a clinical disorder. Those with a high score were more likely to be younger, have previous eating disorder symptoms, to have had a previous miscarriage and their own and partner's employment status was lower. If a woman with an eating disorder wishes to be become pregnant she would best be advised to wait until her eating is under better control if possible.

Consequences

The literature regarding the consequences of eating disorders in relation to pregnancy and childbirth is mixed, as there are differing samples and sample sizes, varying study designs and differences in how the findings are interpreted. A comprehensive review is provided by Astrachan-Fletcher *et al* (2008).

Several studies report that symptoms improve during pregnancy (Namir *et al*, 1986; Lemberg & Phillips, 1989; Abraham, 1998; Morgan *et al*, 1999; Rocco *et al*, 2005), although they may relapse again after delivery. A follow-up study of 54 women with bulimia nervosa and anorexia nervosa who reported 82 pregnancies found that women with bulimia had reduced severity of symptoms during pregnancy and for 9 months afterwards. Women with anorexia had reduced symptoms during pregnancy but these returned to pre-pregnancy levels by 6 months postpartum (Blais *et al*, 2000). Others find an increased rate of relapse, for example a single case study (Conrad *et al*, 2003) and 22% in a small prospective case–control study (Kouba *et al*, 2005). There is also a report of a woman who induced abortion by self-imposed starvation and excessive exercising (Bulik *et al*, 1994).

A large-scale community study found recall of parental mental health problems and early unwanted sexual experiences to be independently associated with laxative use, vomiting and marked concern over shape and weight during pregnancy (Senior *et al*, 2005). Hyperemesis appears to be more common in women with eating disorders (Abraham, 1998; Conti *et al*, 1998; Stewart *et al*, 1987), although it is not clear whether this is the case or whether women with bulimia merely find this a more acceptable explanation for their behaviour.

Whether the eating disorder is treated or not may make a difference. Carter *et al* (2003) found that women with bulimia who had recently received treatment were less symptomatic in relation to childbirth and in the year after than those women who had not had a child. However, women with eating disorders do seem to be at increased risk of having a postnatal depressive episode (Abraham, 1998; Morgan *et al*, 1999; Franko *et al*, 2001; Morgan *et al*, 2006).

Several studies point to poorer outcomes for women with anorexia or bulimia who are symptomatic during pregnancy. They appear to have an elevated rate of pregnancy termination (Abraham, 1998; Blais *et al*, 2000), preterm delivery and perinatal mortality (Brinch *et al*, 1988; Morgan *et al*, 2006), hyperemesis (Kouba *et al*, 2005), gestational diabetes (Morgan *et al*, 2006), be more likely to deliver a low-birth-weight infant (Lacey & Smith, 1987; Stewart *et al*, 1987; Waugh & Bulik, 1999; Sollid *et al*, 2004; Kouba *et al*, 2005; Micali *et al*, 2007) and may also be at greater risk of having a Caesarean section (Abraham, 1998; Franko *et al*, 2001). There is an increased risk of delivering a small-for-gestational-age baby or an infant with a smaller head circumference or microcephaly (Kouba *et al*, 2005). The rate of miscarriage also appears to be increased (Abraham, 1998; Bulik *et al*, 1999; Morgan *et al*, 2006; Micali *et al*, 2007). Other studies, however, report good outcomes (e.g. Lemberg & Phillips, 1989).

Predictors for a low-birth-weight preterm infant include vomiting during pregnancy and low maternal weight prior to pregnancy (Conti *et al*, 1998). Poor foetal growth has been observed during the last trimester in women with anorexia but their infants demonstrated accelerated postnatal growth (Treasure & Russell, 1988). Mothers with eating disorders seem to have more difficulty maintaining breastfeeding (Waugh & Bulik, 1999).

Two large studies include one of 302 women previously hospitalised with eating disorders and controls recruited from Danish population registers (Sollid *et al*, 2004), and one from the UK (Micali *et al*, 2007).

The Danish study reported ORs in the eating disorder group for a low-birth-weight infant as 2.2; for preterm delivery, OR=1.7; and small for gestational age, OR=1.8. Women with anorexia showed lower pregnancy weight gain; women with an eating disorder were more likely to be anaemic and to experience hyperemesis. Low birth weight was found in women with anorexia only, whereas reduced head circumference occurred in women with bulimeia or anorexia. The UK study reported higher rates of miscarriage in women with a history of bulimia (RR=2.0) and significantly higher risk of low-birth-weight infants in women with anorexia. There were no differences in rates of preterm delivery. However, a large study of women who had recovered from anorexia did not have a higher rate of birth complications than the general population (Ekéus et al, 2006).

There are a number of possible mechanisms for these findings: weight-controlling behaviour by restricting intake, excessive exercise, vomiting, using diuretics or laxatives may lead to compromised flow of nutrients via the placenta. Undernourishment can impair the immune system which could lead to an increased risk of maternal infection with adverse consequences for the foetus. The use of laxatives and diuretics can lead to metabolic disturbances and may also exert a teratogenic effect.

Management

There is a great deal of shame and secrecy around eating disorders. Pregnant women may be very reluctant to disclose their problem to health professionals perhaps because they fear being forced to gain weight (Lemberg & Phillips, 1989; Johnson et al, 2001). The following may be a useful guide.

- Any woman booking for antenatal care with a body mass index of 19 or less requires further evaluation.
- In anorexia there may be: hypotension, bradycardia, intolerance of cold, carotenemia, dry skin, brittle hair or lanugo.
- Women with bulimia may be of normal weight but self-induced vomiting may cause:
  - oral mucosa damage and dental erosion
  - calluses or abrasions on knuckles (Russell's sign)
  - parotid gland enlargement.

In addition to the above, laxative or diuretic abuse may lead to abdominal cramps or diarrhoea, and metabolic disturbances.

The Eating Disorders Examination (Cooper et al, 1989) is too time-consuming for routine clinical use but questions from it may be used as screening questions. The use of simple questions to detect bulimia in a primary care setting has been demonstrated: 'Are you satisfied with your eating patterns?' and 'Do you eat in secret?' have been by found to have high specificity and sensitivity in differentiating women with bulimia from controls (Freund et al, 1993).

Franko & Spurrell (2000) suggest that the following are three warning signs that merit further assessment:

- lack of weight gain over two consecutive visits in the second trimester
- history of an eating disorder
- hyperemesis gravidarum.

Caring for pregnant women with an eating disorder requires a team approach with regular communication between maternity services, dieticians and mental health professionals. More frequent monitoring will be required during pregnancy. Maternity staff may need to be made aware of the lengths women with eating disorders may go to conceal their true weight when being weighed and take care that this is done in scanty clothing, with nothing in their pockets and if possible without having the opportunity to 'tank up' by drinking excessive amounts of water before being weighed. However, a critical manner must be avoided. Give information but avoid scare tactics. Systematic enquiry about purging and self-induced vomiting, use of laxatives, diuretics, diet pills and the frequency of these must be carried out. For some women a desire to protect the foetus can prove motivating, help in improving eating and reduce restricting or other behaviours.

However, pregnancy-related improvement may not persist into the postnatal period. Close postpartum surveillance is required with attention to eating disorder symptoms and mood owing to the increased likelihood of depression.

Video feedback during meal times focusing on mother–infant interaction has been shown in a RCT to reduce mealtime conflict and increase infant autonomy in mother–infant pairs where the mother suffers from bulimia (Stein *et al*, 2006).

Learning disability

There has been considerable debate about parenting in the learning disability population. A number of court cases in the last 20 years focusing on the sterilisation of young women with learning disabilities brought to public attention issues such as the right to and consent to sexual relationships, contraception and the right to be a parent where previously it was often assumed that such things were not important. However, there is a balance to be found between normalisation and the protection of vulnerable adults from potential abuse. As women with moderate to severe learning disabilities are less likely to become pregnant, most of the issues relate to those with mild or borderline learning disability.

According to Campion (1995) the relevant factors to consider that influence parenting ability are not IQ (unless this is <55–60) but rather child characteristics such as age and birth order, gender and temperament;

the size of the family (three or more is more stressful); whether or not the partner has mental health problems and the quality of relationship; available support; and whether or not criticism and conflict are present – much the same factors as pertain in populations without learning disabilities.

Problems may not be due to the learning disability per se, but to poverty, poor housing, discrimination and lack of support, or these factors may magnify any difficulties in parenting competence arising from learning disability. The main risks are of maltreatment, developmental delay and behaviour disorders. Abuse is rare and if present is often perpetrated by another person associated with the mother rather than by the mother herself. Where abuse does occur, neglect is the most common form.

Interventions

Feldman (1994) reviewed 20 studies of educational input for parents with learning disabilities. He found that the most effective interventions were performance- rather than knowledge-based and used practice, modelling, feedback and praise, and he pointed out that if not carried out in the home, training should be provided in an environment as 'home-like' as possible. Interventions should focus on supervision of children, positive-based child behaviour management, stress and anger management, non-corporal punishment and age-appropriate cognitive stimulation. The school-age or adolescent children of parents with learning disabilities might need specific counselling or tutoring themselves. However, the professionals providing such interventions should have been appropriately trained and it should not be assumed that community nurses working with parents with learning disabilities have the necessary skills (Culley & Genders, 1999).

Personality disorder

Many people with personality disorder can parent adequately, whereas others cannot and diagnosis is not helpful in discriminating between the two. Key factors are their ability to meet their child's needs and what goes on in the wider environment that the child and family are exposed to – similar issues to those of parents with learning disabilities, and their ability to engage in constructive parenting such as providing emotional warmth and consistent and fair disciplinary practices. Personality disorder is one of the predictors of discharge from a mother and baby unit under some form of social services supervision (Howard et al, 2003). When associated with chaotic lifestyles, substance misuse and comorbidity (commonly depression), a multidisciplinary approach is required.

Assessment and admission of mothers

When an adult requires a mental health assessment (perhaps after self-harm), input from a crisis or home treatment team, or admission to hospital, whether or not she or he has parental responsibility and the whereabouts of their children are an essential part of the assessment. Whether or not other agencies are involved and whether children are known to social services or are on the Child Protection Register should be established. Local social services (and out-of-working hours, the emergency duty team) can provide this information if you have the child's full name and date of birth.

The Code of Practice for the Mental Health Act 1983 (Department of Health, 2008) insists that if parent and child are separated by admission, the hospital should have a policy about visiting and that children should only visit if after review this is deemed to be in their best interest and safe. If a woman has no partner and no other carer for her child or children, then short-term fostering may be required.

Relevant professionals should be involved in care plan reviews and discharge planning. This might include maternity staff if the woman is pregnant, a health visitor if there are children under the age of five and social services if they are involved.

Assessing parenting capacity in serious mental illness

Chapter 6 outlines the ways in which parental mental disorder might pose a risk to infants and children.

Adult psychiatrists may be asked to provide an opinion regarding the parenting capacity of a woman with severe mental illness, most often for social services or the family law courts. Health professionals must remain aware that a child or children's well-being is paramount and the challenge is to be able to safeguard this while maintaining a therapeutic relationship with their patient (most often the mother) which includes an awareness and advocacy of their rights. Other professionals, focusing their attention on the child's needs, parent–child relationships, perhaps observation of interaction, possible risks and family functioning, including the capacity for change, will need to be appraised of the mother's diagnosis, current treatment and prognosis.

Some mother and baby units have, in recent years, begun to undertake planned parenting assessments of women with serious mental illness funded by social services. About 50% of such women admitted for such assessments go home without their babies or are subject to social services supervision (Kumar *et al*, 1995; Howard *et al*, 2003), whereas only 12% of mothers admitted with an acute illness require supervision on discharge.

Poor outcomes are associated with a diagnosis of schizophrenia, behavioural disturbance, low social class, psychiatric illness in the woman's partner, a poor relationship with their partner (Howard *et al*, 2003; Salmon *et al*, 2003) and single marital status (Howard *et al*, 2003). The latter study found that the diagnoses associated with social services supervision on discharge were schizophrenia and personality disorder.

Only half of women with schizophrenia are judged as having good parenting outcomes by staff. However, those of higher social class with a mentally well partner and supportive relationships do better (Abel *et al*, 2005). Legal status on admission and duration of admission do not influence outcome. Mowry & Lennon (1998) in an Australian sample found the only predictor of someone other than the mother caring for the baby on discharge was 'maternal hostility' rather than diagnosis or any socio-demographic variable.

Assessing parenting skills involves considering not only the mother's mental illness and the impact that it has on her ability to care for and nurture her child but also the presence or absence of physical illness or disability and substance misuse. The social and physical environment that the mother and infant are located in and the presence or absence of a partner and any difficulties they might have are highly relevant (Nair & Morrison, 2000).

All assessments should be systematic and follow the 'Framework for Assessing Children in Need and their Families' guidance (Department of Health, 2000). Such assessments should be multidisciplinary and involve both direct observation of the mother and infant plus medical and psychiatric assessment of the parents, occupational therapy assessment of daily living skills, assessment of the social setting, relationships and supports in the family and wider networks, and paediatric assessment of any medical or developmental problems the infant might have.

Referrals for parenting assessments can be triggered by potential risks or follow an incident. Ideally, the possibility of parenting problems should be considered when a woman with serious mental health problems becomes pregnant, so that pre-birth planning, and if necessary a child protection case conference can be held and referral made for residential assessment as early as possible. Women referred to one UK centre waited on average 6 months for admission (Seneviratne *et al*, 2003).

Interventions

There are numerous parenting programmes targeted at the general population or 'at risk' groups such as the socially disadvantaged, but they are unlikely to meet the specific needs of mothers with serious mental illness. There are service descriptions in the literature (reviewed by Craig, 2004) but few outcome data. Brunette & Dean (2002) reviewed seven studies of nurse home visitation models that they thought might be relevant to mothers with serious mental illness. These involved four components: a supportive home visitor; education and training about child development and parenting skills; modelling and feedback; and links to other services and supports. Longer-term interventions appear to be more successful than those delivered in less than a year. Phelan *et al* (2006) describe their 'parenting and mental illness group' programme, which is open to parents of children aged 2–10 years and consists of a

6-week group intervention followed by four weekly individual home visits. The group sessions include:

- positive parenting and the causes of child behaviour problems
- mental health and parenting
- developing positive relationships with children
- promoting children's' development
- managing misbehaviour
- implementing routines and strategies.

Two-thirds of the parents who started the programme completed it (the majority were female) and positive outcomes reported by the evaluation were in children's behaviour and positive parenting, and the participants viewed the intervention favourably. Further work is needed to replicate this in other settings and populations.

Conclusion

There are many obstacles to good outcomes for mother and infant if the mother has an enduring or recurrent mental illness or a learning disability. We have shown in this chapter that proactive management and multidisciplinary and multiagency working with an appreciation of the reproductive and parenting needs of women with mental disorder can reduce the impact of these obstacles.

References

Abel, K. M., Webb, R. T., Salmon, M.P ., et al (2005) Prevalence and predictors of parenting outcomes in a cohort of mothers with schizophrenia admitted for joint mother and baby psychiatric care in England. *Journal of Clinical Psychiatry*, **66**, 781–789.

Abraham, S. (1998) Sexuality and reproduction in bulimia nervosa patients over 10 years. *Journal of Psychosomatic Research*, **44**, 491–502.

Ahuja, N., Vasudev, K. & Lloyd, A. (2008a) Hyperprolactinemia and delusion of pregnancy. *Psychopathology*, **41**, 65–68.

Ahuja, N., Moorhead, S., Lloyd, A. J., et al (2008b) Antipsychotic-induced hyperprolactinemia and delusion of pregnancy. *Psychosomatics*, **49**, 163–167.

Akdeniz, F., Vahip, S., Pirildar, S., et al (2003) Risk factors associated with childbearing-related episodes in women with bipolar disorder. *Psychopathology*, **36**, 234–238.

Altshuler, L., Richards, M. & Yonkers, K. (2003) Treating bipolar disorders during pregnancy. *Current Psychiatry*, **2**, 14–26.

Astrachan-Fletcher, E., Veldhuis, C., Lively, N., et al (2008) The reciprocal effects of eating disorders and the postpartum period: a review of the literature and recommendations for clinical care. *Journal of Women's Health*, **17**, 227–239.

Bandelow, B., Sojka, F., Broocks, A., et al (2006) Panic disorder during pregnancy and postpartum period. *European Psychiatry*, **21**, 495–500.

Bánhidy, F., Ács, N., Puhó, E., et al (2006) Association between maternal panic disorders and pregnancy complications and delivery outcomes. *European Journal of Obstetrics and Gynecology and Reproductive Biology*, **124**, 47–52.

Berle, J. Á., Mykletun, A., Daltveit, A. K., et al (2005) Neonatal outcomes in offspring of women with anxiety and depression during pregnancy. *Archives of Women's Mental Health*, **8**, 181–189.

Bennedsen, B. E., Mortensen, P. B., Olesen, A. V. *et al* (1999) Preterm birth and intrauterine growth retardation among children of women with schizophrenia. *British Journal of Psychiatry*, **175**, 239–245.

Bennedsen, B. E., Mortensen, P. B., Olesen, A. V. *et al* (2001) Congenital malformations, stillbirths and infant deaths among children of women with schizophrenia. *Archives of General Psychiatry*, **58**, 674–679.

Blais, M. A., Becker, A. E., Burwell, R. A., *et al* (2000) Pregnancy: outcome and impact on symptomatology in a cohort of eating-disordered women. *International Journal of Eating Disorders*, **27**, 140–149.

Blehar, M. C., DePaulo Jr, J. R., Gershon, E. S., *et al* (1998) Women with bipolar disorder: findings from the NIMH Genetics Initiative sample. *Psychopharmacology Bulletin*, **34**, 239–243.

Brinch, M., Isager, T. & Tolstrup, K. (1988) Anorexia nervosa and motherhood: reproduction pattern and mothering behaviour of 50 women. *Acta Psychiatrica Scandinavica*, **77**, 611–617.

Brockington, I. (1996) *Motherhood and Mental Health*. Oxford University Press.

Brunette, M. F. & Dean, W. (2002) Community mental health care for women with severe mental illness who are parents. *Mental Health Journal*, **38**, 153–165.

Bulik, C. M., Carter, F. A. & Sullivan, P. F. (1994) Self-induced abortion in a bulimic woman. *International Journal of Eating Disorders*, **15**, 297–299.

Bulik, C. M., Sullivan, P. F., Fear, J. L., *et al* (1999) Fertility and reproduction in women with anorexia nervosa: a controlled study. *Journal of Clinical Psychiatry*, **60**, 130–135.

Campion, M. J. (1995) Mentally handicapped parents. In *Who's Fit to be a Parent?*, pp. 151–167. Routledge.

Carter, F. A., McIntosh, V. V., Joyce, P. R., *et al* (2003) Bulimia nervosa, childbirth, and psychopathology. *Journal of Psychosomatic Research*, **55**, 357–361.

Cohen, L. S., Sichel, D. A., Dimmock, J. A., *et al* (1994) Postpartum course in women with preexisting panic disorder. *Journal of Clinical Psychiatry*, **55**, 289–292.

Cohen, L., Sichel, D., Robertson, L., *et al* (1995) Postpartum prophylaxis for women with bipolar disorder. *American Journal of Psychiatry*, **152**, 1641–1645.

Cohen, L. S., Sichel, D. A., Faraone, S. V. *et al* (1996) Course of panic disorder during pregnancy and the puerperium: a preliminary study. *Biological Psychiatry*, **39**, 950–954.

Conrad, R., Schablewski, J., Schilling, G., *et al* (2003) Worsening of symptoms of bulimia nervosa during pregnancy. *Psychosomatics*, **44**, 76–78.

Conti, J., Abraham, S. & Taylor, A. (1998) Eating behavior and pregnancy outcome. *Journal of Psychosomatic Research*, **44**, 465–77.

Cooper, Z., Cooper, P. & Fairburn, C. (1989) The validity of the eating disorder examination and its subscales. *British Journal of Psychiatry*, **154**, 807–812.

Craig, E. (2004) Parenting programmes for women with mental illness who have young children: a review. *Australian and New Zealand Journal of Psychiatry*, **38**, 923–938.

Crandon, A. J. (1979) Maternal anxiety and obstetric complications. *Journal of Psychosomatic Research*, **23**, 109–111.

Culley, L. & Genders, N. (1999) Parenting by people with learning disabilities: the educational needs of the community nurse. *Nurse Education Today*, **19**, 502–505.

Curran, S., Nelson, T. E. & Rodgers, R. J. (1995) Resolution of panic disorder on pregnancy. *Irish Journal of Psychological Medicine*, **12**, 107–108.

Dannon, P. N., Iancu, I., Lowengrub, K., *et al.* (2006) Recurrence of panic disorder during pregnancy: a 7-year naturalistic follow-up study. *Clinical Neuropharmacology*, **29**, 132–137.

Davies, A., McIvor, R. J. & Kumar, R. C. (1995) Impact of childbirth on a series of schizophrenic mothers: a comment on the possible influence of oestrogen on schizophrenia. *Schizophrenia Research*, **16**, 25–31.

Department of Health (2000) *Framework for the Assessment of Children in Need and their Families*. TSO (The Stationary Office).

Department of Health (2008) *Code of Practice: Mental Health Act 1983*. TSO (The Stationery Office).

Dipple, H., Smith, S., Andrews, H., *et al* (2002) The experience of motherhood in women with severe and enduring mental illness. *Social Psychiatry and Psychiatric Epidemiology*, **37**, 336–340.

Ekéus, C., Lindberg, L., Lindblad, F., *et al* (2006) Birth outcomes and pregnancy complications in women with a history of anorexia nervosa. *British Journal of Obstetrics & Gynaecology*, **113**, 925–929.

Feldman, M. A. (1994) Parenting education for parents with intellectual disabilities: a review of outcome studies. *Research in Developmental Disabilities*, **15**, 299–332.

Field, T., Sandberg, D., Quetel, T. A., *et al* (1985) Effects of ultrasound feedback on pregnancy anxiety, fetal activity, and neonatal outcome. *Obstetrics and Gynecology*, **66**, 525–528.

Franko, D. L., Spurrell, E. B. (2000) Detection and management of eating disorders during pregnancy. *Obstetrics and Gynecology*, **95**, 942–946.

Franko, D. L., Blais, M. A., Becker, E., *et al* (2001) Pregnancy complications and neonatal outcomes in women with eating disorders. *American Journal of Psychiatry*, **158**, 1461–1466.

Freeman, M. P., Gracious, B. L. & Wisner, K. L. (2002*a*) Pregnancy outcomes in schizophrenia. *American Journal of Psychiatry*, **159**, 1609.

Freeman, M. P., Smith, K. W., Freeman, S. A., *et al* (2002*b*) The impact of reproductive events on the course of bipolar disorder in women. *Journal of Clinical Psychiatry*, **63**, 284–287.

Freund, K. M., Graham, S. M., Lesky, L. G. (1993) Detection of bulimia in a primary care setting. *Journal of General and Internal Medicine*, **8**, 236–242.

Geller, P. A., Klier, C. M. & Neugebauer, R. (2001) Anxiety disorders following miscarriage. *Journal of Clinical Psychiatry*, **62**, 432–438.

Gold, K. J., Dalton, V. K., Schwenk, T. L., *et al* (2007) What causes pregnancy loss? Preexisting mental illness as an independent risk factor. *General Hospital Psychiatry*, **29**, 207–213.

Grimm, E. R. & Venet, W. R. (1966) The relationship of emotional attitudes to the course and outcome of pregnancy. *Psychosomatic Medicine*, **28**, 34–49.

Grof, P., Robbins, W., Alda, M., *et al* (2000) Protective effect of pregnancy in women with lithium-responsive bipolar disorder. *Journal of Affective Disorders*, **61**, 31–39.

Guler, O., Koken, G. N., Emul, M., *et al*, (2008) Course of panic disorder during the early postpartum period: a prospective analysis. *Comprehensive Psychiatry*, **49**, 30–34.

Harlow, B. L., Vitonis, A. F., Sparen, P., *et al* (2007) Incidence of hospitalization for postpartum psychotic and bipolar episodes in women with and without prior prepregnancy or prenatal psychiatric hospitalizations. *Archives of General Psychiatry*, **64**, 42–48.

Hendrick, V. C. & Altshuler, L. L. (1997) Management of breakthrough panic disorder symptoms during pregnancy. *Journal of Clinical Psychopharmacology*, **17**, 228–229.

Henriksson, K. M. & McNeil, T. F. (2004) Health and development in the first 4 years of life in offspring of women with schizophrenia and affective psychoses: Well-Baby Clinic information. *Schizophrenia Research*, **70**, 39–48.

Hertzberg, T. & Wahlbeck, K. (1999) The impact of pregnancy and puerperium on panic disorder: a review. *Journal of Psychosomatic Obstetrics and Gynaecology*, **20**, 59–64.

HM Government (2006*a*) *Working Together to Safeguard Children. A Guide to Inter-Agency Working to Safeguard and Promote the Welfare of Children*. TSO (The Stationery Office).

HM Government (2006*b*) *What to do if you're Worried a Child is being Abused*. TSO (The Stationery Office).

Howard, L., Shah, N., Salmon, M., *et al* (2003) Predictors of social services supervision of babies of mothers with mental illness after admission to a psychiatric mother and baby unit. *Social Psychiatry and Psychiatric Epidemiology*, **38**, 450–455.

Howard, L. M. (2005) Fertility and pregnancy in women with psychotic disorders. *European Journal of Obstetrics and Gynecology and Reproductive Biology*, **119**, 3–10.

Howard, L. M, Kumar, R. & Thornicroft, G. (2001) Psychosocial characteristics and needs of mothers with psychotic disorders. *British Journal of Psychiatry*, **178**, 427–432.

Howard, L. M., Kumar, C., Leese, M., *et al* (2002) The general fertility rate in women with psychotic disorders. *American Journal of Psychiatry*, **159**, 991–997.

Howard, L. M., Goss, C., Leese, M. *et al* (2004) The psychosocial outcome of pregnancy in women with psychotic disorders. *Schizophrenia Research*, **71**, 49–60.

Hrdlička, M. (1998) Delusion of maternity. *Psychopathology*, **31**, 270–273.

Hunt, N. & Silverstone, T. (1995) Does puerperal illness distinguish a subgroup of bipolar patients? Journal of Affective Disorders, 34, 101–107.

Hutchinson, G., Bhugra, D., Mallett, R, *et al* (1999) Fertility and marital rates in first onset schizophrenia. *Social Psychiatry and Psychiatric Epidemiology*, **34**, 617–621.

Jablensky, A. V., Morgan, V., Zubrick, S. R., *et al* (2005) Pregnancy, delivery, and neonatal complications in a population cohort of women with schizophrenia and major affective disorders. *American Journal of Psychiatry*, **162**, 79–91.

Johnson, J. G., Spitzer, R. L. & Williams, J. B. W. (2001) Health problems, impairment and illnesses associated with bulimia nervosa and binge-eating disorder among primary care and obstetric gynecology patients. *Psychological Medicine*, **31**, 1455–1466.

Jones, I. & Craddock, N. (2001) Familiality of the puerperal trigger in bipolar disorder: results of a family study. *American Journal of Psychiatry*, **158**, 913–917.

Kaplan, P. W. (2004) Reproductive health effects and teratogenicity of antiepileptic drugs. *Neurology*, **63**, S13–S23.

Kendell, R. E., Chalmers, J. C. & Platz, C. (1987) Epidemiology of puerperal psychoses. *British Journal of Psychiatry*, **150**, 662–673.

King, M. B. (1989) Eating disorders in a general practice population: prevalence, characteristics and follow-up at 12–18 months. *Psychological Medicine Monograph*, **14(Suppl.)**, 1–34.

King-Hele, S. A., Abel, K. M., Webb, R. T. *et al* (2007) Risk of sudden infant death syndrome with parental mental illness. *Archives of General Psychiatry*, **64**, 1323–30.

Kjaer, D., Horvath-Puho, E., Christensen, J., *et al* (2008) Antiepileptic drug use, folic acid supplementation, and congenital abnormalities: a population-based case–control study. *British Journal of Obstetrics and Gynaecology*, **115**, 98–103.

Koren, G., Cohn, T., Chitayat, D., *et al* (2002) Use of atypical antipsychotics during pregnancy and the risk of neural tube defects in infants. *American Journal of Psychiatry*, **159**, 136–137.

Kornischka, J. & Schneider, F. (2003) Delusion of pregnancy. A case report and review of the literature. *Psychopathology*, **36**, 276–278.

Kouba, S., Hallstrom, T., Lindholm, S., *et al* (2005) Pregnancy and neonatal outcomes in women with eating disorders. *Obstetrics and Gynecology*, **105**, 255–260.

Kumar, R., Marks, M., Platz, C., *et al* (1995) Clinical survey of a psychiatric mother and baby unit: characteristics of 100 consecutive admissions. *Journal of Affective Disorders*, **33**, 11–22.

Lacey, J. H. & Smith, G. (1987) Bulimia nervosa. The impact on mother and baby. *British Journal of Psychiatry*, **150**, 777–781.

Laming, W. H. (2003) *The Victoria Climbié Inquiry: Report of an Inquiry by Lord Laming*. TSO (The Stationery Office).

Lemberg, R. & Phillips, J. (1989) The impact of pregnancy on anorexia nervosa and bulimia. *International Journal of Eating Disorders*, **8**, 285–295.

Lewis, G. (2007) *Saving Mothers' Lives. Reviewing Maternal Deaths to make Motherhood Safer – 2003–2005. The Seventh Report on Confidential Enquiries into Maternal Deaths in the United Kingdom.* Confidential Enquiries into Maternal and Child Health.

Littleton, H. L., Breitkjopf, C. R. & Berenson, A. B. (2007) Correlates of anxiety symptoms during pregnancy and association with perinatal outcomes. A meta-analysis. *American Journal of Obstetrics and Gynecology*, **196**, 424–432.

Loveland Cook, C. A., Flick, L. H., Homan, S. M., *et al* (2004) Posttraumatic stress disorder in pregnancy: prevalence, risk factors, and treatment. *Obstetrics and Gynecology*, **103**, 710–717.

Manoj, P. N., John, J. P., Gandhi, A., *et al* (2004) Delusion of test-tube pregnancy in a sexually abused girl. *Psychopathology*, **37**, 152–154.

McCool, W. F., Dorn, L. & Susman, E. (1994) The relation of cortisol reactivity and anxiety to perinatal outcome in primiparous adolescents. *Research in Nursing and Health*, **17**, 411–420.

McGrath, J. J., Hearle, J., Jenner, L., *et al* (1999) The fertility and fecundity of patients with psychoses. *Acta Psychiatrica Scandinavica*, **99**, 441–446.

McLennan, J. D. & Ganguli, R. (1999) Family Planning and parenthood needs of women with severe mental illness: clinicians' perspective. *Community Mental Health Journal*, **35**, 369–380.

Micali. N., Simonoff, E. & Treasure, J. (2007) Risk of major adverse perinatal outcomes in women with eating disorders. *British Journal of Psychiatry*, **190**, 255–259.

Miller, L. J. (1990) Psychotic denial of pregnancy: phenomenology and clinical management. *Hospital and Community Psychiatry*, **41**, 1233–1237.

Miller, L. J. (1997) Sexuality, reproduction, and family planning in women with schizophrenia. *Schizophrenia Bulletin*, **23**, 623–635.

Miller, W. H., Bloom, J. D., Resnick, M. P. (1992) Chronic mental illness and perinatal outcome. *General Hospital Psychiatry*, **14**, 171–176.

Morgan, J. F., Lacey, J. H. & Sedgwick, P. M. (1999) Impact of pregnancy on bulimia nervosa. *British Journal of Psychiatry*, **174**, 135–140.

Morgan, J. F., Lacey, J. H. & Chung, E. (2006) Risk of postnatal depression, miscarriage, and preterm birth in bulimia nervosa: retrospective controlled study. *Psychosomatic Medicine*, **68**, 487–492.

Mowry, B. J. & Lennon, D. P. (1998) Puerperal psychosis: associated clinical features in a psychiatric hospital mother–baby unit. *Australian & New Zealand Journal of Psychiatry*, **32**, 287–290.

Mulder, E. J. H., Robles de Medina, P. G., Huizink, A. C., *et al* (2002) Prenatal maternal stress: effects on pregnancy and the (unborn) child. *Early Human Development*, **70**, 3–14.

Nair, S. & Morrison, M. F. (2000) The evaluation of maternal competency. *Psychosomatics*, **41**, 523–530.

Namir, S., Melman, K. N. & Yager, J. (1986) Pregnancy in restrictor-type anorexia nervosa: a study of six women. *International Journal of Eating Disorders*, **5**, 837–845.

Nilsson, E., Lichtenstein, P., Cnattingius, S., *et al* (2002) Women with schizophrenia: pregnancy outcome and infant death among their offspring. *Schizophrenia Research*, **58**, 221–229.

Northcott, C. J. & Stein, M. B. (1994) Panic disorder in pregnancy. *Journal of Clinical Psychiatry*, **55**, 539–542.

Parry, B. (1989) Reproductive factors affecting the course of affective illness in women. *Psychiatric Clinics of North America*, **12**, 207–219.

Phelan, R., Lee, L., Howe, D., *et al* (2006) Parenting and mental illness: a pilot group programme for parents. *Australasian Psychiatry*, **14**, 399–402.

Reich, T. & Winokur, G. (1970) Postpartum psychosis in patients with manic depressive disease. *Journal of Nervous and Mental Disease*, **151**, 60–68.

Robertson, E., Jones, I., Haque, S., *et al* (2005) Risk of puerperal and non-puerperal recurrence of illness following bipolar affective puerperal (post-partum) psychosis. *British Journal of Psychiatry*, **186**, 258–259.

Rocco, P. L., Orbitello, B., Perini, L., *et al* (2005) Effects of pregnancy on eating attitudes and disorders: a prospective study. *Journal of Psychosomatic Research*, **59**, 175–179.

Rogal, S. S., Poschman, K., Belanger, K., *et al* (2007) Effects of posttraumatic stress disorder on pregnancy outcomes. *Journal of Affective Disorders*, **10**, 137–143.

Salmon, M., Abel, K., Cordingley, L., *et al* (2003) Clinical and parenting skills outcomes following joint mother–baby psychiatric admission. *Australian & New Zealand Journal of Psychiatry*, **37**, 556–562.

Sands, R. G., Koppelman, N. & Solomon, P. (2004) Maternal custody status and living arrangements of children of women with severe mental illness. *Health and Social Work*, **29**, 317–325.

Schmitz, K. & Reif, L. A. (1994) Reducing prenatal risk and improving birth outcomes: the public health nursing role. *Public Health Nursing*, **11**, 174–180.

Seneviratne, G., Conroy, S. & Marks, M. (2003) Parenting assessment in a psychiatric mother and baby unit. *British Journal of Social Work*, **33**, 535–555.

Seng, J. S., Oakley, D. J., Sampselle, C. M., *et al* (2001) Posttraumatic stress disorder and pregnancy complications. *Obstetrics and Gynecology*, **97**, 17–22.

Senior, R., Barnes, J., Emberson, J. R., *et al* (2005) Early experiences and their relationship to maternal eating disorder symptoms, both lifetime and during pregnancy. *British Journal of Psychiatry*, **187**, 268–273.

Serretti, A., Olgiati, P. & Colombo, C. (2006) Influence of postpartum onset on the course of mood disorders. *BMC Psychiatry*, **6**, 4.

Shah, N. & Howard, L. (2006) Screening for smoking and substance misuse in pregnant women with mental illness. *Psychiatric Bulletin*, **30**, 294–297.

Sharma, V. &. Persad, E. (1995) Effect of pregnancy on three patients with bipolar disorder. *Annals of Clinical Psychiatry*, **7**, 39–42.

Sharma, V., Smith, A. & Mazmanian, D. (2006) Olanzapine in the prevention of postpartum psychosis and mood episodes in bipolar disorder. *Bipolar Disorders*, **8**, 400–404.

Sollid, C. P., Wisborg, K., Hjort, J., *et al* (2004) Eating disorder that was diagnosed before pregnancy and pregnancy outcome. *American Journal of Obstetrics and Gynecology*, **190**, 206–210.

Stein, A., Woolley, H., Senior, R., *et al* (2006) Treating disturbances in the relationship between mothers with bulimic eating disorders and their infants: a randomized, controlled trial of video feedback. *American Journal of Psychiatry*, **163**, 899–906.

Stewart, D. E., Raskin, J., Garfinkel, P. E., *et al* (1987) Anorexia nervosa, bulimia, and pregnancy. *American Journal of Obstetrics and Gynecology*, **157**, 1194–1198.

Teixeira, J. M. A., Fisk, N. M. & Glover, V. (1999) Association between maternal anxiety in pregnancy and increased uterine artery resistance index: cohort based study. *BMJ*, **318**, 153–157.

Terp, I. M. & Mortensen, P. B. (1998) Post-partum psychoses. Clinical diagnoses and relative risk of admission after parturition. *British Journal of Psychiatry*, **172**, 521–526.

Treasure, J. L. & Russell, G. F. M. (1988) Intrauterine growth and neonatal weight gain in babies of women with anorexia nervosa. *BMJ*, **296**, 1038.

Turton, P., Hughes, P., Bolton, H., *et al* (1999) Incidence and demographic correlates of eating disorder symptoms in a pregnant population. *International Journal of Eating Disorders*, **26**, 448–452.

Uguz, F., Gezginc, K., Zeytini, I. E., *et al* (2007) Obsessive–compulsive disorder in pregnant women during the third trimester. *Comprehensive Psychiatry*, **48**, 441–445.

Vie, J. & Bobe, J. (1932) *Encéphale*, **28**, 272.

Viguera, A. C. & Cohen, L. S. (1998) The course and management of bipolar disorder during pregnancy. *Psychopharmacology Bulletin*, **34**, 339–346.

Viguera, A. C., Nonacs, R., Cohen, L. S., *et al* (2000) Risk of recurrence of bipolar disorder in pregnant and nonpregnant women after discontinuing lithium maintenance. *American Journal of Psychiatry*, **157**, 179–184.

Viguera, A. C., Cohen, L. S., Bouffard, S., *et al* (2002*a*) Reproductive decisions by women with bipolar disorder after prepregnancy psychiatric consultation. *American Journal of Psychiatry*, **159**, 2102.

Viguera, A. C., Cohen, L. S., Baldessarini, R. J., *et al* (2002*b*) Managing bipolar disorder during pregnancy: weighing the risks and benefits. *Canadian Journal of Psychiatry*, **47**, 426–436.

Wan, M., Moulton, S. & Abel, K. (2008) A review of mother–child relational interventions and their usefulness for mothers with schizophrenia. *Archives of Women's Mental Health*, **11**, 171–179.

Waugh, E. & Bulik, C. M. (1999) Offspring of women with eating disorders. *International Journal of Eating Disorders*, **25**, 123–133.

Webb, R., Abel, K., Pickles, A., *et al* (2005) Mortality in offspring of parents with psychotic disorders: a critical review and meta-analysis. *American Journal of Psychiatry*, **162**, 1045–1056.

Webb, R. T., Pickels, A. R., Appleby, L., *et al* (2007) Death by unnatural causes during childhood and early adulthood in offspring of psychiatric inpatients. *Archives of General Psychiatry*, **64**, 345–352.

Williams, K. E. & Koran, L. M. (1997) Obsessive–compulsive disorder in pregnancy, the puerperium, and the premenstruum. *Journal of Clinical Psychiatry*, **58**, 330-334.

Wisner, K. L., Peindl, K. & Hanusa, B. H. (1994) Symptomatology of affective and psychotic illnesses related to childbearing. *Journal of Affective Disorders*, **30**, 77–87.

Wisner, K. L., Peindl, K. S. & Hanusa, B. H. (1996) Effects of childbearing on the natural history of panic disorder with comorbid mood disorder. *Journal of Affective Disorders*, **41**, 173–180.

Wisner, K. L., Hanusa, B. H., Peindl, K. S., *et al* (2004) Prevention of postpartum episodes in women with bipolar disorder. *Biological Psychiatry*, **56**, 592–596.

Yoldas, Z., Iscan, A.,Yoldas, T. *et al* (1996) A woman who did her own Caesarean section. *Lancet*, **348**, 135.

Zimmer-Gembeck, M. J. & Helfand, M. (1996) Low birthweight in a public prenatal care program: Behavioral and psychosocial risk factors and psychosocial intervention. *Social Science and Medicine*, **43**, 187–197.

Further reading

Apfel, R. J. & Handel, M. H. (1993) *Madness and Loss of Motherhood: Sexuality, Reproduction and Longterm Mental Illness*. American Psychiatric Press.

Ostler, T. (2008) *Assessment of Parenting Competency in Mothers with Mental Illness*. Brookes.

Reder, P., Dincan, S. & Lucey, C. (2003) *Studies in the Assessment of Parenting*. Brunner-Routledge.

Royal College of Psychiatrists. *Patients as Parents. Addressing the Needs, Including the Safety of Children whose Parents have Mental Illness* (College Report CR105). Royal College of Psychiatrists.

Wolfe, B. E. (2005) Reproductive health in women with eating disorders. *Journal of Obstetric, Gynecologic and Neonatal Nursing*, **34**, 255–263.

Guidelines and policy

Refer to the appropriate clinical guidelines for the management of the specific mental disorder in question (www.nice.org.uk) and read it in conjunction with this chapter.

For the latest guidance and policy relating to safeguarding children, see www.everychildmatters.gov/safeguarding/

CHAPTER 5

Substance misuse[*]

This chapter will address use, misuse, harmful use and dependence of drugs (including nicotine) and alcohol in relation to pregnancy, childbirth and the postpartum period. It is particularly pertinent as the number of young women of reproductive age smoking, drinking alcohol and using illicit drugs increases (Crome & Kumar, 2007). The 2002–2004 CEMD (Lewis & Drife, 2004) found that, when all deaths up to 1 year from delivery were taken into account, 8% were caused by substance misuse.

Definitions

Harmful use

Refers to a pattern of substance use which is causing physical or mental damage to health.

Dependence syndrome (or addiction)

Is referred to if three of the following are present:

- a strong desire or compulsion to take the substance
- difficulties in controlling use
- a withdrawal state if use of the substance ceases and which is relieved by the substance
- evidence of tolerance
- neglect of alternative activities
- persistent use despite adverse consequences.

Women who are dependent on drugs or alcohol are likely to have additional problems arising from the need to maintain their supply and often turn to crime, particularly theft and prostitution, to finance it. Self-neglect is common and leads to undernutrition and neglect of health, well-being and social networks. A chaotic lifestyle often leads to poor antenatal care and late presentations. Women who are experiencing violence from their partners have more severe social and psychiatric problems.

[*]Ilana Crome and Khaled Ismail are co-authors of this chapter.

Screening and assessment

Most pregnancies in women who misuse substances are unplanned. Screening usually takes place when a woman books for antenatal care. However, women may book late because services may be too difficult to attend owing to their location, or because usual referral procedures (which rely on GP initiation) are not possible if a woman does not have a GP, is being moved on from practice to practice every few weeks, or is homeless. Lifestyles can be very chaotic with multiple competing demands and women may perceive services to be judgemental or hostile and that losing their children may be a risk.

Hence, specialised services for women who misuse drugs have been developed which have easier access and are staffed by non-judgemental staff who are skilled in the management of substance misuse and can deal with the multiple needs that pregnant substance misusers often have in one consultation, offering easy referral to other services where appropriate.

More detailed questions regarding smoking, alcohol and drug use during pregnancy are more likely to yield accurate reporting than 'yes/no' tick box style assessment (Clark *et al*, 1999), although a structured interview is more reliable at detecting cannabis exposure than opiates or cocaine (Ostrea *et al*, 2001).

If a woman admits to substance misuse, then a full assessment of which substance she uses, the pattern of use – how long, by which route, how much the substance costs and how this is financed – is required in addition to information about a partner if she has one and other supports including professional agencies that she is involved with. If she already has children, their details and their care arrangements must be sought and a full social history including housing, income, debt and benefits, any outstanding charges or prosecutions and whether or not she is involved in prostitution must be noted. As with any other pregnant woman, information regarding the pregnancy and whether or not it was planned, wanted or unwanted and her relationship with the father should be obtained.

An assessment of physical health is required with particular care devoted to the detection of problems related to drug or alcohol use.

Nicotine

In the USA and Western Europe, the prevalence of smoking in young women has declined in recent decades, particularly in highly educated women. However, there are variations within Europe as rates appear to be increasing in the former Eastern Block countries and the rate in different ethnic minority communities within countries also varies (Cnattingius, 2004). Women with schizophrenia or an affective psychosis are more likely to smoke during pregnancy than healthy controls, 31% and 24% respectively compared with 12% in controls (Henriksson & McNeil, 2006).

Estimating the prevalence of smoking during pregnancy can be difficult. Most estimates are based on self-report, and when this has been compared with biochemical markers it has been found in most but not all studies that some women conceal their smoking. Hence, reported prevalences are most likely to be underestimates. A recent British study reported that 21% of mothers in the Millennium Cohort Study continued to smoke during pregnancy (Kiernan & Pickett, 2006). Those who do tend to be younger, less well-educated, White mothers without partners and with no employment outside the home.

Women who stop smoking during pregnancy (around 20–40% of smokers) usually cite fears for the health of their baby as the reason. They tend to stop early in pregnancy but around half will recommence smoking at some point before delivery and most will start again within 6 months after delivery (Coleman & Joyce, 2003). Several studies have found that having a partner who also smokes is associated with failure to stop.

It is abundantly clear from the literature that smoking during pregnancy leads to significant adverse outcomes for both mother and infant (Box 5.1).

In addition, there are a host of studies reporting other adverse outcomes such as increased rates of gestational diabetes, Caesarean section (Urato *et al*, 2005), poor maternal weight gain (Albuquerque *et al*, 2001), autonomic dysfunction in infants (Browne *et al*, 2000), bilateral cryptorchidism (Thorup *et al*, 2006), neonatal excitability and hypertonia (Law *et al*, 2006), increased blood pressure in early childhood (Blake *et al*, 2000), a variety of childhood behaviour disorders and poor school performance. A systematic review including nine studies of nicotine during pregnancy found a greater risk of attention-deficit hyperactivity disorder (ADHD) symptoms in 4–7-year-old children of mothers who smoked during pregnancy (Linnet *et al*, 2003), while Williams & Ross's (2007) systematic review concludes that nicotine exposure is associated with poor academic performance and heavy use with a diminished IQ. There are also data linking maternal smoking with conduct disorder in late adolescence (Fergusson *et al*, 1998) and criminal behaviour in men (Brennan *et al*, 1999).

Studies suggesting links between maternal smoking and various childhood cancers have produced conflicting results, as did studies examining the relationship between smoking and miscarriage. A large Danish study of over 24 000 pregnancies found no association between smoking and miscarriage (Wisborg *et al*, 2003).

A good review of studies on how low to moderate exposure to nicotine, alcohol and cannabis relates to inattention, impulsivity, increased externalising behaviour, reduced cognitive functioning, and learning and memory deficits on tasks has been undertaken by Huizink & Mulder (2006). Using a smokeless tobacco alternative to cigarettes (snuff) does not appear to be safe as it is also associated with an increased risk of preterm delivery and pre-eclampsia (England *et al*, 2003).

Box 5.1 Maternal and infant outcomes following smoking during pregnancy

Maternal
- Placenta previa
- Ectopic pregnancy
- Premature rupture of membranes (Castles *et al*, 1999)
- Miscarriage
- Stillbirth (Gold *et al*, 2007)
- Reduced risk of pre-eclampsia (Castles *et al*, 1999; Conde-Agudelo *et al*, 1999)
- Increased risk of pre-eclampsia (Hammoud *et al*, 2005; England & Zhang, 2007)
- Placental abruption (Ananth *et al*, 1999; Castles *et al*, 1999)
- Preterm delivery (Shah & Bracken, 2000; Hammoud *et al*, 2005; Raatikainen *et al*, 2007; Malik *et al*, 2008)
- Sudden intrauterine unexplained death (Froen *et al*, 2002)
- Perinatal death (Raatikainen *et al*, 2007)

Infant
- Low birth weight (Okah *et al*, 2005; Steyn *et al*, 2006; Malik *et al*, 2008)
- Small for gestational age (Raatikainen *et al*, 2007)
- Small head circumference for gestational age (Källen, 2000)
- Intrauterine growth retardation (Hammoud *et al*, 2005)
- Cardiac septal defects (Malik *et al*, 2008)
- Oral clefts (Wyszynski *et al*, 1997)
- Digital anomalies (Man & Chang, 2006)
- Parental reports of cyanotic episodes (Ponsonby *et al*, 1997)
- Hospitalised for more days over first 5 years of life and greater health costs (Petrou *et al*, 2005)
- Sudden infant death syndrome (Mitchell, 1995; Blair *et al*, 1996; Froen *et al*, 2002; Chong *et al*, 2004; Smith & White, 2006)

Possible mechanisms for some of these adverse events are suggested by reports of increased resistance in uterine, umbilical and middle cerebral arteries (Albuqueruqe *et al*, 2004) and changes in the placentas of smokers which might provide a route to impaired foetal growth (Zdravkovic *et al*, 2005). Impaired arousal from sleep may contribute to the strong relationship between sudden infant death syndrome and maternal smoking (Horne *et al*, 2004).

Smoking cessation

Smoking is one of the few potentially modifiable predictors of some of the adverse events described. Pregnancy is a motivating factor for many women, hence there have been numerous strategies devised aiming at cessation. These include giving information about the risks, advice to stop, individual or group counselling, more specific therapies sometimes using rewards, peer support, nicotine replacement therapy and a host of leaflets, books and computer-based programmes. There have also been public education programmes. Much of the research on these interventions has been conducted in private healthcare settings and therefore cannot necessarily be generalised to public healthcare settings, although a few studies are now beginning to emerge. For example, telephone counselling when compared with usual cessation advice in a publicly funded antenatal clinic with an ethnically diverse population was superior in achieving cessation (Dornelas et al, 2006).

A Cochrane review (Lumley et al, 2004) found a significant reduction in smoking following the interventions in the 48 included trials and a reduction in low-birth-weight infants, preterm birth and an increase in mean birth weight. The intervention that was most likely to result in cessation was rewards plus social support. An RCT of telephone counselling using CBT and motivational interviewing methods (mean=five calls lasting 68 min over 2 months) was not superior to brief counselling (Rigotti et al, 2006) and a brief 10–15 min intervention based on motivational interviewing by a midwife was not effective (Hajek et al, 2001).

Although interventions might be effective during pregnancy, the effects may not persist postpartum (e.g. Lawrence et al, 2005). Trials of relapse prevention in pregnant and postpartum ex-smokers have not been shown to be effective (Hajek et al, 2005).

Pharmacological interventions

Nicotine replacement therapy is widely used in smoking cessation and the exposure to nicotine via replacement therapy is less than the exposure to nicotine through continued smoking. Pregnant women metabolise nicotine more quickly but the aim should be to use the lowest effective dose for the shortest possible time and as early in pregnancy as possible. A recent large population study in Denmark found no increase in congenital malformations in the infants of mothers who smoked during pregnancy but that there was a 60% increased risk (relative prevalence ratio, 1.61) of malformations (particularly skeletal) in non-smoking mothers using nicotine replacement therapy (Morales-Suarez-Varela et al, 2006). A health technology assessment funded RCT comparing the efficacy and safety of nicotine replacement therapy with placebo is underway (Coleman et al, 2007).

The clinical and cost effectiveness of bupropion in smoking cessation has been established and there are studies in pregnant populations (e.g. Miller et al, 2003). However, reported side-effects include seizures, about 0.1% of smokers suffer severe hypersensitivity reactions (e.g. angioedema, dyspnoea/bronchospasm and anaphylactic shock), and a further 3% suffer milder reactions such as rash, urticaria or pruritis. The most common adverse events are insomnia and dry mouth. Therefore, currently, the National Institute for Health and Clinical Excellence (NICE) states that 'women who are pregnant or breastfeeding should not use bupropion' but permits the use of nicotine replacement therapy if an assessment by a health professional has been made (National Institute for Health and Clinical Excellence, 2002). A good review of drug therapy for smoking cessation in pregnancy is Benowitz & Dempsey (2004).

Why are women reluctant to engage in cessation?

Ussher *et al* (2004) surveyed 206 women who had been identified as smokers at their antenatal booking visit. The majority (87%) said they wanted to stop smoking and expressed a preference for face-to-face behavioural support and self-help materials. Around half were interested in telephone support, half in having an exercise plan and a third of the total sample in having a 'buddy'. Most preferred individual rather than group appointments and interest was highest in those in professional or managerial professions and in the heaviest smokers.

Ussher *et al* (2006) explored barriers to interventions in a group of 491 pregnant smokers or ex-smokers. The most frequently endorsed barriers were 'being afraid of disappointing myself if I failed' (54%) and not tending to seek help for 'this sort of thing' (41%). However, the women did also perceive benefits such as advice about cravings (71%) and praise and encouragement about quitting (71%).

An Australian study identified addiction to nicotine, scepticism about the claims of nicotine replacement therapy and smoking behaviour of partners as barriers. Some women were concerned about the safety of nicotine patches and preferred to continue smoking (Hotham *et al*, 2002). A pilot study of nicotine patches by the same group found a low interest in participation and high withdrawal rate which the participants attributed to 'too much hassle' and it not being 'a good time to quit' (Hotham *et al*, 2006).

There appears to be a high prevalence of depressive disorders in women seeking smoking cessation (Blalock *et al*, 2005). Untreated depression may be one factor making it hard for women to stop or increasing the likelihood of relapse if they do stop, so mood should be assessed in those requesting smoking cessation.

Who should provide the intervention?

Health professionals providing maternity care vary in their attitudes towards smoking cessation and how much they are personally involved. Almost all US obstetricians/gynaecologists surveyed perceived that smoking had negative consequences for the foetus and would ask pregnant patients about smoking when assessing them (Jordan *et al*, 2006). However, only 62% always documented smoking status in the medical record and only 66% always advised their patient to stop smoking. Less than a half reported always assessing whether their patients were willing to stop and only 29% suggested using problem-solving methods for cessation as indicated in national guidelines. Only 2% reported always prescribing nicotine replacement therapy and 6% always provided a referral to a smoking cessation service. In Jordan, a high proportion of obstetricians and gynaecologists are smokers and only 54.3% provide any cessation counselling. Those who do not smoke are more likely to record their patients smoking habits (Amarin, 2005).

Midwives in many countries, including the UK, have the primary role in maternity care and the most frequent contact with pregnant women. There is documented evidence that interventions given by them can be effective in stopping smoking (e.g. Heggard *et al*, 2003; McLeod *et al*, 2004) and many will agree that it is important and part of the midwife's role. However, the literature indicates that many are reluctant or unable to engage in this work (e.g. Condliffe *et al*, 2005). Possible reasons are lack of time, concern about interfering with their therapeutic relationship, lack of expertise and lack of knowledge (e.g. about nicotine replacement therapy or where to refer women to for specialist services). Specific training and agreed procedures are likely to be required before staff will regularly deliver smoking cessation interventions but midwives and doctors appear to respond differently to training. Midwives are more likely to take it up and to provide more smoking cessation interventions at follow-up (Cooke *et al*, 2001).

Alcohol

Alcohol has long been recognised to have a detrimental effect on pregnancy and foetal development. One of the earliest studies was that of Lemoine *et al* (1968), who observed unusual facial characteristics, short stature, frequent malformations and what they referred to as 'psychomotor disturbance' in 127 children of parents with alcohol dependency. Ulleland (1972) reported low birth weight occurring more frequently in mothers dependent on alcohol than in controls. In 1973, Jones *et al* described the morphological features of the children of mothers who misused alcohol as foetal alcohol syndrome. This is now well-documented as the most severe consequence of maternal drinking during pregnancy and occurs in 0.5–3 per 1000 births (and higher in some indigenous populations where heavy drinking occurs). Exposed children may lack the classical triad of poor growth (evidenced by small height and small head size), central nervous system (CNS) disorders (including cognitive deficits) and abnormal facial features of foetal alcohol syndrome (Box 5.2) but exhibit other congenital anomalies, developmental, behavioural and social deficits which is known as foetal alcohol-spectrum disorder. The probability of the latter disorder depends on the level of alcohol exposure and there are other associated factors such as advanced maternal age, high gravity and parity, smoking, drug misuse, low socio-economic status and having a partner with alcohol problems. Alcohol-related neurodevelopmental disorder refers to CNS dysfunction without the facial or growth abnormalities. Useful reviews of the disorders and their sequelae are reported in O'Leary (2004), Riley & McGee (2005) and Mukherjee *et al* (2006).

Box 5.2 Diagnostic criteria for foetal alcohol syndrome

A. Confirmed maternal alcohol exposure

B. Evidence of a characteristic pattern of facial anomalies that includes features such as short palpebral fissures and abnormalities in the premaxillary zone (e.g. flat upper lip, flattened philtrum and flat midface)

C. Evidence of growth retardation, as in at least one of the following:
- low birth weight for gestational age
- decelerating weight over time not owing to nutrition
- disproportional low weight to height

D. Evidence of CNS neurodevelopmental abnormalities, as in at least one of the following:
- decreased cranial size at birth
- structural brain abnormalities (e.g. microcephaly, partial or complete agenesis of the corpus callosum, cerebellar hypoplasia)
- neurological hard or soft signs (as age appropriate) such as impaired fine motor skills, neurosensory hearing loss, poor tandem gait, poor eye–hand coordination

Reproduced with permission from Stratton *et al*, 1996

Recent statistics for England found that 9% of women were drinking more than the safe limits per week as were 39% of the 16–24 age group (Information Centre, 2006). Similar figures have been reported from the USA (Nayak & Kaskutas, 2005).

Between a quarter and a half of all pregnant women will drink some alcohol while pregnant, with 27% drinking not more than once a month and 15% drinking two to four times per month (Göransson *et al*, 2003). Estimates of the prevalence of drinking above safe limits for pregnancy range from 15.3% to 33.2% (Göransson *et al*, 2003; Houet *et al*, 2005; Alvik *et al*, 2006; Chambers *et al*, 2006), depending on the definition of safe limits used and the population studied.

Data from a large representative US population study found 2.3% of pregnant women to be alcohol dependent, 1.3% were defined as misusing alcohol, 16.7% binge-drinking and 38.8% as drinkers without binges (Caetano *et al*, 2006). Other recent US data indicate that 10% of pregnant women drink and 1.9–4% binge drink (Morbidity and Mortality Weekly Report, 2004; Anderson *et al*, 2006).

In 1995, UK guidance suggested limiting intake to one or two units once or twice a week (Department of Health, 1995) and this advice remained the same in *The Pregnancy Book* (Department of Health, 2006). The NICE guideline on antenatal care of the low-risk woman stated 'no more than one standard unit per day' (National Collaborating Centre for Women's and Children's Health, 2003) and the US Surgeon General advised in 2005 that pregnant women should not consume alcohol. In March 2008, NICE revised its guidance, stating that:

> 'Pregnant women and women planning to become pregnant should be advised to avoid drinking alcohol in the first 3 months of pregnancy, because there may be an increased risk of miscarriage. Women should be advised that if they choose to drink alcohol while they are pregnant they should drink no more than 1–2 units once or twice a week ... women should be advised not to get drunk or binge drink (drinking more than 7.5 units of alcohol on a single occasion) while they are pregnant because this can harm their unborn baby.'

A survey of over 4000 pregnant women in the USA found that younger, less well-educated, single and unemployed women were more likely to use alcohol while pregnant and that those who had a past history of sexual abuse, current or past physical abuse, smoked or used drugs, lived with or had partners or friends who misused substances were at particularly high risk (Leonardson & Loudenburg, 2003). Women who are older (>30 years compared with <30 years), those who report a history of physical abuse and those who use drugs have also been reported as being more likely to use and misuse alcohol during pregnancy (Haynes *et al*, 2003). Those who misuse alcohol while pregnant are more likely to also smoke and smoke heavily (Burns *et al*, 2006a).

Alcohol may impair fertility in both women and men, and alcohol intake during the week of conception increases the risk of a miscarriage (Henriksen *et al*, 2004). Maternal and infant sequelae of drinking during pregnancy are listed in Box 5.3.

Testa *et al* (2003) undertook a meta-analysis of the effects of foetal alcohol exposure and infant mental development. There appeared to be no effect on 6–8- or 18–24-month-old children but a linear association with scores on the Mental Development Index (MDI) of the Bayley Scales of Infant Development in 12–13-month-old children. There may, of course, also be more subtle or specific cognitive effects not detected by global measures like the MDI and several studies report increased behavioural problems in children exposed *in utero*. One study has identified that binge-drinking in early pregnancy, even when not followed by continued drinking, led to children at 7–9 months of age showing more social disinhibition than infants of control mothers (Nulman *et al*, 2004).

For many of the outcomes there is a dose–response association with the risk of sequelae increasing with increased alcohol consumption. For outcomes such as stillbirth this is related to increased foeto–placental dysfunction with increased alcohol intake. It is also related to reduced transfer across the placenta to the foetus of essential fatty acids. These are essential precursors of prostacyclins, prostaglandins, thromboxanes and leukotrienes, and important for foetal development (Haggarty *et al*, 2002). Animal studies have shown that foetal exposure to alcohol increases HPA axis activity and impairs immune system functioning (Zhang *et al*, 2005).

Box 5.3 Maternal and infant outcomes following alcohol consumption during pregnancy

Maternal
- First trimester miscarriage (Kesmodel *et al*, 2002a; Rasch, 2003; Henriksen *et al*, 2004; Nielsen *et al*, 2006; Gold *et al*, 2007)
- Seek antenatal care later in pregnancy
- Arrive for delivery unbooked (Burns *et al*, 2006a)
- Induction of labour for intrauterine growth retardation or premature rupture of membranes
- Caesarean section for foetal distress
- Epidural pain relief
- General anaesthesia (Burns *et al*, 2006a)
- Preterm delivery (Albertsen *et al*, 2004)
- Stillbirth (Kesmodel *et al*, 2002b; Gold *et al*, 2007)

Infant
- Low birth weight (Burns *et al*, 2006a; Mariscal *et al*, 2006)
- Small for gestational age (Whitehead & Lipscomb, 2003; Burns *et al*, 2006a)
- Lower APGAR scores (Burns *et al*, 2006a)
- Neonatal intensive care admission (Burns *et al*, 200a)
- Congenital anomalies (Baumann *et al*, 2006)
- Orofacial clefts (Munger *et al*,1997)
- Poor visual acuity (Carter *et al*, 2005)
- Early onset atopic dermatitis (Linneberg *et al*, 2004)
- Greater activity of stress response systems (cortisol, heart rate and affect)
- Lower scores on MDI of the Bayley Infant Development Scale at 12–13 months (Testa *et al*, 2003)

Cognitive deficits in 7-year-old (Burden *et al*, 2005) and 10-year-old children (Richardson *et al*, 2002; Wilford *et al*, 2006) have been found to be related to maternal drinking during pregnancy, but studies that have examined the relationship between foetal alcohol exposure and ADHD have produced conflicting results (Linnet *et al*, 2003). Alcohol and coffee consumption while pregnant is associated with childhood acute and non-acute lymphoid leukaemia (Menegaux *et al*, 2005).

Young adults whose mothers took part in a large prospective study and who were exposed to one or more binge episodes during foetal life had double the odds of somatoform disorders, substance misuse or dependence, and paranoid, passive–aggressive and antisocial personality disorders (Barr *et al*, 2006). Drinking during pregnancy is also associated with alcohol disorders in the adult offspring (Alati *et al*, 2006). Binge-drinking, rather than the total amount of exposure, was associated with IQ scores for learning disablity range and clinically significant behavioural problems in 7-year-olds (Bailey *et al*, 2004).

Postnatal heavy alcohol consumption is associated with sudden infant death syndrome (Alm *et al*, 1999).

Breastfeeding

Alcohol can have effects on the breastfeeding mother and her infant. It diffuses passively into breast milk and within 30–60 min of ingestion reflects levels in maternal blood. The latter is affected by maternal weight, percentage of body fat, stomach contents when the alcohol was consumed, the rate at which it was consumed and the strength of the alcoholic drink. Alcohol can suppress lactation via its inhibitory action on oxytocin and there does appear to be a reduction in milk yield in both animals and humans.

Clearly, infants exposed to alcohol via breast milk will absorb it. Human research data on the impact of alcohol on infants' growth, development, sleep–wake cycles and behaviour are limited for ethical reasons but there is sufficient evidence which when reviewed systematically suggests that consumption even within limits regarded as 'safe' for non-lactating women may have adverse effects (Giglia & Binns, 2006).

Screening and detection

As with smoking, routine antenatal assessment is unlikely to detect all problem drinkers, as women who are drinking may not easily admit to this because of social pressure, embarrassment or anxiety, but an adequate assessment should be undertaken in all pregnant women. There is also no laboratory test for chronic, persistent drinking as blood, urine and breath tests mainly test recent consumption. Although there is interest in developing biomarkers, this remains experimental.

Hence, various brief screening instruments developed for the detection of problem alcohol consumption in other settings could be used in antenatal care settings. A review in 1997 identified the CAGE (cut down, annoyed, guilty, eye-opener), Alcohol Use Disorder Identification Test (AUDIT) and the TWEAK (tolerance, worried, eye-opener, amnesia, cut down) as being the optimal questionnaires to use in women, with lower cut-off scores being used than those employed when screening men (Bradley et al, 1998). A modified version of the AUDIT, the AUDIT–C, focuses solely on consumption and includes the follwoing questions.

- During the past 12 months about how often did you drink ANY alcoholic beverage?
- Counting all types of alcohol combined, how many drinks did you usually have on days when you drank during the past 12 months?
- During the past 12 months, about how often did you drink FIVE OR MORE drinks in a single day?

Scores range from 0 to 4 on each question and the cut-off for identifying problem drinking is 3 or more. This has demonstrated good sensitivity and specificity in US samples of pregnant and non-pregnant women from a variety of racial and ethnic groups. The T–ACE (Box 5.4), a four-item

---

Box 5.4 The T–ACE questionnaire

T Tolerance: how many drinks does it take to make you feel high?

A Have people annoyed you by criticising your drinking?

C Have you ever felt you ought to cut down on your drinking?

E Eye-opener: have you ever had a drink first thing in the morning to steady your nerves or get rid of a hangover

Reproduced with permission from Sokol *et al*, 1989

---

antenatal alcohol-use, self-administered screening questionnaire, has also been found to outperform clinician questioning about consumption (Chang *et al*, 1998).

Whether or not a screening questionnaire is used, the actual number of units of alcohol consumed, the drinking pattern, associated problems and presence or absence of dependence should be ascertained.

Most women spontaneously reduce or stop drinking once they discover they are pregnant (Tough *et al*, 2006) but others will need help to do so. Those who continue drinking are more likely to also smoke.

Interventions

Psychosocial interventions with the aim of reducing alcohol intake during pregnancy are usually brief and often based on education and motivational interviewing. They can be one-off or consist of several contacts either face to face or by telephone and may involve the use of manuals or workbooks. Those involving multiple contacts are more likely to achieve reduction in consumption and can be incorporated into the antenatal care schedule. There is a good evidence base for this approach in women of childbearing age and growing data to support the approach in pregnant women (see below).

Chang *et al* (1999) reported on an RCT of brief intervention addressing alcohol use during pregnancy. Women in the intervention and control arms both received the same assessment and then those randomised to intervention received the following:

- review of general health and pregnancy course to date
- review of lifestyle changes made since pregnancy
- participant asked to articulate drinking goals while pregnant
- participant asked to identify situations and triggers which might lead to drinking
- identify alternatives to drinking
- summary of the session and provided with manual to take home.

105

Women in both groups reduced their alcohol intake but there was no significant difference between them. Those who abstained before assessment were more likely to remain abstinent if they had received the intervention.

Handmaker & Wilbourne (2001) reviewed motivational interviewing in antenatal care settings. They advocated a stepped approach in which women were screened and assessed if alcohol appeared to be a problem. The assessment categorises women into 'low-risk' or 'high-risk' groups. Advice is offered to the low-risk group and those in the high-risk group are offered intervention.

The Protecting the Next Pregnancy Project is an intervention that targets women identified as drinking high levels of alcohol during their last pregnancy. The goal of this approach is to reduce alcohol use during future pregnancies. Following the intervention, these women not only drank significantly less than those in a control group during their later pregnancies, they also had fewer low-birth-weight infants and fewer premature deliveries (Hankin & Sokol, 1995; Hankin et al, 2000). Moreover, children born to women in the brief intervention group had better neurobehavioural performance at 13 months when compared with control group children (Hankin et al, 2000).

Similarly, initial results of a clinical trial of an RCT using a motivational intervention in women exposed to alcohol and likely to become pregnant are promising, though follow-up was only for 1 month (Ingersoll et al, 2004). There is also evidence for the efficacy of CBT (Peterson & Lowe, 1992).

As women with alcohol problems are likely to face other difficulties, such as trauma and abuse, to smoke and suffer from depression or anxiety, there is a need for interventions aimed at reducing alcohol intake to be integrated with other health and social care strategies.

Detoxification

If a pregnant woman with alcohol dependence has to be withdrawn from alcohol it must be remembered that the foetus will be withdrawing also. The British Association for Psychopharmacology (Lingford-Hughes et al, 2004) advise that if withdrawal symptoms are present, a short reducing course of diazepam will prevent maternal convulsions which carry a great risk of foetal anoxia; for example, 10 mg three times daily reducing by 5 mg each day and rotating the dose to be reduced. Vitamin replacement should also be given.

Withdrawal should be carried out in parallel with management as described above under close medical supervision and preferably as an in-patient.

There are no safety data for the use of acamprosate, naltrexone or disulfiram in pregnant or lactating women, so they should be avoided and the focus instead should be on psychosocial interventions.

Drug misuse and dependence

Prevalence

Sherwood *et al* (1999) demonstrated by testing urine samples positive for pregnancy in a UK inner city population, that around 16% of women had taken one or more illicit substances, with cannabis accounting for the majority. Meconium sampling revealed 7.9% positive for illicit drugs (mostly opiates and cocaine) in a study carried out in Barcelona, Spain (Pichini *et al*, 2005). A nationally representative sample of pregnant women surveyed in the USA revealed 2.8% reported that they had misused drugs in the past month, the most common being cannabis (Ebrahim & Gfroerer, 2003), whereas when the drug and alcohol CAGE questionnaires were used to screen pregnant women, 6% scored positive for drug misuse in the year before they knew they were pregnant (Kelly *et al*, 2001).

Cannabis is the most common illicit drug used by women, with 57% of young Australian women reporting ever having used it, 17% using it currently and 31% using it in addition to other drugs (Turner *et al*, 2003).

Over 12 000 pregnant women in the Avon Longitudinal Study of Pregnancy and Childhood (ALSPAC) were asked about cannabis consumption before and during pregnancy. Five per cent reported having taken the drug and were also more likely to smoke, use alcohol and other drugs (Fergusson *et al*, 2002).

The incidence of methamphetamine use rose in the 1990s in the UK and USA and this inevitably raised concerns regarding pregnancy exposures. A recent US study estimates that 5.2% of women used methamphetamine at some point during their pregnancy often in addition to alcohol and tobacco (Arria *et al*, 2006).

Volatile substances or solvents are a wide group of substances that can be sniffed or ingested orally and which cause CNS stimulation and disinhibitions similar to those seen with alcohol. Volatile substance misuse is commonly referred to as 'glue sniffing' and has been problematic in the UK since the 1980s. Substances misused in this way are often easily accessible and cheap. They include deodorant, antifreeze, pain relief, air freshener and hairspray aerosols, cigarette lighter fuel, gas for mobile homes (butane or propane) and petrol (more commonly used in the USA and in indigenous populations in Australia where alternatives are less easily available). Adhesives containing toluene are responsible for most of the UK deaths caused by volatile substance misuse. Fire extinguishers, typewriter correction fluid and solvents, and degreasing agents have also been implicated in deaths. Less often used are alkyl nitrites and volatile anaesthetic drugs or propellants.

Most women who misuse drugs come from disadvantaged backgrounds. Polydrug use is common, as is alcohol use, smoking and mental illness such as depression, anxiety and PTSD. Lifetime and current rates of physical, emotional and sexual abuse are high (Horrigan *et al*, 2000; Velez *et al*, 2006), and poor nutrition and infection common, all of which have an adverse effect on the pregnancy and foetus.

Pregnancy and infant outcomes

It is clear that several adverse outcomes are associated with illicit drug use during pregnancy (Table 5.1) and drug misuse that continues into the postpartum period leads to worse developmental outcomes in infants (Schuler et al, 2003). However, it is extremely difficult, if not impossible, to isolate specific drug effects from the multiple risk factors that pregnant drug users and their infants are exposed to, including stress, poor nutrition and deprivation.

Particularly vulnerable women are those who are homeless and misuse substances. A Canadian study identified that being homeless was associated with an OR of 2.9 for preterm delivery, 6.9 for having a low-birth-weight infant and 3.3 for having an infant that is small for gestational age. The odds were increased if the woman was both homeless and misusing substances (Little et al, 2005).

The neonatal abstinence syndrome consists of:

- gastrointestinal disturbances
- high-pitched cry
- irritability
- hyperactivity and hyperreflexia
- feeding and sleeping disturbances
- autonomic hyperactivity
- seizures (rarely).

Table 5.1 Adverse outcomes associated with pregnancy exposure to illicit drugs

Outcome	Odds ratio[1]
Placental abruption	2.53
Antepartum haemorrhage	1.41
Preterm birth	2.63
Small for gestational age	1.79
Congenital anomalies	1.52
Neonatal nursery care >7 days	4.07
Stillbirth	2.54
Neonatal death	2.92
Polyhydramnios	28.6% v. 3.9%*[2]

*$P<0.005$.
1. Kennare et al, 2005.
2. Panting-Kemp et al, 2002.

The timing of neonatal abstinence syndrome onset depends on the drug. Alcohol withdrawal can start within 2 days of birth, heroin within 48–72 h and methadone around 7–14 days as it has a longer half-life.

Opiates

Opiate use during pregnancy increases the risk of neonatal mortality, with a relative risk of 3.27 for heroin and 6.37 for methadone when used together, though risks approach unity if the drug is considered in isolation (Hulse *et al*, 1998*a*). There is also an increased risk of antepartum haemorrhage (OR=2.33) (Hulse *et al*, 1998*b*) and a decrease in birth weight with heroin compared with methadone (RR=4.61) (Hulse *et al*, 1997*b*). Preterm delivery also seems to be more likely. However, confounding variables are likely to be responsible for at least some of these effects.

Stimulants

Amphetamine

Amphetamines are CNS stimulants that can be injected, snorted or ingested orally. Some women use them to control weight. There is no evidence that they are linked with an increase in congenital anomalies but there are reports of a withdrawal syndrome in exposed infants. An expert panel concluded that although animal studies showed some evidence of developmental toxicity in rats, there are insufficient data in humans. However, the animal studies raise concern about the neurobehavioural consequences of prenatal exposure to amphetamines (Golub *et al*, 2005).

Methyenedioxymethamphetamine (ecstasy)

Infants exposed *in utero* to methamphetamine are 3.5 times more likely to be small for gestational age (Smith *et al*, 2006) and this might be due to the vasoconstrictive effect of amphetamines, appetite suppression in the mother or the cluster of risk factors associated with methamphetamine use such as being young, single and misusing alcohol, tobacco and other drugs. There are also reports of a possible association with ventricular septal defect (Bateman *et al*, 2004). The use of amphetamines during pregnancy has been reviewed by Vritsios & Deltsidou (2005).

Cocaine

A systematic review controlling for confounders has rebutted the notion that cocaine is associated with any specific adverse developmental outcomes that cannot be accounted for by other risk factors (Frank *et al*, 2001) but other meta-analyses have confirmed an association with premature rupture of membranes and abruption placentae (Hulse *et al*, 1997*a*; Addis *et al*, 2001). Subsequently, a prospective controlled study confirmed no effect on full-scale, verbal or performance IQ but an increased risk of specific cognitive impairments (Singer *et al*, 2004). Cone-Wesson (2005) reviewed the literature relating to children's speech and hearing in addition to cognition. She concluded that exposed children might be liable to language delay or disorder and that cocaine did not appear to increase the risk of sensorineural hearing impairment but that newborns at least might have some central auditory processing problems. However, lower birth weight cocaine-exposed infants seem to be at risk of poorer developmental outcomes (Frank *et al*, 2002) and mothers who smoke in addition to misusing cocaine might be particularly liable to have growth-retarded infants. Impairment of growth appears to persist into later childhood and the effect is more marked in children born to mothers over the age of 30 (Covington *et al*, 2002).

Cocaine intoxication can cause cardiac dysrythmias and ischaemia, and its toxic effects are enhanced by pregnancy. Hence, there must be a high index of suspicion in any woman known to be using cocaine, as toxicity can mimic pregnancy-induced hypertension. Studies have linked cocaine with thrombocytopaenia, which can lead to excessive bleeding (e.g. Kain *et al*, 1995), but a more recent case–control study disputed this (Miller & Nolan, 2001).

Infants exposed to cocaine *in utero* have been reported to exhibit more central and autonomic nervous system symptoms, high-pitched cries, irritability, excessive suck, hyperalertness and autonomic instability, suggesting neonatal abstinence syndrome. They also appear to have more infections including hepatitis, syphilis and HIV exposure (Bauer *et al*, 2005).

Hallucinogens

Lysergic acid diethylamide (LSD) is a hallucinogen and is often mixed with amphetamines. High doses can provoke psychotic episodes. There have been a variety of congenital anomalies associated with LSD use in the literature including skeletal dysplasia, hydrocephaly, ocular abnormalities and anopthalmia, neuroblastoma and Fallot's tetralogy. However, the small numbers and confounding factors involved mean larger studies are required to substantiate a link between LSD and any specific anomalies.

Benzodiazepines

As reducing the dose of benzodiazepines rapidly or stopping them can cause seizures, this is not advisable during pregnancy. Therefore, either low-dose maintenance or very gradual withdrawal and discontinuation should be negotiated. Women taking very short-acting drugs should be transferred to the equivalent dose of diazepam.

Cannabis

The ALSPAC study found no association with increased perinatal morbidity or mortality but regular cannabis use may be associated with a small reduction in birth weight (Fergusson *et al*, 2002). However, a systematic review in 1997 did not find any evidence to support an association between cannabis and birth weight (English *et al*, 1997).

Maternal cannabis use pre-conception, during pregnancy or in the postpartum is not associated with sudden infant death syndrome when smoking and other relevant variables are accounted for, but paternal cannabis use at all these time periods is (Klonoff-Cohen & Lam-Kruglick, 2001). Maternal use of cannabis during pregnancy has been shown in several studies to have adverse effects in children on sleep, cognitive development, behaviour, performance on memory, attention and executive functioning tests, and is associated with increased depression and anxiety. It is also a predictor of cannabis use in children at age 14 (Day *et al*, 2006).

Volatile substance misuse

Several of the compounds used in volatile substance misuse have been implicated in animal studies as behavioural and developmental teratogens. The first reports of a syndrome similar to foetal alcohol syndrome emerged in the late 1970s. However, a systematic review of pregnancy exposure to volatile substance misuse and pregnancy outcomes (Medrano, 1996) could not determine from the evidence whether a discrete foetal solvent syndrome existed. There does appear to be an increased risk of pregnancy-induced hypertension, hydramnios and lower APGAR scores (Hewitt & Tellier, 1998).

There is a case report of ethylene glycol intoxication in a woman who was 26 weeks pregnant presenting with symptoms which are very similar to those of eclampsia, including convulsions, hyperventilation and coma with both mother and infant experiencing a severe metabolic acidosis but both surviving (Kralova *et al*, 2006). The diagnosis was made by osmolality gap analysis and the detection of oxalate crystals in the urine.

Another case-report describes a 32-week pregnant woman found lying almost suffocated by a plastic bag containing 'household solvents'. The infant was successfully delivered by Caesarean section and the mother then admitted to regular volatile substance misuse (Kuczkowski, 2003).

Screening and detection

Self-report as a measure of drug use is unreliable and leads to underestimation of substance misuse. Biological markers are more reliable (Markovic *et al*, 2000), with the most accurate being analysis of meconium, but this is not routinely used in the UK. Urine analysis can lead to false negatives as it is dependent upon the time the sample is taken in relation to last drug use. Hair analysis has a high sensitivity for opiates and cocaine but low for cannabis and a 13% false positive rate for cocaine and opiates that may have been caused by passive exposure (Ostrea *et al*, 2001).

There are increased risks of infection such as bacterial endocarditis, abscesses and tuberculosis, in addition to blood-borne viruses such as hepatitis B, C and HIV, and sexually transmitted diseases in illicit drug users (Bauer *et al*, 2002). Conditions such as endocarditis and deep vein thrombosis must be identified as these may indicate the need for antibiotic cover in labour or anticoagulation, and the presence of HIV infection and hepatitis have implications for delivery and aftercare. Dentition may be poor and anaemia present.

Management during pregnancy

This depends on the drug being used. For example, if there is no substitution therapy (e.g. cocaine, cannabis) or substitution therapy is not yet established (amphetamine), the aim is to stop use.

Aiming towards greater stability is more important in those dependent upon opiates to avoid the cycle of intoxication and withdrawal, which can have a greater adverse impact on the foetus. Insistence upon abstinence may also drive women away from services and several studies have shown that maintaining women on methadone enables them to receive more antenatal care and achieve better outcomes (e.g. Burns *et al*, 2006*b*).

Detoxification

If mothers do not wish to take methadone throughout pregnancy (partly to avoid neonatal withdrawal) it is recommended that detoxification is undertaken in the second trimester at a rate of 1 mg/day methadone or 2–5 ml weekly or every 2 weeks or what is manageable for the patient (Kendall *et al*, 1999). If gradual, this can be carried out as an out-patient or more rapidly as an in-patient. Detoxification in the first trimester may be associated with increased risk of spontaneous abortion and in the third trimester there may be increased risk of premature labour and foetal death. So, if possible, it should be avoided in the first trimester and carried out very cautiously in the third.

Substitution and maintenance

Methadone maintenance treatment decreases illicit opioid use, maternal mortality and morbidity, criminality, drug-seeking behaviour and prostitution, sexually transmitted diseases and the incidence of obstetric complications. It increases foetal stability and ensures improved adherence with obstetric care. Methadone can be taken orally, is difficult to inject, has a low street value and a long half-life, so can be taken daily, although it may be helpful in some cases to split the daily dose. It reduces withdrawal in the foetus.

Disadvantages associated with methadone are: it is an addictive opiate; it is associated with neonatal withdrawal; and it can (albeit rarely) cause neonatal thrombocytopaenia.

Methadone dose does not always correlate with neonatal abstinence syndrome. Three studies have investigated the relationship between maternal methadone dosage and neonatal withdrawal (Berghella *et al*,

2003; Dashe *et al*, 2004; McCarthy *et al*, 2005). Berghella *et al* (2003) demonstrated that maternal methadone dosage does not correlate with neonatal withdrawal, whereas Dashe *et al* (2004) showed the opposite. This might be related to the cut-off threshold, or to the fact that the neonate may be exposed to low maternal methadone serum levels, despite high methadone doses.

A daily dose may vary between 50 and 150 mg methadone but clearance increases from the first to the third trimester (Wolff *et al*, 2005); more may be required in the third trimester. Methadone dose needs to be taken into account when pain relief is assessed during labour. Clearance will decline rapidly after delivery and the mother may become over-sedated if the dose is not adjusted downwards.

Neonatal withdrawal may not emerge until 48 h after delivery. Data to date suggest that methadone-exposed infants function normally at 1–2 year cognitive evaluation (Kaltenbach & Finnegan, 1989).

Higher doses of methadone may be associated with less heroin supplementation (Dashe *et al*, 2004) but at the cost of greater neonatal withdrawal (Bergella *et al*, 2003; McCarthy *et al*, 2005).

Buprenorphine

Buprenorphine has become available relatively recently and a number of small-scale studies have been undertaken (Fischer *et al*, 2000, 2006; Johnson *et al*, 2001; Lacroix *et al*, 2004; Jones *et al*, 2005; Lejeune *et al*, 2006). At this stage it is not clear whether there is any advantage over methadone. Fischer *et al* (2006) found that retention was greater with buprenorphine, but less illicit drug use occurred with methadone. Forty-three per cent of neonates in both groups did not require treatment for neonatal abstinence syndrome, but there was earlier onset of the syndrome in the methadone group than in the buprenorphine group.

A high level of suspicion of acute toxicity is required if a pregnant woman known to use drugs presents with altered perception of sensory stimuli, loss of coordination, headache, nausea or vomiting, or reduced respiration. However, clinicians must also be aware of medical disorders that might present in a similar way, especially eclampsia, and seek an urgent obstetric opinion.

Postnatal care

After delivery, mothers and babies should go to the postnatal ward. Some infants with severe neonatal abstinence syndrome may require admission to a neonatal unit for treatment.

Methadone is excreted in breast milk in small amounts and is related to the amount the mother is receiving. It appears insufficient to prevent neonatal abstinence syndrome despite reports that it can ameliorate the syndrome, so an infant suffering from this might still require specific treatment. Small amounts of buprenorphine are also excreted into breast milk but data are only available from one patient (Elkader & Sproule, 2005). A mother who is HIV positive or at high risk of becoming so should not breastfeed; other women can be encouraged to do so but they will require considerable support if they have an irritable baby who has difficulty latching on. A good review of the issues relating to methadone and lactation is provided by Jansson *et al* (2004).

Management should start before postnatal discharge and include consideration of contraception during pregnancy. Long-acting progestagen delivered by depot injection, implant or intrauterine system is suitable and can be commenced in the postpartum period.

Conclusion

Substance misuse in pregnant and postpartum women is clearly an issue of growing concern and associated with significant morbidity and mortality both acute and chronic for the mother, her baby and family. Interventions for substance misuse in the general population are likely to be beneficial and there is accumulating evidence for some specific treatments.

There is a need for easily accessible comprehensive services with trained staff where proper detection and assessment, efficacious and cost-effective management and follow-up can be provided. Such services can be a focus for continued research.

References

Addis, A., Moretti, M. E., Ahmed Syed, F., *et al* (2001) Fetal effects of cocaine: an updated meta-analysis. *Reproductive Toxicology*, **15**, 341–369.

Alati, R., Al Mamum, A., Williams, G. M., *et al* (2006) In utero alcohol exposure and prediction of alcohol disorders in early adulthood: a birth cohort study. *Archives of General Psychiatry*, **63**, 1009–1006.

Albertsen, K., Andersen, A.-M. N., Olsen, J., *et al* (2004) Alcohol consumption during pregnancy and the risk of preterm delivery. *American Journal of Epidemiology*, **159**, 155–161.

Albuquerque, C. A., Doyle, W., Hales, K., *et al* (2001) Influence of cigarette smoking on maternal body mass index and fetal growth. *Obstetrics and Gynecology*, **97**, S70–S71.

Albuquerque, C. A., Smith, K. R., Johnson, C., *et al* (2004) Influence of maternal tobacco smoking during pregnancy on uterine, umbilical and fetal cerebral artery blood flows. *Early Human Development*, **80**, 31–42.

Alm, B., Wennergren, G., Norvenius, G., *et al* (1999) Caffeine and alcohol as risk factors for sudden infant death syndrome. Nordic Epidemiological SIDS Study. *Archives of Disease in Childhood*, **81**, 107–111.

Alvik, A., Heyerdahl, S., Haldorsen, T., *et al* (2006) Alcohol use before and during pregnancy. *Acta Obstetricia et Gynecologica Scandinavica*, **85**, 1292–1298.

Amarin, Z. O. (2005) Obstetricians, gynecologists and the anti-smoking campaign: a national survey. *European Journal of Obstetrics and Gynecology and Reproductive Biology*, **119**, 156–160.

Ananth, C. V., Smulian, J. C. & Vintzileos, A. M. (1999) Incidence of placental abruption in relation to cigarette smoking and hypertensive disorders during pregnancy: a meta-analysis of observational studies. *Obstetrics and Gynecology*, **93**, 622–628.

Anderson, J. E., Ebrahim, S., Floyd, L., *et al* (2006) Prevalence of risk factors for adverse pregnancy outcomes during pregnancy and the preconception period – United States, 2002–2004. *Maternal and Child Health Journal*, **10(5 Suppl.)**, 101–106.

Arria, A. M., Derauf, C., LaGasse, L. L., *et al* (2006) Methamphetamine and other substance use during pregnancy: preliminary estimates from the Infant Development, Environment, and Lifestyle (IDEAL) study. *Maternal and Child Health Journal*, **10**, 293–302.

Bailey, B. N., Delaney-Black, V., Covington, C. Y., *et al* (2004) Prenatal exposure to binge drinking and cognitive and behavioral outcomes at age 7 years. *American Journal of Obstetrics and Gynecology*, **191**, 1037–1043.

Barr, H., Bookstein, F. L., O'Malley, K. D., *et al* (2006) Binge drinking during pregnancy as a predictor of psychiatric disorders on the structured clinical interview for DSM–IV in young adult offspring. *American Journal of Psychiatry*, **163**, 1061–1065.

Bateman, D. N., McElhatton, P. R., Dickinson, D., *et al* (2004) A case–control study to examine the pharmacological factors underlying ventricular septal defects in the north of England. *European Journal of Clinical Pharmacology*, **60**, 635–641.

Bauer, C. R., Shankaran, S., Bada, H. S., *et al* (2002) The maternal lifestyle study: drug exposure during pregnancy and short-term maternal outcomes. *American Journal of Obstetrics and Gynecology*, **186**, 487–495.

Bauer, C. R., Langer, J. C., Shankaran, S., *et al* (2005) Acute neonatal effects of cocaine exposure during pregnancy. *Archives of Pediatrics & Adolescent Medicine*, **159**, 824–834.

Baumann, P., Schild, C., Hume, R. F. *et al* (2006) Alcohol abuse – a persistent and preventable risk for congenital anomalies. *International Journal of Gynecology and Obstetrics*, **95**, 66–72.

Benowitz, N. L. & Dempsey, D. A. (2004) Pharmacotherapy for smoking cessation during pregnancy. *Nicotine and Tobacco Research*, **6**, S189–S202.

Berghella, V., Lim, P. J., Hill, M. K., *et al* (2003) Maternal methadone dose and neonatal withdrawal. *American Journal of Obstetrics and Gynecology*, **189**, 312–317.

Blair, P. S., Fleming, P. J., Bensley, D., *et al* (1996) Smoking and the sudden infant death syndrome: results from 1993–5 case–control study for confidential inquiry into stillbirths and deaths in infancy. Confidential Enquiry into Stillbirths and Deaths Regional Coordinators and Researchers. *BMJ*, **313**, 195–198.

Blake, K. V., Gurrin, L. C., Evans, S. F., *et al* (2000) Maternal cigarette smoking during pregnancy, low birth weight and subsequent blood pressure in early childhood. *Early Human Development*, **57**, 137–147.

Blalock, J. A., Fouladi, R. T., Wetter, D. W., *et al* (2005) Depression in pregnant women seeking smoking cessation. *Addictive Behaviours*, **30**, 1195–1208.

Bradley, K. A., Boyd-Wickizer, J., Powell, S. H., *et al* (1998) Alcohol screening questionnaires in women: a critical review. *JAMA*, **280**, 166–171.

Brennan, P. A., Grekin, E. R. & Mednick, S. A. (1999) Maternal smoking during pregnancy and adult male criminal outcomes. *Archives of General Psychiatry*, **56**, 215–219.

Browne, C. A., Colditz, P. B., Dunster, K. R. (2000) Infant autonomic function is altered by maternal smoking during pregnancy. *Early Human Development*, **59**, 209–218.

Burden, M. J., Jacobson, S. W. & Jacobson, J. L. (2005) Relation of prenatal alcohol exposure to cognitive processing speed and efficiency in childhood. *Alcoholism: Clinical and Experimental Research*, **29**, 1473–1483.

Burns, L., Mattick, R. P. & Cooke, M. (2006a) Use of record linkage to examine alcohol use in pregnancy. *Alcoholism: Clinical and Experimental Research*, **30**, 642–648.

Burns, L., Mattick, R. P., Lim, K., *et al* (2006b) Methadone in pregnancy: treatment retention and neonatal outcomes. *Addiction*, **102**, 264–270.

Caetano, R., Ramisetty- Mikler, S., Floyd, L. R., *et al* (2006) The epidemiology of drinking among women of child-bearing age. *Alcoholism: Clinical and Experimental Research*, **30**, 1023–1030.

Carter, R. C., Jacobson, S. W., Molteno, C. D., *et al* (2005) Effects of prenatal alcohol exposure on infant visual acuity. *Journal of Pediatrics*, **147**, 473–479.

Castles, A., Adams, E. K., Melvin, C. L., *et al* (1999) Effects of smoking during pregnancy: Five meta-analyses. *American Journal of Preventive Medicine*, **16**, 208–215.

Chambers, C. D., Kavteladze, L., Joutchenko, L., *et al* (2006) Alcohol consumption patterns among pregnant women in the Moscow region of the Russian Federation. *Alcohol*, **54**, 133–137.

Chang, G., Wilkins-Haug, L., Berman, S., *et al* (1998) Alcohol use and pregnancy: improving identification. *Obstetrics and Gynecology*, **91**, 892–898.

Chang, G., Wilkins-Haug, L., Berman, S., *et al* (1999) Brief intervention for alcohol use in pregnancy: a randomized trial. *Addiction*, **94**, 1499–1508.

Cnattingius, S. (2004). The epidemiology of smoking during pregnancy: smoking prevalence, maternal characteristics, and pregnancy outcomes. *Nicotine Tobacco Research*, **6(Suppl. 2)**, S125–S140.

Chong, D. S., Yip, P. S. & Karlberg, J. (2004) Maternal smoking: an increasing unique risk factor for sudden infant death syndrome in Sweden. *Acta Paediatrica*, **93**, 471–478.

Clark, K. A., Dawson, S. & Martin, S. L. (1999) The effect of implementing a more comprehensive screening for substance use among pregnant women in North Carolina. *Maternal and Child Health Journal*, **3**, 161–166.

Coleman, T., Thornton, J., Britton, J., *et al* (2007) Protocol for the Smoking, Nicotine and Pregnancy (SNAP) trial: double-blind, placebo-randomised, controlled trial of nicotine replacement therapy in pregnancy. *BMC Health Services Research*, **7**, 2.

Colman, G. J. & Joyce, T. (2003) Trends in smoking before, during, and after pregnancy in ten states. *American Journal of Preventive Medicine*, **24**, 29–35.

Conde-Agudelo, A., Althabe, F., Belizàn, J. M., *et al* (1999) Cigarette smoking during pregnancy and risk of preeclampsia: A systematic review. *American Journal of Obstetrics and Gynecology*, **181**, 1026–1035.

Condliffe, L., McEwen, A. & West, R. (2005) The attitude of maternity staff to, and smoking cessations with, childbearing women in London. *Midwifery*, **21**, 233–240.

Cone-Wesson, B. (2005) Prenatal alcohol and cocaine exposure: Influences on cognition, speech, language, and hearing. *Journal of Communication Disorders*, **38**, 279–302.

Cooke, M., Mattick, R. P. & Walsh, R. A. (2001) Differential uptake of a smoking cessation programme disseminated to doctors and midwives in antenatal clinics. *Addiction*, **96**, 495–505.

Covington, C. Y., Nordstrom-Klee, B., Ager, J., *et al* (2002) Birth to age 7 growth of children prenatally exposed to drugs: a prospective cohort study. *Neurotoxicology and Teratology*, **24**, 489–496.

Crome, I. B. & Kumar, M. J. (2007) Epidemiology of drug and alcohol use in young women. *Seminars in Fetal and Neonatal Medicine*, **12**, 98–105.

Dashe, J. S., Sheffield, J. S., Olscher, D. A., *et al* (2004) Relationship between maternal methadone dosage and neonatal withdrawal. *Obstetrics and Gynecology*, **100**, 1244–1249.

Day, N. L., Goldschmidt, L. & Thomas, C. A. (2006) Prenatal marijuana exposure contributes to the prediction of marijuana use at age 14. *Addiction*, **101**, 1313–1322.

Department of Health (1995) *Sensible Drinking: Report of an Interdepartmental Working Group*. Department of Health.

Department of Health (2006). *The Pregnancy Book: 2006 Edition*. Department of Health.

Dornelas, E. A., Magnavita, J., Beazoglu, T., *et al* (2006) Efficacy and cost-effectiveness of a clinic-based counselling intervention tested in an ethnically diverse sample of pregnant smokers. *Patient Education and Counseling*, **64**, 342–349.

Ebrahim, S. H. & Gfroerer, J. (2003) Pregnancy-related substance use in the United States during 1996–1998. *Obstetrics and Gynecology*, **101**, 374–379.

Elkader, A. & Sproule, B. (2005) Buprenorphine: Clinical pharmacokinetics in the treatment of opioid dependence. *Clinical Pharmacokinetics*, **44**, 661–680.

England, L. & Zhang, J. (2007) Smoking and risk of pre-eclampsia: a systematic review. *Frontiers in Bioscience*, **12**, 2471–2483.

England, L. J., Levine, R. J., Mills, J. L., *et al* (2003) Adverse pregnancy outcomes in snuff users. *American Journal of Obstetrics and Gynecology*, **189**, 939–943.

English, D. R., Hulse, G. K., Milne, E., *et al* (1997) Maternal cannabis use and birth weight: a meta-analysis. *Addiction*, **92**, 1553–1560.

Fergusson, D. M., Woodward, L. J. & Horwood, L. J. (1998) Maternal smoking during pregnancy and psychiatric adjustment in late adolescence. *Archives of General Psychiatry*, **55**, 721–727.

Fergusson, D. M., Horwood, L. J. & Northstone, K. (2002) Maternal use of cannabis and pregnancy outcome. *British Journal of Obstetrics and Gynaecology*, **109**, 21–27.

Fischer, G., Johnson, R. E., Eder, H., *et al* (2000) Treatment of opioid-dependent pregnant women with buprenorphine. *Addiction*, **95**, 239–244.

Fischer, G., Ortner, R., Rohrmeister, K., *et al* (2006) Methadone versus buprenorphine in pregnant addicts: a double-blind, double-dummy comparison study. *Addiction*, **101**, 275–281.

Frank, D. A., Augustyn, M., Knight, W. G., *et al* (2001) Growth, development, and behaviour in early childhood following prenatal cocaine exposure: a systematic review. *JAMA*, **285**, 1613–1625.

Frank, D. A., Jacobs, R. R., Beeghly, M., *et al* (2002) Level of prenatal cocaine exposure and scores on the Bayley Scales of Infant Development: Modifying effects of caregiver, early intervention, and birth weight. *Pediatrics*, **110**, 1143–1152.

Froen, J. F., Arnestad, M., Vege, A., *et al* (2002) Comparative epidemiology of sudden infant death syndrome and sudden intrauterine unexplained death. *Archives of Disease in Childhood Fetal and Neonatal Edition*, **87**, 118–121.

Giglia, R. & Binns, C. (2006) Alcohol and lactation: a systematic review. *Nutrition and Dietetics*, **63**, 103–116.

Gold, K. J., Dalton, V. K., Schwenk, T. L., *et al* (2007) What causes pregnancy loss? Preexisting mental illness as an independent risk factor. *General Hospital Psychiatry*, **29**, 207–213.

Golub, M., Costa, L., Crofton, K., *et al* (2005) NTP–CERHR Expert Panel Report on the reproductive and developmental toxicity of amphetamine and methamphetamine. *Birth Defects Research. Part B Developmental and Reproductive Toxicology*, **74**, 471–584.

Göransson, M., Magnusson, Å., Bergman, H., *et al* (2003) Fetus at risk: prevalence of alcohol consumption during pregnancy estimated with a simple screening method in Swedish antenatal clinics. *Addiction*, **98**, 1513–1520.

Haggarty, P., Abramovich, D. R. & Page, K. (2002) The effect of maternal smoking and ethanol on fatty acid transport by the human placenta. *British Journal of Nutrition*, **87**, 247–252.

Hajek, P., West, R., Lee, A., *et al* (2001) Randomized controlled trial of a midwife-delivered brief smoking intervention during pregnancy. *Addiction*, **96**, 485–494.

Hajek, P., Stead, L. F., West, R., *et al* (2005) Relapse prevention interventions for smoking cessation. *Cochrane Database of Systematic Reviews*, **1**, CD003999.

Hammoud, A. O., Bujold, E., Sorokin, Y., *et al* (2005) Smoking in pregnancy revisited: findings from a large population-based study. *American Journal of Obstetrics and Gynecology*, **192**, 1856–1862.

Handmaker, N. S. & Wilbourne, P. (2001) Motivational interventions in prenatal clinics. *Alcohol Research and Health*, **25**, 219–229.

Hankin, J. R. & Sokol, R. J. (1995) Identification and care of problems associated with alcohol ingestion in pregnancy. *Seminars in Perinatology*, **19**, 286–292.

Hankin, J., McCaul, M. E. & Heussner, J. (2000) Pregnant, alcohol abusing women. *Alcoholism: Clinical and Experimental Research*, **24**, 1276–1286.

Haynes, G., Dunnagan, T. & Christpher, S. (2003) Determinants of alcohol use in pregnant women at risk for alcohol consumption. *Neurotoxicology and Teratology*, **25**, 659–666.

Heggard, H., Kjærgaard, H., Møller, L., *et al*, (2003) Multimodal intervention raises smoking cessation rates during pregnancy. *Acta Obstetricia et Gynecologica Scandinavica*, **82**, 813–819.

Henriksen, T. B., Hjollund, N. H., Jensen, T. K., *et al* (2004) Alcohol consumption at the time of conception and spontaneous abortion. *American Journal of Epidemiology Baltimore*, **160**, 661–667.

117

Henriksson, K. M. & McNeil, T. F. (2006) Smoking in pregnancy and its correlates among women with a history of schizophrenia and affective psychosis. *Schizophrenia Research*, **81**, 121–123.

Hewitt, J. B. & Tellier, L. (1998) Risk of adverse outcomes in pregnant women exposed to solvents. *Journal of Obstetric, Gynecologic and Neonatal Nursing*, **27**, 521–531.

Horne, R. S. C., Franco, P., Adamson, T. M., et al (2004) Influences of maternal cigarette smoking on infant arousability. *Early Human Development*, **79**, 49–58.

Horrigan, T. J., Schroeder, A. V. & Schaffer, R. M. (2000) The triad of substance abuse, violence, and depression are interrelated in pregnancy. *Journal of Substance Abuse Treatment*, **18**, 55–58.

Hotham, E. D., Atkinson, E. R. & Gilbert, A. L. (2002) Focus groups with pregnant smokers; barriers to cessation, attitudes to nicotine patch use and perceptions of counselling by care providers. *Drug and Alcohol Review*, **21**, 163–168.

Hotham, E. D., Gilbert, A. L. & Atkinson, E. R. (2006) A randomised controlled trial of nicotine patches in pregnant women. *Addictive Behaviours*, **31**, 641–648.

Houet, T., Vabret, F., Herlicoviez, M., et al (2005) Comparison of women's alcohol consumption before and during pregnancy from a prospective series of 150 women. *Journal de Gynecologie, Obstetrique et Biologie de la Reproduction*, **7**, 687–693.

Huiznik, A. C. & Mulder, E. J. H. (2006) Maternal smoking, drinking or cannabis use during pregnancy and neurobehavioural and cognitive functioning in human offspring. *Neuroscience and Behavioral Reviews*, **30**, 24–41.

Hulse, G. K., Milne, E., English, D. R., et al (1997a) Assessing the relationship between maternal cocaine use and abruption placentae. *Addiction*, **92**, 1547–1551.

Hulse, G. K., Milne, E., English, D. R., et al (1997b) The relationship between maternal use of heroin and methadone and birth weight. *Addiction*, **92**, 1571–1579.

Hulse, G. K., Milne, E., English, D. R., et al (1998a) Assessing the relationship between maternal opiate use and neonatal mortality. *Addiction*, **93**, 1033–1042.

Hulse, G. K., Milne, E., English, D. R., et al (1998b) Assessing the relationship between maternal opiate use and antepartum haemorrhage. *Addiction*, **93**, 1533–1558.

Information Centre (2006) Statistics on alcohol in England. *Health and Social Care Statistical Bulletin*, **11**, 3–8.

Ingersoll, K. S., Knisely, J. S., Dawson, K. S., et al (2004) Psychopathology and treatment outcome of drug dependent women in a perinatal program. *Addictive Behaviours*, **29**, 731–741.

Jansson, L. M., Velez, M. & Harrow, C. (2004) Methadone maintenance and lactation: a review of the literature and current management guidelines. *Journal of Human Lactation*, **20**, 62–71.

Johnson, R. E., Jones, H. E., Jasinski, D. R., et al (2001) Buprenorphine treatment of pregnant opioid-dependent women: maternal and neonatal outcomes. *Drug and Alcohol Dependence*, **63**, 97–103.

Jones, H. E., Johnson, R. E., Jasinski, D. R., et al (2005) Buprenorphine versus methadone in the treatment of opioid-dependent patients: effects on the neonatal abstinence syndrome. *Drug and Alcohol Dependence*, **79**, 1–10.

Jones, K. L., Smith, D. W., Ulleland, C. N., et al (1973) Pattern of malformation in offspring of chronic alcoholic mothers. *Lancet*, **1**, 1267–1271.

Jordan, T. R., Dake, J. A. & Price, J. H. (2006) Best practices for smoking cessation in pregnancy: do obstetrician/gynecologists use them in practice? *Journal of Women's Health*, **15**, 400–441.

Kain, Z., Mayes, L., Pakes, J., et al (1995) Thrombocytopenia in pregnant women who use cocaine. *American Journal of Obstetrics and Gynecology*, **173**, 885–890.

Källen, K. (2000) Maternal smoking during pregnancy and infant head circumference at birth. *Early Human Development*, **58**, 197–204.

Kaltenbach, K. A. & Finnegan, L. P. (1989) Prenatal narcotic exposure: perinatal and developmental effects. *Neurotoxicology*, **10**, 597–604.

Kelly, R. H., Zatick, D. & Anders, T. F. (2001) The detection and treatment of psychiatric disorders and substance use among pregnant women cared for in obstetrics. *American Journal of Psychiatry*, **158**, 213–219.

Kendall, S. R., Doberczak, T. M., Jantumen, M., *et al* (1999) The methadone maintained pregnancy. *Clinics in Perinatology*, **26**, 173–183.

Kennare, R., Heard, A. & Chan, A. (2005) Substance use during pregnancy: risk factors and obstetric and perinatal outcomes in South Australia. *Australian and New Zealand Journal of Obstetrics and Gynaecology*, **45: 220–225.**

Kesmodel, U., Wisborg, K., Olsen, S., *et al* (2002*a*) Moderate alcohol intake in pregnancy and the risk of spontaneous abortion. *Alcohol and Alcoholism*, **37**, 87–92.

Kesmodel, U., Wisborg, K., Olsen, S. F., *et al* (2002*b*) Moderate alcohol intake during pregnancy and the risk of stillbirth and death in the first year of life. *American Journal of Epidemiology*, **155**, 305–312.

Kiernan, K. & Pickett, K. E. (2006) Marital status disparities in maternal smoking during pregnancy, breastfeeding and maternal depression. *Social Science and Medicine*, **63**, 335–346.

Klonoff-Cohen, H. & Lam-Kruglick, P. (2001) Maternal and paternal recreational drug use and sudden infant death syndrome. *Archives of Pediatric and Adolescent Medicine*, **155**, 765–770.

Kralova, I., Stepanak, Z. & Dusek, J. (2006) Ethylene glycol intoxication misdiagnosed as eclampsia. *Acta Anaesthesiologica Scandinavica*, **50**, 385–387.

Kuczkowski, K. M. (2003) Solvents in pregnancy: an emerging problem in obstetrics and obstetric anaesthesia. *Anaesthesia*, **58**, 1036–1037.

Lacroix, I., Bribe, A., Chaumerliac, C., *et al* (2004) Buprenorphine in pregnant opioid-dependent women: first results of a prospective study. *Addiction*, **99**, 209–214.

Law, K. L., Stroud, L. R., LaGasse, L. L., *et al* (2003) Smoking during pregnancy and newborn neurobehavior. *Pediatrics*, **111**, 1318–1323.

Lawrence, T., Aveyard, P., Cheng, K.K., *et al* (2005) Does stage-based smoking cessation advice in pregnancy result in long-term quitters? 18-month postpartum follow-up of a randomized controlled trial. *Addiction*, **100**, 107–116.

Lejeune, C., Simmat, D., Gourarier, L., *et al* (2006) Prospective multicenter observational study of 260 infants born to 259 opiate-dependent mothers on methadone or high-dose buprenorphine substitution. *Drug and Alcohol Dependence*, **82**, 250–257.

Lemoine, P., Harousseau, H., Borteyru, J. P., *et al* (1968) Les enfants des parents alcooliques: anomalies observées à propos de 127 cas. *Ouest Medical*, **21**, 476–482.

Leonardson, G. R. & Loudenburg, R. (2003) Risk factors for alcohol use during pregnancy in a multistate area. *Neurotoxicology and Teratology*, **25**, 651–658.

Lewis, G. & Drife, J. (2004) *Why Mothers Die 2000–2002. The Sixth Report of the Confidential Enquiries into Maternal Death in the United Kingdom*. RCOG Press.

Lingford-Hughes, A. R., Welch, S. & Nutt, D. J. (2004) Evidence-based guidelines for the pharmacological management of substance misuse, addiction and comorbidity: recommendations from the British Association for Psychopharmacology. *Journal of Psychopharmacology*, **18**, 293–335.

Linneberg, A., Petersen, J., Gronbaek, M., *et al* (2004) Alcohol during pregnancy and atopic dermatitis in the offspring. *Journal of Allergy and Clinical Immunology*, **34**, 1678–1683.

Linnet, K. M., Dalsgaard, S., Obel, C., *et al* (2003) Maternal lifestyle factors in pregnancy risk of attention deficit hyperactivity disorder and associated behaviors: review of the current evidence. *American Journal of Psychiatry*, **160**, 1028–1040.

Little, M., Shah, R., Vermeulen, M. J., *et al* (2005) Adverse perinatal outcomes associated with homelessness and substance misuse in pregnancy. *Canadian Medical Association Journal*, **173**, 615–618.

Lumley, J., Oliver, S. S., Chamberlain, C., *et al* (2004) Interventions for promoting smoking cessation during pregnancy. *Cochrane Database of Systematic Reviews*, **4**, CD001055.

Malik, S., Cleves, M. A., Honein, M. A., *et al* (2008) Maternal smoking and congenital heart defects. *Pediatrics*, **121**, e810–e816.

Man, L. X. & Chang, B. (2006) Maternal cigarette smoking during pregnancy increases the risk of having a child with a congenital digitial anomaly. *Plastic and Reconstructive Surgery*, **117**, 301–308.

Mariscal, M., Palma, S., Llorca, J., *et al* (2006) Pattern of alcohol consumption during pregnancy and risk for low birth weight. *Annals of Epidemiology*, **16**, 432–438.

Markovic, N., Ness, R. & Cefilli, D. (2000) Substance use measures among women in early pregnancy. *American Journal Obstetrics & Gynecology*, **183**, 627–632.

McCarthy, J. J., Leamon, M. H., Parr, M. S., *et al* (2005) High dose methadone maintenance in pregnancy: maternal and neonatal outcomes. *American Journal of Obstetrics and Gynecology*, **193**, 606–610.

McLeod, D., Pullon, S., Benn, C., *et al* (2004) Can support and education for smoking cessation and reduction be provided effectively by midwives within primary maternity care? *Midwifery*, **20**, 37–50.

Medrano, M. A. (1996) Does a discrete fetal solvent syndrome exist? *Alcoholism Treatments Quarterly*, **14**, 59–79.

Menegaux, F., Steffen, C., Bellec, S., *et al* (2005) Maternal coffee and alcohol consumption during pregnancy, parental smoking and risk of childhood acute leukaemia. *Cancer Detection and Prevention*, **29**, 487–493.

Miller, H., Ranger-Moore, J. & Hingten, M. (2003) Bupropion SR for smoking cessation in pregnancy: a pilot study. *American Journal of Obstetrics and Gynecology*, **189**, S133.

Miller, J. & Nolan, T. (2001) Case–control study of antenatal cocaine use and platelet levels. *American Journal of Obstetrics and Gynecology*, **184**, 434–437.

Mitchell, E. A. (1995) Smoking: the next major modifiable risk factor. In *Sudden Infant Death Syndrome: New Trends in the Nineties* (ed. T. O. Rognum), pp. 114–118. Scandinavian University Press.

Morales-Suarez-Varela, M. M., Bille, M., Christensen, K., *et al* (2006) Smoking habits, nicotine use and congenital malformations. *Obstetrics and Gynecology*, **107**, 51–57.

Morbidity and Mortality Weekly Report (2004) Notice to readers: Surgeon General's advisory on alcohol use in pregnancy. Centers for Disease Control and Prevention (http://www.cdc.gov/mmwr/preview/mmwrhtml/mm5409a6.htm).

Mukherjee, R. A., Hollins, S. & Turk, J. (2006) Fetal alcohol spectrum disorder: an overview. *Journal of the Royal Society of Medicine*, **99**, 298–302.

Munger, R. G., Romitti, P. A., Daack-Hirsch, S., *et al* (1997) Maternal alcohol use and risk of orofacial birth defects. *International Journal of Pediatric Otorhinolaryngology*, **40**, 217–212.

National Collaborating Centre for Women's and Children's Health (2003) *Antenatal Care: Routine Care for the Healthy Pregnant Woman*. RCOG Press.

National Institute for Health and Clinical Excellence (2002) *Guidance on the Use of Nicotine Replacement Therapy (NRT) and Bupropion for Smoking Cessation*. NICE.

Nayak, M. B. & Kaskutas, L. A. (2004) Risky drinking and alcohol use patterns in a national sample of women of childbearing age. *Addiction*, **99**, 1393–1402.

Nielsen, A., Hannibal, C. G., Linekilde, B. E., *et al* (2006) Maternal smoking predicts the risk of spontaneous abortion. *Acta Obstetricia et Gynecologica Scandinavica*, **85**, 1057–1065.

Nulman, I., Rovet, J., Kennedy, D., *et al* (2004) Binge alcohol consumption by non-alcohol-dependent women during pregnancy affects child behaviour, but not general intellectual functioning; a prospective controlled study. *Archives of Women's Mental Health*, **7**, 173–181.

Okah, F. A., Cai, J. & Hoff, G. L. (2005) Term-gestation low birth weight and health-compromising behaviors during pregnancy. *Obstetrics and Gynecology*, **105**, 543–550.

O'Leary, C. M. (2004) Fetal alcohol syndrome: diagnosis, epidemiology, and developmental outcomes. *Journal of Paediatrics and Child Health*, **40**, 2–7.

Ostrea, J., Enrique, M., Knapp, D. K., *et al* (2001) Estimates of illicit drug use during pregnancy by maternal interview, hair analysis, and meconium analysis. *Journal of Pediatrics*, **138**, 344–348.

Panting-Kemp, A., Nguyen, T. & Castro, L. (2002) Substance abuse and polyhydramnios. *American Journal of Obstetrics and Gynecology*, **187**, 602–605.

Peterson, P. L. & Lowe, J. B. (1992) Preventing fetal alcohol exposure: a cognitive behavioral approach. *International Journal of the Addictions*, **27**, 613–626.

Petrou, S., Hockley, C., Mehta, Z., *et al* (2005) The association between smoking during pregnancy and hospital inpatient costs in childhood. *Social Science and Medicine*, **60**, 1071–1085.

Pichini, S., Puig, C., Zuccaro, P., et al (2005) Assessment of exposure to opiates and cocaine during pregnancy in a Mediterranean city: preliminary results of the 'Meconium Project'. *Forensic Science International*, **153**, 59–65.

Ponsonby, A. L., Dwyer, T. & Couper, D. (1997) Factors related to infant apnoea and cyanosis: a population-based study. *Journal of Paediatrics and Child Health*, **33**, 317–323.

Raatikainen, K., Huurinainen, P. & Heinonen, S. (2007) Smoking in early gestation or through pregnancy: a decision crucial to pregnancy outcome. *Preventive Medicine*, **44**, 59–63.

Rasch, V. (2003) Cigarette, alcohol, and caffeine consumption: risk factors for spontaneous abortion. *Acta Obstetricia et Gynecologica Scandinavica*, **82**, 182–188.

Richardson, G. A., Ryan, C., Willford, J., et al (2002) Prenatal alcohol and marijuana exposure: effects on neuropsychological outcomes at 10 years. *Neurotoxicology and Teratology*, **24**, 309–320.

Rigotti, N. A., Park, E. R., Regan, S., et al (2006) Efficacy of telephone counselling for pregnant smokers: a randomised controlled trial. *Obstetrics and Gynecology*, **108**, 83–92.

Riley, E. P. & McGee, C. L. (2005) Fetal alcohol spectrum disorders: an overview with emphasis on changes in brain and behavior. *Experimental Biology and Medicine*, **230**, 357–365.

Schuler, M. E., Nair, P. & Kettinger, L. (2003) Drug-exposed infants and developmental outcome. *Archives of Pediatrics and Adolescent Medicine*, **157**, 133–138.

Shah, N. R. & Bracken, M. B. (2000) A systematic review and meta-analysis of prospective studies on the association between maternal cigarette smoking and preterm delivery. *American Journal of Obstetrics and Gynecology*, **182**, 465–472.

Sherwood, R. A., Keating, V., Kavvadia, A., et al (1999) Substance misuse in early pregnancy and relationship to fetal outcome. *European Journal of Pediatrics*, **158**, 488–492.

Singer, L. T., Minnes, S. & Short, E. (2004) Cognitive outcomes of preschool children with prenatal cocaine exposure. *JAMA*, **291**, 2448–2456.

Smith, G. C. & White, I. R. (2006) Predicting the risk for sudden infant death syndrome from obstetric characteristics: a retrospective cohort study of 505,011 live births. *Pediatrics*, **117**, 60–66.

Smith, L. M., La Gasse, L. L., Derauf, C., et al (2006) The infant development, environment, and lifestyle study: effects of prenatal methamphetamine exposure, polydrug exposure, and poverty on intrauterine growth. *Pediatrics*, **118**, 1149–1156.

Sokol, R. J., Martier, S. S. & Ager, J. W. (1989) The T–ACE questions: practical prenatal detection of risk-drinking. *American Journal of Obstetrics and Gynecology*, **160**, 863–871.

Steyn, K., de Wet, T., Salooje, Y., et al (2006) The influence of maternal smoking, snuff use and passive smoking on pregnancy outcomes: the Birth To Ten Study. *Paediatric and Perinatal Epidemiology*, **20**, 90–99.

Sratton, K., Howe, C. & Battaglia, F. C. (eds) (1996) *Fetal Alcohol Syndrome: Diagnosis, Epidemiology, Prevention, and Treatment*. National Academy Press.

Testa, M., Quigley, B. M. & Eiden, R. D. (2003) The effects of prenatal alcohol exposure on infant mental development: a meta-analytical review. *Alcohol and Alcoholism*, **38**, 295–304.

Thorup, J., Cortes, D. & Petersen, B. L. (2006) The incidence of bilateral cryptorchidism is increased and the fertility potential is reduced in sons born to mothers who have smoked during pregnancy. *Journal of Urology*, **176**, 734–737.

Tough, S., Tofflemire, K., Clarke, M., et al (2006) Do women change their drinking behaviors while trying to conceive? An opportunity for preconception counseling. *Clinical Medicine and Research*, **4**, 97–105.

Turner, C., Russell, A. & Brown, W. (2003) Prevalence of illicit drug use in young Australian women, patterns of use and associated risk factors. *Addiction*, **98**, 1419–1426.

Ulleland, C. N. (1972) The offspring of alcoholic mothers. *Annals of the New York Academy of Sciences*, **197**, 167–169.

Urato, A., Craigo, S., Collins, J., et al (2005) Maternal smoking and pregnancy outcomes. *American Journal of Obstetrics and Gynecology*, **193**, S121.

Ussher, M., West, R, & Hibbs, N. (2004) A survey of pregnant smokers' interest in different types of smoking cessation support. *Patient Education and Counselling*, **54**, 67–72.

121

Ussher, M., Etter, J-F. & West, R. (2006) Perceived barriers to and benefits of attending a stop smoking course during pregnancy. *Patient Education and Counselling*, **61**, 467–472.

Velez, M. L., Montoya, I. D., Jansson, L. M., *et al* (2006) Exposure to violence among substance-dependent pregnant women and their children. *Journal of Substance Abuse Treatment*, **30**, 31–38.

Vritsios, J. & Deltsidou, A. (2005) Amphetamines and LSD use during pregnancy. *Review of Clinical Pharmacology and Pharmacokinetics, International Edition*, **19**, 99–104.

Whitehead, N. & Lipscomb, L. (2003) Patterns of alcohol use before and during pregnancy and the risk of small-for-gestational-age birth. *American Journal of Epidemiology*, **158**, 654–662.

Wilford, J. A., Leech, S. L. & Day, N. L. (2006) Moderate prenatal alcohol exposure and cognitive status of children at age 10. *Alcoholism: Clinical and Experimental Rsearch*, **30**, 1051–1059.

Williams, J. H. & Ross, L. (2007). Consequences of prenatal toxin exposure for mental health in children and adolescents: a systematic review. *European Child and Adolescent Psychiatry*, **16**, 243–253.

Wisborg, K., Kesmodel, U., Henriksen, T. B., *et al* (2003) A prospective study of maternal smoking and spontaneous abortion. *Acta Obstetricia et Gynecologica Scandinavica*, **82**, 936–41.

Wolff, K., Boys, A., Rostami-Hodjegan, A., *et al* (2005) Changes to methadone clearance during pregnancy. *European Journal of Clinical Pharmacology*, **61**, 763–768.

Wyszynski, D. F., Duffy, D. L. & Beatty, T. H. (1997) Maternal cigarette smoking and oral clefts: a meta-analysis. *Cleft Palate-Craniofacial Journal*, **34**, 206–210.

Zdravkovic, T., Genbacev, O., McMaster, M. T., *et al* (2005) The adverse effects of maternal smoking on the human placenta: a review. *Placenta*, **26**, S81–S86.

Zhang, X., Sliwowska, J. H. & Weinberg, J. (2005) Prenatal alcohol exposure and fetal programming: effects on neuroendocrine and immune function. *Experimental Biology and Medicine*, **230**, 376–388.

Further reading

Kassim, Z. & Greenough, A. (2006) Neonatal abstinence syndrome: identification and management. *Current Paediatrics*, **16**, 172–175.

Klee, H., Jackson, M. & Lewis, S. (2002) *Drug Misuse and Motherhood*. Routledge.

Rayburn, W. F. & Bogenschurtz, M. P. (2004) Pharmacotherapy for pregnant women with addictions. *American Journal of Obstetrics and Gynecology*, **191**, 1885–1897.

Royal College of Obstetricians and Gynaecologists (2006) *Alcohol Consumption and the Outcomes of Pregnancy (Statement No. 5)*. Royal College of Obstetricians and Gynaecologists.

Williams, J. H. G. & Ross, L. (2007) Consequences of prenatal toxin exposure for mental health in children and adolescents. *European Child and Adolescent Psychiatry*, **16**, 243–253.

CHAPTER 6

Perinatal mental illness, children and the family

Perinatal psychiatry is a rapidly developing field with increasing knowledge about the causation, presentation and management of parental mental health problems during pregnancy and the year following delivery. As our understanding of perinatal mental illness has grown and developed so has our recognition of the impact of parental psychopathology during this period on the health and well-being of the unborn baby and infant (Federenko & Wadhwa, 2004). In addition, there is an awareness that early life experiences may influence the health of an individual across their lifespan and that it is important to pay attention to infant mental health (Carter *et al*, 2004).

No book on perinatal psychiatry therefore would be complete without an examination of the impact of maternal and paternal mental health problems in the perinatal period on their children both in the short and longer term.

The birth of a child represents a significant life event, particularly if it is a first child. In the main it is expected that this is a joyful time but nevertheless it represents a time of enormous transition for all concerned. It is not surprising, therefore, that for some it is overwhelming and associated with increased levels of stress and anxiety. It is important to consider the effects of this as well as the impact of formal mental illness on the preparedness of parents for the birth of their infant and on the infant (Maldonado-Durán *et al*, 2000). Severe mental health problems in parents will usually be detected and treated. It is likely, however, that there is a significant body of subclinical parental psychopathology that although not severe enough to necessitate referral to specialist mental health services, nevertheless has the potential to adversely affect developing parent–child relationships and the well-being of the child. It is not uncommon for parents presenting with their children at child and adolescent mental health services to describe parental (most usually maternal) mental health problems, frequently untreated, early in the child's life.

Parental mental illness may affect children in a number of ways, including effects on all aspects of development, mental health and increased vulnerability to abuse and neglect. The parent's illness will exert direct effects and in addition associated risk factors may further compromise the child's outcome.

Fundamental to child outcome is the relationship between the child and their primary caregivers. Relationships are bidirectional and it is important to explore the nature of parent–child interactions from the child and the parent perspective. Disruption in either direction may potentially affect outcome (Brockington, 1996; Main, 1996).

Any illness that disrupts the physical and psychological processes of pregnancy has implications for the physical and psychological well-being of the foetus and infant. There are therefore some illness effects that can be generalised across the range of mental health problems. In addition, particular diagnoses are associated with particular risks and effects, many of which are described elsewhere in this book. Although the bulk of this book explores the parent's experience of mental illness, the focus of this chapter is on the experience of the foetus and infant. The aim is to highlight the potential risks posed by parental perinatal mental illness. The existing evidence for the effects of perinatal mental illness on the main indicators of child outcome will be considered and the role of intervention reviewed. The emphasis will be on the management of perinatal mental illness in routine clinical practice.

Pregnancy

Parental psychological adjustment

The process of pregnancy involves both physical and psychological aspects. Thus, while mother and father progress through the physical changes of pregnancy, both are also undergoing psychological changes in preparation for the arrival of their baby and their new role as parents (Stern, 1999). This 'psychological pregnancy' may be influenced by a range of factors including normal fears and anxieties, maternal and paternal physical and mental illness, and environmental stressors such as financial and housing worries and domestic violence. Previous perinatal loss is a risk factor in that it is associated with increased levels of pregnancy-specific anxiety and depression (Cote-Arsenault, 2003), with mothers having more symptoms than fathers. That is to say, understandably, parents who have lost a baby are more concerned about their baby during a subsequent pregnancy.

Parents' previous experiences of being parented are also important in this process. A conflicted past may have a significant effect on a parents' emerging relationship with their child both *in utero* and postnatally. Fraiberg *et al* (1987) describe maternal negative recollections of childhood relationships with parents as 'ghosts in the nursery' which may adversely affect parent–infant relationships. The ghosts vary in their tenacity, some being transient intruders while others become more firmly established. It is important to note, however, that many parents who have experienced neglect, cruelty and abuse do not revisit this on their own children.

Parents form expectations about what their baby will be like in terms of temperament, personality, abilities and about their future. In addition, there are cultural expectations and beliefs about babies and how they should behave. Babies may be conceived for specific reasons, for example to replace a lost child, save a marriage, to be a boy or a girl, or so that a parent might feel loved by someone (Maldonado-Durán et al, 2000). Stern (1999) describes the 'imagined' baby and the conflicts that may arise after birth if the real and imagined babies do not match up. Factors such as preterm delivery or physical handicaps may immediately raise conflicts. In the case of preterm delivery it is important to remember that the parents are also 'preterm' in their preparation for the arrival of their child. Conflicts may arise because of discrepancies between the real and imagined babies in terms of their temperament and behaviour.

The psychoanalytic literature provides perspectives that are of use in understanding new parents' experiences and reactions. Joan Raphael-Leff (1985), Dana Breen (1975) and Helen Deutsch (1947) describe unconscious and developmental processes in the perinatal period that may provide insights into vulnerability to mental health problems and attachment difficulties during this time.

This process of psychological adjustment, therefore, includes the development of an attachment to and a relationship with the foetus. Various factors are recognised to potentially influence this. Factors such as supportive family relationships and being psychologically well are associated with higher levels of maternal–foetal attachment, while mental health problems such as depression, anxiety and substance misuse are associated with poorer attachment. There is, however, a lack of robust research in this area (Alhusen, 2008). Although it might have been expected that previous perinatal loss would affect prenatal attachment, this does not appear to be the case (Armstrong, 2002).

Feeling the baby move and seeing ultrasound pictures enhance parental attachment and parents' developing image of their baby (Sedgman et al, 2006). It is interesting that the addition of three- or four-dimensional ultrasound scans does not add any additional emotional impact or affect prenatal attachment to that seen with two-dimensional scans (Rustico et al, 2005; Sedgman et al, 2006).

The psychological adjustment to pregnancy may not always be positive. In such cases there must be immediate concerns about the well-being of the unborn child. Having an unwanted pregnancy or being ambivalent about pregnancy may be associated with some risk to the foetus in terms of preterm delivery and low birth weight (Mohllajee et al, 2007). Knowing both parents' attitudes to the pregnancy is important (Korenman et al, 2002). Having an unwanted pregnancy may be associated with later rejection of the baby (Brockington et al, 2006). Similarly, denial of pregnancy and concealed pregnancies are associated with risks to the foetus related to lack of antenatal care.

Denial and concealment of pregnancy may result from inexperience and a lack of awareness of the physical changes of pregnancy. Denial of pregnancy is also recognised to occur in the context of psychological conflict, stress, trauma, dissociative states, psychotic illness and learning disability. Denial may also occur where a mother wishes to have a baby but is worried that the baby may be taken away because of concerns about her ability to look after it. There are also occasions where mothers know they are pregnant but behave as though they are not (Friedman *et al*, 2007). The immediate physical risks to the baby are in terms of inadequate antenatal care and the sudden unexpected arrival of the baby (Maldonado-Durán *et al*, 2000). The available evidence suggests that there may be some association between concealed pregnancy and increased risk of preterm delivery (Nirmal *et al*, 2006), but in general it seems that following delivery women are often able to care for their babies (Friedman *et al*, 2007).

There is a paucity of information about the occurrence of and factors associated with foetal abuse (Kent *et al*, 1997). The concept of foetal abuse encompasses a range of potential insults from physical assault to abuse with alcohol and drugs (Condon, 1986). Maternal–foetal attachment may be important in foetal abuse (Pollock & Percy, 1999) and further investigation in this area is essential to understanding and identifying mothers and fathers who may harm their unborn child.

Intimate partner violence during pregnancy may be responsible for as many as 16 per 1000 foetal deaths (Boy & Salihu, 2004). Here again there is a lack of information about the relationship between the nature of intimate partner violence and pregnancy outcome. Mothers who are abused are at increased risk of delivering low-birth-weight and/or preterm babies; risk of foetal death is also increased (Sharps *et al*, 2007). Mothers who are abused are also more likely to present to services with infections and to have poor antenatal care. Ultimately, mothers who are victims of intimate partner violence are at risk of being murdered (Chambliss, 2008). There may be an association between intimate partner violence and unintended pregnancy, with the further risk of unplanned children being born into violent families (Pallitto *et al*, 2005).

Antenatal mental health problems

There is now a considerable body of evidence that shows an association between maternal mental health problems during pregnancy and adverse outcome for the child, including their emotional, cognitive, physical health and development (Hollins, 2007). Much less information is available about paternal antenatal mental health problems. Research also looks at the effects on the developing foetus. Measuring these effects is challenging and usually confined to physical effects, although there is increasing interest in foetal perception and responses, and neurobehavioural development (Kurjak, *et al*, 2006). The need to measure foetal neurobehavioural development is driven by a recognition that the antenatal period is important in the development of differences in later functioning (DiPietro, 2005). Although to date there is some evidence for the effects of antenatal mental health problems on foetal neurobehavioural development, this is limited and the bulk of evidence explores the physical risks associated with complications of pregnancy and delivery.

Although maternal depression was at one time thought to be primarily a postnatal phenomenon, it is now widely recognised that in some cases depression begins in the antenatal period. In addition, babies are also born to women with established depressive or bipolar disorders. There is evidence of increased risks of complications of pregnancy, delivery and early neonatal problems, including foetal distress, in mothers who have major affective disorders (Jablensky et al, 2005). Mothers with prenatal depression have been shown to be at increased risk of preterm delivery (Dayan et al, 2006). The mechanism for this link between prenatal depression and adverse outcome is unclear as depression occurs against a background of other risk and protective factors (Alder et al, 2007).

Antenatal anxiety and psychosocial stress are associated with greater levels of foetal activity and higher rates of preterm birth and perinatal complications (Alder et al, 2007). There is an association between maternal stress during pregnancy and an increased risk of low birth weight. A range of stressors have been implicated including pregnancy denial, getting back with a partner, being unhappy about and having an unplanned pregnancy (Sable & Wilkinson, 2000).

There are some immediate risks to the foetus associated with eating disorders. Reported risks linked to anorexia include low infant birth weight together with prematurity, increased perinatal mortality and congenital malformations. Bulimia is linked with intrauterine growth retardation and congenital malformations (Morrill & Nickols-Richardson, 2001). It is important to note, however, that the evidence base in respect of these disorders and foetal outcome is limited (Park et al, 2003).

Mothers with a diagnosis of schizophrenia are at increased risk of complications such as antepartum haemorrhage, placental abnormalities, foetal distress and low birth weight (Jablensky et al, 2005).

The harmful effects of maternal substance misuse on foetal development are widely accepted. Chiriboga (2003) provides as review of this subject. In general terms, substance misuse is associated with a range of foetal effects including growth retardation, physical abnormalities and neurobehavioural changes. It is noteworthy that the two most commonly available substances of misuse, nicotine and alcohol, are associated most clearly with adverse foetal outcome; nicotine with the highest risk of foetal growth retardation, and alcohol with learning disability (foetal alcohol syndrome). The direct foetal effects of other substances of misuse are less clear.

For a more detailed examination of the impact of mental disorder and substance misuse on pregnancy and foetal outcomes see Chapters 3 and 5.

Foetal experiences

It is important to remember that as parents are progressing through the psychological and physical changes of pregnancy, the foetus continues to grow and develop. Maldonado-Durán *et al* (2000) describe the foetus as a 'real presence' and a 'contributor' to the pregnancy who is 'immersed ... in an emotional field that may be more or less conducive to healthy development'. In this way we are interested in the foetus' experiences *in utero* and to what extent these influence later development (Lecanuet *et al*, 1996; Lickliter, 2000). With modern imaging/scanning techniques we are able to observe the foetus in some detail. Studies have examined foetal neurobehavioural development as well as foetal response to various maternal states and stimuli. Most of the evidence in relation to foetal perception is from the third trimester of pregnancy. There is evidence that the foetus experiences taste (Mennella *et al*, 2001) and that these experiences may influence the enjoyment of flavours postnatally. There is also evidence that the foetus responds to sound and that with increasing maturity can discriminate the mother's voice (Kisilevsky *et al*, 2003).

Foetal experience of pain is of particular interest in view of the developing fields of foetal medicine and surgery, with interventions for medical and surgical conditions being performed *in utero*. It is thought that the foetus cannot recognise pain as a noxious stimulus until functional thalamocortical fibres are in place. Such fibres do not begin to develop until 23 weeks gestation (Lee *et al*, 2005). The extent of our current knowledge therefore suggests that the foetus does not experience pain until 29–30 weeks gestation. An important aspect of foetal pain perception lies in the potential impact of the physiological response to pain on the developing brain and subsequent neurological outcome (Lowery *et al*, 2007).

An association has been demonstrated between maternal psychological state during pregnancy and foetal neurobehavioural function (DiPietro *et al*, 2002). Foetuses whose mothers describe their lives as stressful and who experience more 'hassles' in relation to their pregnancy are more active throughout pregnancy. By contrast, the foetuses of mothers who are more positive and perceive their pregnancy as 'up-lifting' are less active. It is not clear what such findings mean in terms of the postnatal development of the foetus, although some studies have examined the associations between foetal neurobehavioural functioning and infant temperament (DiPietro *et al*, 1996). Foetuses that were more active tend to be more difficult and unpredictable infants. The suggestion is that foetal neurobehavioural functioning may predict differences in infant regulation and reactivity.

Perhaps the most widely explored maternal psychological state in relation to foetal experience is maternal stress. There is a significant body of evidence describing the adverse effects of maternal stress in terms of pregnancy complications (e.g. pre-eclampsia, preterm delivery, miscarriage and foetal distress). In addition, there is evidence that maternal stress during pregnancy is associated with adverse physical and mental health outcomes for the foetus and infant and indeed throughout life (for a review see Van den Bergh *et al*, 2005). The mechanism by which maternal stress leads to these adverse outcomes is complex and still to be clearly elucidated. The evidence suggests, however, that the effects are mediated through a mechanism of foetal programming (Knackstedt *et al*, 2005) via the HPA and neurotransmitter systems (Kapoor *et al*, 2006; Talge *et al*, 2007).

Pregnancy, therefore, is a time of great change and a time of great challenges for parents and the developing child. Even in the best of circumstances this can be difficult but it is more so when there are other problems such as parental mental illness or psychosocial stressors, all of which potentially affect the baby either directly or indirectly.

Attachment

The preceding information illustrates that a relationship is emerging between the foetus and parents antenatally. This may be compromised by a range of factors including parental mental illness, stressors such as worry and anxiety, preterm delivery and time in neonatal intensive care units. This emerging relationship can be considered to be part of the attachment process (Main, 1996).

The term 'attachment' has entered common parlance where it is used in general terms to describe the relationship between parents and their infant children. However, the term was first used by Sears to describe children's relationships with their parents (Sears, 1943). Bowlby later used the term in association with his work in relation to the affectional ties being described by animal ethologists (Bowlby, 1958). Bowlby considered the attachment of human infants to their mother to be largely biologically based and to represent a safety mechanism in which the infant stays close to the mother for protection. The mother in turn provides a secure base from which the infant can explore the world. Bowlby considered that the relationship between parent and child formed the basis for the child's later psychological development (Bowlby, 1982). This early parent–child relationship is thought to be essential to the child's developing sense of themselves and their understanding of relationships (Stern, 2002).

Ainsworth (1963) further developed Bowlby's ideas and much of our current understanding of attachment behaviour is based on her seminal work. The first studies of attachment involved examining the infants' reactions to separation from their mother. From this work, Ainsworth identified three stages of attachment during infancy (undiscriminating social responsiveness, discriminating social responsiveness and active initiation). Ainsworth & Wittig (1969) developed a laboratory experiment to examine children's response to separation from their parents (the 'strange situation') and described different styles of attachment as a result (securely attached, anxiously attached and anxious avoidant). A fourth category of attachment was identified by Main & Solomon (1986). They

129

described disorganised attachment in which the infant shows attachment behaviour that is confused or incomplete.

Psychoanalytical theory describes the importance of early parent–child relationships in an individual's development, including their personality and their future relationships (Freud, 1963). Anna Freud described the importance of a mother recognising and responding sensitively to her infant in relation to the child's further psychological development (Freud, 1970). The emphasis is on 'emotional reciprocity', a theme that is further explored by the object relations theorists who discuss the importance of parent–infant relationships in the child's future interpersonal relationships (Winnicott, 1970).

Most of the research to date has focused on the role of mothers in attachment. This is not to say, however, that fathers are not important or that infants do not form attachments to their fathers. Infants do demonstrate attachment behaviours to their fathers, for example infants cry at separation from their fathers and greet them on return. However, there may be differences in attachment behaviour, for example there is evidence that in stressful situations the infant is more likely to prefer the mother (Lamb, 1976). Attachment behaviours are also seen with other caregivers such as grandparents.

Attachment requires maternal and paternal responsivity. Anything that gets in the way of this can adversely affect attachment with implications for the infant particularly in respect of future relationships. In this way parental perinatal mental illness may pose a threat to the development of attachment by impairing or limiting the extent of the relationship and bonding. A mother or father affected by mental illness may be less available for or able to meet the needs of the developing infant. This in turn will affect the attachment relationship and in extreme cases lead to the development of attachment disorders. Disorders of attachment (reactive attachment disorder and disinhibited attachment disorder) are described in both ICD–10 (World Health Organization, 1992) and DSM–1V (American Psychiatric Association, 1994).

The role of attachment in the development and maintenance of child and adolescent mental health problems is widely recognised. At the extreme of disrupted attachment are those children and young people who have been removed from the care of their parents. Levels of psychopathology are so high in this group of children that specialist mental health services have been developed to address their needs. To a lesser extent, any child who has experienced a compromised attachment relationship will be vulnerable to mental health problems. Rutter et al (2004), in the English and Romanian Adoptees (ERA) Study, have examined the experiences and outcome of children adopted into British families following profoundly deprived early life experiences in Romanian institutions. Their studies have confirmed the validity of the attachment disorder construct (O'Connor & Rutter, 2000) and have highlighted the vulnerability of children deprived in this way to developmental impairment (O'Connor et al, 2000).

Impact of parental mental illness on attachment

Any parental mental health problem may interfere with the formation and maintenance of attachment. Thus, parents with substance misuse disorder who continue to misuse drugs or alcohol following the birth of their child may not be available for the infant. There is, however, experience of mothers who misuse substances being highly motivated during pregnancy and postnatally to reduce and stop their substance misuse in the interests of their child (Pajulo *et al*, 1999). This is in keeping with a commonly expressed desire on the part of parents who have endured adverse experience themselves, 'I want something better for my child than I have had' (Fraiberg *et al*, 1987).

Depression is most commonly identified in the postnatal period but a significant number of women date the onset of their depression to the antenatal period. Depression at this time may have an effect on parental psychological adjustment and preparation for the arrival of the new baby. Pregnancy may be perceived as a dark miserable time and this in turn may affect the parents developing relationship with the unborn child. Parents with depression may also feel guilty about being depressed, recognising the incongruity of their mood with the anticipated joyful event. Here again the risk to the unborn infant is in terms of the potential impact on bonding and attachment (Maldonado-Durán *et al*, 2000).

Schizophrenic and psychotic illnesses are potentially highly disruptive to the psychological aspects of pregnancy and are associated with risks and poor outcome for the child (Bosanac *et al*, 2003). Both pregnancy occurring during the course of an established psychotic illness and new onset of psychosis during the perinatal period may disrupt the attachment process.

Pre-existing anxiety disorders (e.g. generalised anxiety disorder, PTSD, obsessive–compulsive disorder) may be exacerbated during pregnancy and concerns may focus on the well-being and outcome of the baby. It is easy to imagine how mothers and fathers preoccupied by their own anxieties will be unavailable for their infants and thus the attachment relationship is at risk. In acute onset of obsessive–compulsive disorder symptoms during pregnancy or within the first few weeks postpartum, obsessional thoughts are usually about harming the baby. This in turn results in avoidance of situations that evoke the thoughts, which in turn may have implications for family life and attachment (Abramowitz *et al*, 2001).

So far we have considered the impact of treatable mental illness. Many of these illnesses fluctuate and in some cases parents will have periods when they are well, in addition to periods when their mental health deteriorates. Personality disorder in a parent presents different challenges. There is little research evidence to help us in this area but once again the impact during the antenatal period will be on parental conceptualisation of their role as a parent and their ability to manage their pregnancy, and prepare physically and psychologically for the arrival of their child. Postnatally, the risk to

131

the child is in terms of the parents' inability to parent and of impaired attachment relationships (Hobson *et al*, 2005).

Parent–infant relationships

In the preceding section the emphasis has been on the child's relationship with and attachment to the parent and in particular the detrimental effects to the child when this process is compromised. It is also important, however, to explore parent–child relationships from the perspective of the parent and consider what happens when this relationship is disordered. Here again the emphasis is on mother–infant interaction primarily because this has been the focus of research.

The neurobiology of parent–infant relationships and behaviour is being elucidated with studies exploring the neurohormonal and neuroanatomical basis of parents' responses to children (Swain *et al*, 2007). Brockington (1996, 2004) describes the crucial psychological process of the development of the mother's relationship with her infant. He notes that disorders of this process are relatively common and may be extreme with the mother rejecting her child. There are risks of child abuse and neglect and to later child cognitive functioning (Murray *et al*, 1996*b*). Interventions are aimed at helping the mother to enjoy her child.

Risk and resilience

It is important to note that the child is not passive in their relationship with their parent or caregiver. There is an increasing awareness that children's responses to parental mental illness and their outcome vary with some children doing well (Kim-Cohen, 2007). It is also recognised that from birth children have different temperamental styles. This may be important in how the infant responds to adverse factors such as parental mental illness and also in the development of attachment as described above.

The most notable research into infant temperament was undertaken by Thomas *et al* (1968) in the New York Longitudinal Study. They described nine characteristics of infant temperament including: activity level, rhythmicity of biological functions, quality of mood, approach or withdrawal from new experiences, persistence and ease of adaptability. On analysing these characteristics they found that some clustered together and in this way identified three patterns of infant temperament: difficult (biologically irregular, withdraw from new situations, adapt poorly, have negative mood and intense reactions); easy (positive mood, biological regularity, mild intensity, adaptable and react positively to new situations); and slow to warm up (initial withdrawal, slow adaptation and mild intensity). Not surprisingly, infants with the easy temperament had the best outcome and were least likely to develop mental health problems.

From the above it is apparent how infant temperament may compromise developing attachments in the perinatal period. Attachment is a reciprocal process and the infant's response to their parent in turn imparts an effect on the parent's subsequent behaviour. For example, infants who are difficult to soothe and who do not feed or sleep well may undermine parental self-confidence, which in turn affects the way they feel towards the child. In this way, a negative spiral of a deteriorating attachment relationship may develop. It is not uncommon in clinical practice for parents presenting children with emotional and behavioural problems to describe that their child was a 'difficult baby' who did not feed well or settle easily to sleep.

The concept of resilience is increasingly acknowledged as important in child outcome (e.g. O'Connor *et al*, 2000). Although child temperament may be a component of resilience, it is likely that it is more complex than this. Various authors have attempted to operationalise resilience, measuring it in terms of achievement against a range of global markers of outcome (McGloin & Widom, 2001; Daniel, 2006). An awareness of resilience is important in day-to-day clinical practice, a recognition that despite adverse circumstances, such as having a parent with mental illness, some children will do well. Intervention must include an assessment of resilience factors and strategies to promote these as well as treating risk factors.

Child development

Parental mental illness is known to potentially adversely affect child physical, social, emotional, behavioural and cognitive development. In some instances the risks to the physical well-being of the foetus are well recognised, for example substance misuse and domestic violence. Postnatally, infants may be compromised by any mental health problem that impairs a parent's capacity to care for the needs of their child. There is some evidence that compromised or poor interaction between mother and child as in the case of perinatal mental illness is associated with poor physical health outcomes for children (Mantymaa *et al*, 2003). The antenatal and postnatal screening programmes in operation in the UK are designed to alert healthcare professionals to any child at risk both *in utero* and postnatally. Thus, any child who is failing to thrive should be identified and appropriate interventions put in place through child protection and safeguarding processes (Hall & Williams, 2008).

The effects of abuse and various substances of misuse on the developing foetus are well described in the literature and are summarised in Chapter 5. Some of the better known effects include foetal alcohol syndrome and opiate dependency. There may also be immediate effects in the postnatal period with withdrawal symptoms. In addition to the direct physical effects of substance misuse on the foetus, it is important to consider the disruption to the process of pregnancy caused by being addicted. Being addicted diverts attention away from preparing for the arrival of a child. Mothers who misuse substances often neglect themselves and do not attend antenatal care, putting the unborn child at risk. A range of associated environmental and psychosocial factors may also be important or indeed as important to the outcome of the child. For example, recent evidence from systematic reviews has shown that there is no conclusive evidence that prenatal cocaine misuse is associated with adverse developmental outcome that is different from that caused by a variety of environmental factors (Frank *et al*, 2001). Similarly, there is evidence that at 12 months there is no difference in the interaction between cocaine-exposed and non-exposed babies and their mothers (Ukeje *et al*, 2001). There is, however, evidence that cocaine exposure may have different effects on very low-birth-weight infants. Thus, it may be that exposure to substances has differential effects depending on other vulnerability factors (Singer *et al*, 2001). These findings bring us again to the concept of risk and resilience in child outcome.

The effects of maternal stress on the developing foetal brain are described earlier in this chapter. Animal models have demonstrated a link between maternal antenatal stress and later behavioural problems. The effect of excessive maternal stress on the development and functioning of the foetal stress system may in turn have a longer-term effect on aspects of child psychological well-being (Charmandari *et al*, 2003), temperament and behaviour (Wadhwa *et al*, 2001). Talge *et al* (2007) provide a review of the evidence linking antenatal maternal stress and later risk of emotional, behavioural (including ADHD), cognitive and language problems.

Maternal starvation or binging and vomiting as part of an eating disorder can potentially threaten the physical well-being of the developing foetus. The baby may also be at increased risk of being small for gestational age. Postnatally, the mother may have a distorted image/perception of the baby and may worry that it is too fat. This in turn puts the baby at risk of feeding difficulties and failure to thrive (Waugh & Bulik, 1999; Cooper *et al*, 2004). In their review of children of mothers with eating disorders, Park *et al* (2003) explore the effect on feeding in infancy and childhood together with the effects on growth. They describe the lack of systematic controlled studies of mothers with eating disorders and a relative absence of information about the effects of paternal eating problems. Overall, the evidence suggests that children of mothers with eating disorders are at risk of eating problems but that other factors are important in the development of these problems. Eating problems may be present from birth with mothers finding feeding difficult.

The risks posed to children's social, emotional and behavioural development by parental mental illness lie in the effects of illness on a parent's ability to meet their children's emerging developmental needs. Children require different things of their parents at different stages in their development. In the immediate neonatal period the most apparent needs are physical in relation to the child being fed and kept warm and safe. In addition, the parent has a role in responding to the child's emotional state and, for example, soothing the child when they are distressed as a result of being hungry or uncomfortable. The parent has an important role here in helping the child differentiate between different arousal states and this in turn is important in the early development of higher-order executive functions (Kopp, 1982, 1989). Thus, parent–child interaction in infancy is important to the child's later cognitive development. The impact of parental mental illnesss on parent–child interaction cannot be underestimated. Research in this area has focused on the quality of interaction in mothers with depression and schizophrenia (Riordan *et al*, 1999) where mothers are recognised to have difficulties in relating to their infants and to show low responsiveness.

Maternal postnatal depression has been linked with poor infant cognitive outcome. It is likely that the mechanism for this is via impaired mother–infant interaction. Murray *et al* (1996*b*), in a study examining the longer-term influence of postnatal depression on child cognitive function, found that at 5 years of age there was no evidence for adverse effects on child cognitive function. Insensitive mother–child interaction did, however, predict the persistence of poorer cognitive function. Other risk factors may be important in longer-term cognitive outcome, particularly the chronicity of maternal depression, gender (boys are more at risk than girls) and other socio-economic risks (Kurstjens & Wolke, 2001; Grace *et al*, 2003). In general, however, exposure to maternal depression (pre- and postnatally) is a risk factor for child cognitive and language delays (Sohr-Preston & Scaramella, 2006). Evidence suggests that it is chronic and recurrent maternal depression that is important in the longer-term outcome of children.

Child mental health problems

We know that children of parents affected by mental illness are themselves at increased risk of mental health problems. The most likely explanation for this is a complex interaction between a variety of risk conditions (Zeanah *et al*, 1997) including genetic predisposition and environmental influences. There is increasing evidence for a genetic contribution to many of the major psychiatric illnesses seen in adulthood. In this way, being born to a parent with a mental health problem is a risk factor. The potential impact of parental mental illness on attachment and the effect of attachment disorganisation on child psychopathology must also be considered (Green & Goldwyn, 2002). At this stage, however, we do not understand the complexity of the interaction between a child's genetic predisposition and their experience of the environment in which they live regarding mental health problems later in life.

It is important to recognise that not every child whose parent has a mental illness will become mentally ill or present with emotional or behavioural problems. Protective or resiliency factors as discussed above, whether these represent inherent child characteristics, environmental experiences, or both, are important.

135

There is some evidence linking specific parental psychiatric disorders with particular child mental health outcomes. Thus, the most common substance of misuse in pregnancy is nicotine and there is a body of evidence that supports an association between maternal smoking and subsequent child behavioural problems (Wasserman *et al*, 2001). In the early neonatal period there is evidence that babies who were exposed to nicotine *in utero* are more aroused and excitable than non-exposed infants (Law *et al*, 2003). There is some evidence that exposure to alcohol *in utero* contributes to the development of alcohol misuse in later life (Alati *et al*, 2006). In general, it seems children of parents who misuse alcohol are at greater risk of developing alcohol problems. Children of parents with alcohol dependency are at increased risk of behavioural problems but longer-term outcome has been less well studied than the immediate postnatal effects (Johnson & Leff, 1999).

Maternal eating disorder and disturbed eating patterns are associated with child feeding disorders, problems regulating food intake and eating difficulties. There are also effects on growth, with infants of mothers with eating disorders weighing less than controls (Park, *et al*, 2003). It is likely that the development of eating disorders in adolescent girls is influenced by other factors such as sociocultural pressures (Sanftner *et al*, 1996).

Stressful experiences in the later stages of pregnancy have been associated with emotional and behavioural problems in the child (O'Connor *et al*, 2003). Similarly, high levels of maternal antenatal anxiety are associated with higher rates of behavioural and emotional problems in children beyond the immediate perinatal period, highlighting the potential for long-term adverse effects (O'Connor *et al*, 2002).

Both antenatal anxiety and postnatal depression predict child emotional and behavioural problems but do so independently of each other. There may also be an additive effect (O'Connor *et al*, 2002). This might suggest that interventions could usefully be targeted at mothers who have risk factors for anxiety such as domestic violence and previous abuse (Austin, 2004).

Longer term, the risk of psychopathology in children of mothers with depression is recognised but the mechanisms by which this risk is transmitted are unclear (Goodman & Gotlib, 1999). Children are at risk of depression and other mental health problems. Where both parents have depression children are at increased risk of adverse outcome (Burke, 2003). Children of parents who have bipolar disorders are at increased risk of developing bipolar disorders and disruptive behaviour disorders (Singh *et al*, 2007).

Child abuse and neglect

Intimate partner violence during pregnancy can put the foetus at risk as a result of direct physical harm. The continuation of the pregnancy may be compromised and there is a risk of premature labour and delivery (Sharps et al, 2007). Domestic violence is associated with high levels of maternal stress and anxiety that may adversely affect the developing foetus.

The exposure of the infant and child to violence between parents is associated with increased risk of poor mental health and behavioural outcome. Children who have been exposed to domestic violence have higher rates of internalising and externalising disorders including anxiety, depression and PTSD (Kitzmann et al, 2003). In addition, they may be at increased risk of risk-taking behaviour in adolescence (Bair-Merritt et al, 2006). Whitaker et al (2006) have described the cumulative effect of maternal mental health problems, substance misuse and domestic violence on child behaviour problems. Associations between being physically abused as a child, witnessing domestic violence and becoming a perpetrator of domestic violence have been described (Gil-Gonzalez et al, 2008).

Children of parents with mental health problems are at increased risk of abuse and neglect (Sidebotham et al, 2006). Indeed, parental mental health is consistently identified as a risk factor for recurrent maltreatment (Hindley et al, 2006). In this way it is essential that professionals working with parents with mental health problems are alert to the possibilities of child abuse and neglect and are familiar with child protection and safeguarding procedures (Hall & Williams, 2008). An essential component of the management of mental illness during the perinatal period involves considering the capacity of the ill parent to care for their child. In some cases it is obvious that an ill parent will not cope and that it would be unsafe for a child to remain in their care. Ideally, the other parent or another family member such as a grandparent or aunt/uncle will care for the child until the parent is well enough to resume parental responsibilities. Being looked after or accommodated by social services and being fostered by another family are additional risk factors for mental health problems in children and young people (Kerker & Dore, 2006). It is important to remember that having a child put into alternative accommodation is also an adverse risk factor for a parent.

In the majority of cases, parents with mental illness do not set out with the intention of harming their children. Instead, their illness interferes with their ability to provide for the needs of their child. This may manifest as physical or emotional neglect and abuse. Child sexual abuse may also occur in the context of a parental mental illness. Rarely, a parent who is mentally ill may murder their child (Stanton & Simpson, 2006).

Flynn et al (2007) have examined the characteristics of people who kill infants in the context of the National Confidential Inquiry into Suicide and Homicide by People with Mental Illness. Between 1996 and 2001 in England and Wales, 112 people were convicted of infanticide. They found that fathers killed more infants than mothers. At the time of the killing, 24% had a mental illness while 34% had a lifetime history of mental illness and 53% had a history of drug or alcohol misuse; 44% of infants were killed within 3 months of birth and 78% within 6 months. The authors emphasise the need for perinatal assessment and support.

Spinelli (2004) reviews maternal infanticide and highlights the impact of a lack of ICD and DSM categories for postpartum psychiatric disorders in adversely affecting the decisions about treatment and punishment of women who kill their infants in the context of a mental illness. In a further review, Spinelli (2005) addresses the historical, cultural and political views of infanticide.

Paternal mental illness

The bulk of the evidence about the effect of parental mental illness describes the impact of maternal psychopathology. There is relatively little about paternal mental health problems. It is unlikely that paternal mental illness is insignificant in terms of child outcome and our lack of information in this area is simply because, to date, we have tended to focus research interest on mothers. Further research is needed to explore the relationship between paternal psychopathology and child emotional and behavioural outcomes, and to explore the differential effects of maternal and paternal psychopathology (Connell & Goodman, 2002). It is a feature of most cultures that mothers are the primary caregivers of small children. Nevertheless, fathers do have a role and indeed paternal caregiving is being promoted in Western cultures. It is important, therefore, that we consider paternal mental health and the impact of fathers who are mentally ill on children (Currid, 2005). Condon (2006) reviews the psychological adjustment of expectant fathers, their response to having a partner with a mental health problem and the impact of partner relationships and father's mental health on father–infant interaction.

In all aspects of child psychopathology studies, there is a lack of attention to the role fathers play (Phares, 1992; Phares *et al*, 2005). Little attention has been paid to their role in the development and maintenance of child and adolescent psychopathology and also their inclusion in therapeutic work with children. This applies equally to paternal mental illness in the perinatal period.

We do know that, in general, paternal mental illness is important in terms of an association between paternal psychological problems and child externalising problems (Rutter, 1999). Paternal depression in the postnatal period affects children's later emotional and behavioural development (Ramchandani *et al*, 2005).

Phares *et al* (2005) describe that fathers are not included in therapy with children as often as mothers but when they are, there are indirect benefits in terms of retention in treatment, improved interparental relationships and improved long-term outcome.

Adolescents with postnatal mental illness

There is an increased risk of both physical and psychological pregnancy complications in adolescents. Studies have shown rates of postnatal depression of around 50% in adolescents and a similar number admit to consuming alcohol during their pregnancy. Up to 30% will have used marijuana. Additional risk factors include poor housing, nutrition and cognitive and emotional immaturity (Combs-Orme, 1993).

The UK has the highest rate of teenage pregnancy in Europe (Social Exclusion Unit, 1999). Young mothers experience greater levels of the risk factors that we recognise as being associated with poor outcome for both mother and child. In comparison to older mothers, young mothers (less than 20 years of age) are exposed to higher levels of socio-economic deprivation, have more mental health problems and their partners are more unreliable, antisocial and abusive, and less supportive both economically and emotionally (Moffitt *et al*, 2002).

Children of teenage mothers have higher levels of emotional and behavioural problems, poorer educational attainment and are at increased risk of accidents, injuries and illness. However, contrary to the popular perception of teenage pregnancies most teenage parents do care for each other and have known each other for some time (1–4 years) (Barret & Robinson, 1990).

Children of teenage mothers are at increased risk of adverse long-term outcome. In particular, they at risk of early school leaving, unemployment, early parenthood and offending behaviour (Jaffee *et al*, 2001). Social influence and social characteristics both contribute to this risk.

There is less information about adolescent fathers but they also present with increased vulnerability and also represent a risk for the outcome of the child. They are more likely to have experienced adverse family relationships such as parental separation or domestic violence and in this respect may not have a positive role model of parenting on which to draw (Tan & Quinlivan, 2006).

As with teenage mothers, teenage fathers are at risk of increased levels of psychological symptoms including anxiety and depression (Quinlivan & Condon, 2005). Teenage expectant fathers are stressed about the pending birth. Many are concerned about how they are going to support the baby and the mother, finish school and get a job, as well as the well-being of the mother and child. Most want to be involved with their children and where they are involved this is associated with better behavioural and cognitive outcome for the child (Barret & Robinson, 1990).

Thus, having teenage parents represents an added vulnerability for the child with potentially adverse consequences for their shorter- and longer-term outcome. This group is also vulnerable because of the likelihood of suboptimal antenatal and postnatal care. Clinically, this is a group to be vigilant of in ante- and postnatal monitoring for both maternal and child outcome.

Family aspects

When a mother or father has mental health problems there is an impact on family functioning and dynamics. The roles and responsibilities of the ill parent in general and specifically in relation to childcare may have to be taken over to varying degrees by the other parent, other family members, friends or professionals. This is disruptive for all concerned. Burke (2003) has reviewed the effect of maternal depression on family relationships and described that men may become depressed, particularly if their partner had postnatal depression. Also there are increased levels of conflict and discord.

Other family members and friends will also be affected. The other parent will have to take over all parenting responsibilities which in turn may comprise their other roles (e.g. work). There may also be effects on their own mental health because of the worry and stress associated with having an ill partner. Grandparents and siblings also often take on childcare responsibilities and this is associated with negative effects on their own mental health. Grandparents describe the stress of having to look after young children at a time of life when they had not expected to do so. In addition, they may also take on responsibilities for caring for the ill parent (Gopfert *et al*, 2004). Similarly, older children who take on the role of carer for the ill parent as well as assuming childcare responsibilities are a vulnerable group (Aldridge & Becker, 2003). The effect of this on the ill parent must also be recognised. Many describe feeling guilty about the burden they feel they represent to their family and struggle with their loss of role.

Perinatal mental health in gay and lesbian couples

Increasingly, same-gender couples are entering into parenthood although there is little research addressing the perinatal mental health in gay men and lesbians.

Ross (2005) discusses the issues facing lesbians and highlights that many of the challenges associated with moving into parenthood are equally applicable to same-gender couples but that there may be additional vulnerabilities such as lack of the usual social and familial supports compounded by the negative impact of discrimination.

Intervention

The primary focus for treatment in perinatal mental illness is the ill parent. The natural assumption is that if the parent's mental illness is treated and they recover then the effects on the child will be minimised or at least by treating the parent the risk to the child is removed or lessened. The aim must be to restore the parent to normal day-to-day functioning which will then facilitate their parenting. Increasingly, it is recognised that it is important to consider the outcome of the child in their own right and that the specific needs of the child must be included in any treatment plan. Some interventions have been developed with the aim of promoting positive child outcome; however, there continues to be a paucity of evidence about the effect of routine treatment in terms of child outcome.

There are challenges in the definition and measurement of child outcome in the immediate perinatal period. In the longer term, child outcome can be described by examining social, emotional and behavioural adjustment as well as cognitive function.

Assessment

The recognition of the potentially detrimental effect on child outcome of parental perinatal mental illness suggests a role for early identification and intervention. This in turn requires mechanisms for screening in the perinatal period. There are well-established mechanisms for identifying postnatal depression, such as the EPDS (Cox & Holden, 2003), but probably less robust mechanisms for screening for other mental health problems particularly in the antenatal period. Severe mental illness will in most cases be immediately apparent but still children will be at risk if because of their illness parents do not take up available ante- and postnatal care.

It is important that all staff involved in delivering perinatal services are aware of the range of parental mental health problems and the risk/ vulnerability factors for children. In this way, infants who are potentially at risk of adverse outcome can be identified antenatally and appropriate measures put in place to monitor their well-being.

The measurement of child outcome in the early neonatal period is complicated and is often described in terms of physical parameters such as birth weight and the achievement of milestones. It is clear that a key outcome is the quality of parent–child interaction. Aspects of the attachment relationship can be measured in a number of ways, including self-report, for example the Parenting Stress Index (Abidin, 1986), and observation, for example the Parent–Child Early Relational Assessment (Clark, 1985) and the HOME (Home Observation for the Measurement of the Environment) inventory (Caldwell & Bradley, 1978).

Although measures such as those described above will provide detailed information about parent–child relationships, they are primarily research tools and are difficult to employ in routine day-to-day practice because of the need for training and the time taken to administer and score measures. Self-report measures have limitations in terms of objectivity. The development of clinically appropriate assessment tools that can be used by a range of professionals should be a focus for further work.

In the longer term, a range of outcome measures can be considered including those that examine child cognitive development (e.g. Bayley Infant Development Scales; Bayley, 1993). As children get older, their social, emotional and behavioural adjustment can be assessed by means of parent and nursery teacher self-report scales such as the Strengths and Difficulties Questionnaire (Goodman, 1997).

It is recognised that social, emotional and behavioural problems may present early in life and that if left untreated may have significant implications for long-term prognosis. There is, however, a lack of reliable, clinically useful tools with which to assess mental health problems in infancy and early childhood. This represents a challenge for the emerging specialty of infant mental health (DelCarmen-Wiggins & Carter, 2004).

Treatment

The treatment of the range of perinatal mental illnesses is described throughout this book. The evidence base describing the effect of treatment on child outcome both in the short and longer term is limited. Most of the information available describes the effect of treatment for postnatal depression.

The detail of the various pharmacological interventions for adult mental illness will not be reviewed here as this material is discussed throughout the various chapters of this book. However, the basic principles of pharmacological management in relation to child outcome are illustrated by the case for the pharmacological treatment of perinatal maternal depression. The aim of treatment is to relieve maternal suffering and avoid adverse neurobehavioural outcomes for the child. There is evidence that treatment with SSRIs throughout pregnancy is not associated with any adverse effect on child cognitive and language development or temperament in the pre-school period. Maternal depression is, however, associated with a detrimental effect on child language and cognitive development. The implication, therefore, is that SSRI treatment for depression should be continued throughout pregnancy and in the postnatal period as this is in the best interest of the mother and her child (Nulman *et al*, 2002).

The key consideration in the use of pharmacological agents in relation to child outcome is in terms of potential effects on the foetus and the newborn infant. The psychological aspects of pharmacotherapy for the mother (parents) must also be considered. Parental concerns about the use of medication in relation to their unborn child must be addressed. Parents often raise concerns in the context of a child and adolescent mental health assessment that their child's difficulties may be the result of something they did or a medication they took during pregnancy.

The evidence presented in this chapter suggests that in addition to treating the parent, another potentially useful intervention would be to address parent–child interaction. A range of interventions are used including baby massage and interaction coaching. The use of unqualified staff in delivering such interventions has been explored with some evidence for effectiveness in some domains of functioning (Cooper *et al*, 2002).

There are a range of models of parent–child psychotherapy which can be generalised to parents with mental illness, although most of the evidence for effectiveness relates to evaluations of specific programmes. There is little information available from systematic reviews or RCTs specifically in relation to the use of such interventions in perinatal mental illness.

Parent management training is fashionable at present, with parenting interventions being recommended to address a range of problems. In particular, parent management training has been shown to improve outcome for young children with disruptive behavioural problems (Barlow & Parsons, 2003). There is some evidence that such programmes are also beneficial to maternal psychosocial health (anxiety, depression, self-esteem), although more research is needed in this area (Barlow & Coren, 2004). Parent management training may be useful in supporting parents with mental illness but the generic programmes that are widely available are unlikely to be appropriate and will require modification to meet the specific needs of parents who are mentally ill (Craig, 2004). Residential treatment programmes for expectant mothers misusing substances have been shown to improve the physical outcome of babies in terms of birth weight and length (Little *et al*, 2003). The incorporation of attachment-based parenting interventions into such programmes may improve their effectiveness in terms of parent–child relationships (Suchman *et al*, 2004).

There has been considerable interest in the use of large-scale intensive home-visiting programmes in the promotion of the well-being of children born into adverse circumstances. The majority have included a component of parent training. There is some evidence of positive benefit in terms of maternal mental health and mother–child interaction (Beeber *et al*, 2004). A number of projects have also explored the use of volunteer home visitors (Taggart *et al*, 2000). In this way, home-based intervention programmes may provide large-scale indirect support of parental (especially maternal) mental health.

In addition to the more generic parent training interventions, some programmes specifically address parent–infant interaction, for example 'Minding the Baby' (Slade *et al*, 2005) and 'Watching, Waiting and Wondering' (Muir, 1992). Such interventions aim to work with parents to develop their reflective capacities so that they are able to observe and reflect on their infant's emotional life and follow their lead. Video-feedback of mother–infant interaction with mothers with bulimia has been demonstrated in a controlled trial to improve interaction (Stein *et al*, 2006). Underdown *et al* (2006) found that there was some benefit of baby massage in respect of mother–infant interaction. Therapies targeting mother–child interaction in postnatal depression have been shown to improve relationships (Poobalan *et al*, 2007).

In extreme cases it may not be safe for a child to remain with a parent with severe mental health problems. It is, therefore, essential that multidisciplinary staff working with parents with mental health problems are aware of their responsibilities in terms of child protection. Parents with mental health problems are often aware of the effect of their illness on their parenting and are concerned about this, often feeling guilty and that they are failing their children. This is particularly so when a child is removed and taken into the care of social services or when a parent is hospitalised. Evidence suggests that even when separated, parenting remains important and mothers describe their efforts to maintain meaningful relationships with their children (Savvidou *et al*, 2003; Montgomery *et al*, 2006). The aim is always to rehabilitate the parent and child and in doing this close attention must be paid to addressing the parent's feelings of guilt.

It is clear that perinatal mental illness is complex and has the potential to adversely affect parents and children across multiple domains of functioning. This in turn suggests the need for a multidisciplinary approach to management. However, there are few specialist multidisciplinary services and little comparative evaluation data describing their effectiveness. In day-to-day clinical practice it is important that child mental health services develop close working relationships with their colleagues in adult mental health such that collaborative working can take place where parents are affected by mental health problems. It is estimated that 15–30% of adult mental health patients are parents and we have read earlier in this text that 13% of mothers experience perinatal mental illness. It is remarkable, therefore, that so little joint working takes place routinely. Many adult mental health services do not routinely or reliably collect information about dependent children (Creswell & Brereton, 2000).

Conclusion

It is apparent that perinatal mental illness has implications for the immediate and longer-term well-being of the child. A range of factors influence this and at this stage in our understanding it is difficult to predict outcome for individual children. Why do some children whose parents have mental illness do well and others not? Further work is needed to characterise risk and resilience factors for the child, their parents and the environment. Such information will inform the development and refining of interventions as well as informing us about the most appropriate ways to target preventive interventions.

Much of the evidence available to us focuses on the immediate impact of perinatal mental illness. Some perinatal mental health problems are short term but in many cases they represent more enduring psychopathology. The effects of this on the infant beyond the perinatal period must be considered in terms of the risk to the child's development and general well-being. Equally, a child who is exposed to perinatal mental illness and whose early development is thereby compromised may be exposed to positive experiences later on which may have a self-righting effect.

Children are always part of complex systems the most immediate of which is their family. Parental mental illness affects everyone who is part of that system (grandparents, siblings, partners) and their reaction will in turn have an impact on that system and the child. An awareness of these systemic influences is important in the development and delivery of perinatal mental health interventions and for all practitioners who work with children and families.

The information presented here demonstrates that perinatal mental illness does potentially adversely affect the well-being of the foetus and infant. Therefore, the outcome of the unborn infant is an important consideration in the management of parental mental illness. There is, however, only limited information about the effectiveness of interventions in perinatal mental illness in terms of child outcome. Intervention is complex, requiring the knowledge and skills of both child and adult mental health practitioners. Despite our increasing awareness of the implications of parental mental health for child outcome there is a paucity of collaborative work between child and adult practitioners in the delivery of perinatal and indeed all mental health interventions. Specialist services for families affected by mental illness in the perintatal period are limited. There is a need for closer working between generic child and adult mental health specialists in the day-to-day management of the range of perinatal mental illness and for there to be further evaluation of the effectiveness of interventions both in the short and long term. Work to identify effective models of service delivery incorporating liaison between child and adult mental health services must be a priority.

References

Abidin, R. R. (1986) *Parenting Stress Index Manual* (2nd edn). Pediatric Psychology Press.

Abramowitz, J. A., Moore, K., Carmin, C., *et al* (2001) Acute onset of obsessive–compulsive disorder in males following childbirth. *Psychosomatics*, **42**, 429–431.

Ainsworth, M. D. S. (1963) The development of infant–mother interaction among the Ganda. In *Determinants of Infant Behaviour* (Volume 2) (ed. B.M. Foss), pp. 67–112. Methuen.

Ainsworth, M. D. S. & Wittig, B. A. (1969) Attachment and exploratory behaviour of one-year-olds in a strange situation. In *Determinants of Infant Behaviour* (Volume 2) (ed. B. M. Foss), pp. 111–136. Methuen.

Alati, R., Al Mamun, A. & Williams, G. M. (2006) *In utero* alcohol exposure and prediction of alcohol disorders in early adulthood: a birth cohort study. *Archives of General Psychiatry*, **63**, 1009–1016.

Alder, J., Fink, N., Bitzer, J., *et al* (2007) Depression and anxiety during pregnancy: a risk factor for obstetric, fetal and neonatal outcome? A critical review of the literature. *The Journal of Maternal–Fetal & Neonatal Medicine*, **20**, 189–209.

Aldridge, A. & Becker, S. (2003) *Children Caring for Parents with Mental Illness. Perspectives of Young Carers, Parents and Professionals*. Policy Press.

Alhusen, J. L. (2008) A literature update on maternal fetal attachment. *Journal of Obstetric, Gynecologic and Neonatal Nursing*, **37**, 315–328.

American Psychiatric Association (1994) *Diagnostic and Statistical Manual of Mental Disorders (4th edn) (DSM–IV)*. APA.

Armstrong, D. S. (2002) Emotional distress and prenatal attachment in pregnancy after perinatal loss. *Journal of Nursing Scholarship*, **34**, 339–345.

Austin, M. P. (2004) Antenatal screening and early intervention for 'perinatal' distress, depression and anxiety: where to from here? *Archives of Women's Mental Health*, **7**, 1–6.

Bair-Merritt, M. H., Blackstone, M. & Feudtner, C. (2006) Physical health outcomes of childhood exposure to intimate partner violence: a systematic review. *Pediatrics*, **117**, e278–e290.

Barlow, J. & Coren, E. (2004) Parent-training programmes for improving maternal psychosocial health. *Cochrane Database Systematic Review*, **1**, CD002020.

Barlow, J. & Parsons J. (2003) Group-based parent-training programmes for improving emotional and behavioural adjustment in 0–3 year old children. *Cochrane Database of Systematic Reviews*, **2**, CD003680.

Barret, R. L. & Robinson, B. E. (1990) The role of adolescent father in parenting and childrearing. *Advances in Adolescent Mental Health*, **4**, 189–200.

Bayley, N. (1993) *Bayley Scales of Infant Development* (2nd edn). Psychological Corporation.

Beeber, L. S., Holdithch-Davis, D., Belyea, M. J. et al (2004) In-home intervention for depressive symptoms with low-income mothers of infants and toddlers in the United States. *Health Care Women International*, **25**, 561–580.

Bosanac, P., Buist, A. & Burrows, G. (2003) Motherhood and schizophrenic illnesses: a review of the literature. *Australian and New Zealand Journal of Psychiatry*, **37**, 24–30.

Bowlby, J. (1958) The nature of the child's tie to his mother. *International Journal of Psychoanalysis*, **39**, 350–373.

Bowlby, J. (1982) *Attachment* (Volume 1, 2nd edn). Basic Books.

Boy, A. & Salihu, H. M. (2004) Intimate partner violence and birth outcomes: a systematic review. *International Journal of Fertility and Women's Medicine*, **49**, 159–164.

Breen, D. (1975) *The Birth of a First Child*. Tavistock.

Brockington, I. F. (1996) *Motherhood and Mental Health*. Oxford University Press.

Brockington, I. F. (2004) Postpartum psychiatric disorders. *Lancet*, **363**, 303.

Brockington, I. F., Aucamp, H. M. & Fraser, C. (2006) Severe disorders of mother–infant relationship: definitions and frequency. *Archives of Women's Mental Health*, **9**, 243–251.

Burke, L. (2003) The impact of maternal depression on familial relationships. *International Review of Psychiatry*, **B15**, 243–255.

Caldwell, B. M. & Bradley, R. H. (1978) *Manual for the Home Observation for Measurement of the Environment*. University of Arkansas.

Carter, A. S., Briggs-Gowna, M. J. & Ornstein Davis, N. (2004) Assessment of young children's social-emotional development and psychopathology: recent advances and recommendations for practice. *Journal of Child Psychology and Psychiatry*, **45**, 109–134.

Chambliss, L. R. (2008) Intimate partner violence and its implications for pregnancy. *Clinical Obstetrics and Gynecology*, **51**, 385–397.

Charmandari, E., Kino, T., Souvatzoglou, E., et al (2003) Pediatric stress: hormonal mediators and human development. *Hormone Research*, **59**, 161–179.

Chiriboga, C. A. (2003) Fetal alcohol and drug effects. *Neurologist*, **9**, 267–279.

Clark, R. (1985) *The Parent–Child Early Relational Assessment. Instrument and Manual*. Department of Psychiatry, University of Wisconsin Medical School.

Combs-Orme T. (1993) Effects of adolescent pregnancy: implications for social workers. *Family Society*, **74**, 344–354.

Condon, J. (2006) What about dad? Psychosocial and mental health issues for new fathers. *Australian Family Physician*, **35**, 690–692.

Condon, J. T (1986) The spectrum of fetal abuse in pregnant women. *Journal of Nervous and Mental Disease*, **174**, 509–516.

Connell, A. M. Goodman, S. H. (2002) The association between psychopathology in fathers versus mothers and in children's internalizing behaviour problems: a meta-analysis. *Psychological Bulletin*, **128**, 746–73.

Cooper, P. J., Landman, M., Tomlinson, M., et al (2002) Impact of a mother–infant intervention in an indigent peri-urban South African context: pilot study. *British Journal of Psychiatry*, **180**, 76–81.

Cooper, P. J., Whelan, E., Woolgar, M. *et al* (2004) Association between childhood feeding problems and maternal eating disorder: role of the family and environment. *British Journal of Psychiatry*, **184**, 210–215.

Cote-Arsenault, D. (2003) The influence of perinatal loss on anxiety in multigravidas. *Journal of Obstetric and Gynecological Neonatal Nursing*, **32**, 623–629.

Cox, J. & Holden, J. (2003) *Perinatal Mental Health: A Guide to the Edinburgh Postnatal Depression Scale*. Gaskell Press.

Craig, E. A. (2004) Parenting programmes for women with mental illness who have young children: a review. *Australian and New Zealand Journal of Psychiatry*, **38**, 923–928.

Creswell, C. & Brereton, J. (2000) Community mental health services and the children of service users. *Clinical Psychology Forum*, **144**, 4–6.

Currid, T. J. (2005) Psychological issues surrounding paternal perinatal mental health. *Nursing Times*, **101**, 40–42.

Daniel, B. (2006) Operationalizing the concept of resilience in child neglect: case study research. *Child Care Health Development*, **32**, 303–309.

Dayan, J., Creveuil, C., Marks, M. N., *et al* (2006) Prenatal depression, prenatal anxiety, and spontaneous preterm birth: a prospective cohort study among women with early and regular care. *Psychosomatic Medicine*, **68**, 938–946.

DelCarmen-Wiggins, R. & Carter, A. (eds) (2004) *Handbook of Infant, Toddler and Preschool Mental Health Assessment*. Oxford University Press.

Deutsch, H. (1947) *Psychology of Women: Volume 2 – Motherhood*. Research Books.

DiPietro, J. A. (2005) Neurobehavioural assessment before birth. *Mental Retardation and Developmental Disabilities Research Reviews*, **11**, 4–13.

DiPietro, J. A., Hilton, S. C., Hawkins, M., *et al* (2002) Maternal stress and affect influence fetal neurobehavioural development. *Developmental Psychology*, **38**, 659–668.

DiPietro, J. A., Hodgson, D. M., Costigan, K. A., *et al* (1996) Fetal antecedents of infant temperament. *Child Development*, **67**, 2568–2583.

Federenko, I. S. & Wadhwa, P. D. (2004) Women's mental health during pregnancy influences fetal and infant developmental and health outcomes. *CNS Spectrums*, **9**, 198–206.

Flynn, S. M., Shaw, J. J. & Abel, K. M. (2007) Homicide of infants: a cross-sectional study. *Journal of Clinical Psychiatry*, **68**, 1501–1509.

Fraiberg, S., Adelson, E. & Shapiro, V. (1987) Ghosts in the nursery: a psychoanalytic approach to the problems of impaired infant–mother relationships. In *Selected Writings of Selma Fraiberg* (ed. L. Fraiberg), pp. 100–136. Ohio State University Press.

Frank, D. A., Augustyn, M., Knight, W. G., *et al* (2001) Growth, development, and behavior in early childhood following prenatal cocaine exposure: a systematic review. *JAMA*, **285**, 1613–1625.

Freud, A. (1963) The concept of developmental lines. *Psychoanalytic Study of the Child*, **18**, 245–265.

Freud, A. (1970) The concept of the rejecting mother. In *Parenthood: Its Psychology and Psychopathology* (eds E. J. Anthony & T. Benedek), pp. 376–409. Little, Brown.

Friedman, S. H., Heneghan, A. & Rosenthal, M. (2007) Characteristics of women who deny or conceal pregnancy. *Psychosomatics*, **48**, 117–122.

Gil-Gonzalez, D., Vives-Cases, C., Ruiz, M. T., *et al* (2008) Childhood experiences of violence in perpetrators as a risk factor for intimate partner violence: a systematic review. *Journal of Public Health*, **30**, 14–22.

Goodman, R. (1997) The Strengths and Difficulties Questionnaire: a research note. *Journal of Child Psychology and Psychiatry*, **38**, 581–586.

Goodman, S. H. & Gotlib, H. H. (1999) Risk for psychopathology in the children of depressed mothers: a developmental model for understanding mechanisms of transmission. *Psychological Review*, **106**, 458–90.

Gopfert, M. V., Webster, M. & Seeman, M. V. (eds) (2004) *Parental Psychiatric Disorder: Distressed Parents and Their Families*. Cambridge University Press.

Grace, S. L., Evindar, A. & Stewart, D. E. (2003) The effect of postpartum depression on child cognitive development and behaviour: a review and critical analysis of the literature. *Archives of Women's Mental Health*, **6**, 263–274.

Green, J. & Goldwyn, R. (2002) Annotation: attachment disorganization and psychopathology: new findings in attachment research and their potential implications for developmental psychopathology in childhood. *Journal of Child Psychology and Psychiatry*, **43**, 835–846.

Hall, D. & Williams, J. (2008) Safeguarding, child protection and mental health. *Archives of Diseases in Childhood*, **93**, 11–13.

Hindley, N., Rachmandani, P. G. & Jones, D. P. H. (2006) Risk factors for recurrence of maltreatment: a systematic review. *Archives of Diseases in Childhood*, **91**, 744–752.

Hobson, R. P., Patrick, M., Crandell, L., *et al* (2005) Personal relatedness and attachment in infants and mothers with borderline personality disorder. *Developmental Psychopathology*, **17**, 329–347.

Hollins, K. (2007) Consequences of antenatal mental health problems for child health development. *Current Opinion in Obstetrics and Gynecology*, **19**, 568–572.

Jablensky, A. V., Morgan, V., Zubrick, S. R., *et al* (2005) Pregnancy, delivery, and neonatal complications in a population of women with schizophrenia and major affective disorders. *American Journal of Psychiatry*, **162**, 79–91.

Jaffee, S., Caspi, A., Moffitt, T. E., *et al* (2001) Why are children born to teenage mothers at risk of adverse outcomes in young adulthood? Results from a 20 year longitudinal study. *Developmental Psychopathology*, **13**, 377–397.

Johnson, J. J. & Leff, M. (1999) Children of substance abusers; overview of research findings. *Pediatrics*, **103**, 1085–1099.

Kapoor, A., Dunn, E., Kostaki, A. *et al* (2006) Fetal programming of hypothalamo–pituitary–adrenal function: prenatal stress and glucocorticoids. *Journal of Physiology*, **572**, 31–44.

Kent, L., Laidlaw, J. D. & Brockington, I. F. (1997) Fetal abuse. *Child Abuse and Neglect*, **21**, 181–186.

Kerker, B. D. & Dore, M. M. (2006) Mental health needs and treatment of foster youth: barriers and opportunities. *American Journal of Orthopsychiatry*, **76**, 138–147.

Kim-Cohen, J. (2007) Resilience and developmental psychopathology. *Child and Adolescent Psychiatric Clinics of North America*, **16**, 271–283.

Kisilevsky, B. S., Hains, S. M., Lee, K., *et al* (2003) Effects of experience on fetal voice recognition. *Psychological Science*, **14**, 220–224.

Kitzmann, K. M., Gaylord, N. K., Holt, A. R., *et al* (2003) Child witness to domestic violence: a meta-analytic review. *Journal of Consulting and Clinical Psychology*, **71**, 339–352.

Knackstedt, M. K., Hamelmann, E. & Arck, P. C. (2005) Mothers in stress: consequence for offspring. *American Journal of Reproductive Immunology*, **54**, 63–69.

Kopp, C. B. (1982) Antecedents of self-regulation: a developmental perspective. *Developmental Psychology*, **18**, 199–214.

Kopp, C. B. (1989) Regulation of distress and negative emotions: a developmental view. *Developmental Psychology*, **25**, 343–354.

Korenman, S., Kaestner, R. & Joyce, T. (2002) Consequences of infants of parental disagreement in pregnancy intention. *Perspectives of Sexual and Reproductive Health*, **34**, 198–205.

Kurjak, A., Andonotopo, W., Hafner, T., *et al* (2006) Normal standards for fetal neurobehavioural developments: longitudinal quantification by four dimensional sonography. *Journal of Perinatal Medicine*, **34**, 56–65.

Kurstjens, S. & Wolke, D. (2001) Effects of maternal depression on cognitive development of children over the first seven years of life. *Journal of Child Psychology and Psychiatry*, **42**, 623–636.

Lamb, M. E. (1976) Interactions between eight-month-old children and their fathers and mothers. In *The Role of the Father in Child Development* (ed. M. E. Lamb), pp. 307–327. John Wiley.

Law, K. L., Stroud, L. R., LaGasse, L. L., et al (2003) Smoking during pregnancy and newborn neurobehaviour. *Pediatrics*, **111**, 1318–1323.

Lecanuet, J. P. & Schaal, B. (1996) Fetal sensory competencies. *European Journal of Obstetrics, Gynecology and Reproductive Biology*, **68**, 1–23.

Lee, S. J., Ralston, H. J., Drey, E. A. et al (2005) Fetal pain: a systematic multidisciplinary review of the evidence. *JAMA*, **294**, 947–954.

Lickliter, R. (2000) Atypical perinatal sensory stimulation and early perceptual development: insights from developmental psychopathology. *Journal of Perinatology*, **28**, 45–54.

Little, B. B., Snell, L. M., Van Beveren, T. T., et al (2003) Treatment of substance abuse during pregnancy and infant outcome. *American Journal of Perinatology*, **20**, 255–262.

Lowery C. L., Hardman, M. P., Manning, N., et al, (2007) Neurodevelopmental changes of fetal pain. *Seminars in Perinatology*, **31**, 275–282.

Main, M. (1996) Introduction to the special section on attachment and psychopathology: 2 Overview of the filed of attachment. *Journal of Consulting and Clinical Psychology*, **64**, 237–243.

Main, M. & Solomon, J. (1986) Discovery of an insecure-disorganized/disoriented attachment pattern. In *Affective Development in Infancy* (eds T. B. Brazelton & M. Yogman). Ablex.

Maldonado-Durán, J., Lartigue, T. & Feintuch, M. (2000) Perinatal psychiatry: infant mental health interventions during pregnancy. *Bulletin of the Menninger Clinic*, **64**, 317–340.

Mantymaa, M., Puura, K., Luoma, I., et al (2003) Infant–mother interaction as a predictor of child's chronic health problems. *Child Care Health and Development*, **29**, 181–191.

McGloin, J. M. & Widom, C. S. (2001) Resilience among abused and neglected children grown up. *Developmental Psychopathology*, **13**, 1021–1038.

Mennella, J. A., Jagnow, C. P. & Beauchamp, G. K. (2001) Prenatal and postnatal flavour learning by human infants. *Pediatrics*, **107**, E88.

Moffitt, T. E. & the E-Risk study team (2002) Teen-aged mothers in contemporary Britain. *Journal of Child Psychology and Psychiatry*, **43**, 727–742.

Mohllajee, A. P., Curtis, K. M., Morrow, B., et al (2007) Pregnancy intention and its relationship to birth and maternal outcomes. *Obstetrics and Gynecology*, **109**, 678–686.

Montgomery, P., Tompkins, C., Forhuk, C., et al (2006) Keeping close: mothering with serious mental illness. *Journal of Advanced Nursing*, **54**, 20–28.

Morrill, E. S. & Nickols-Richardson, H. M. (2001) Bulimia nervosa during pregnancy: a review. *Journal of the American Dietetics Association*, **101**, 448–454.

Muir, M. (1992) Watching, waiting and wondering: applying psychoanalytic principles to mother–infant intervention. *Infant Mental Health Journal*, **13**, 319–328.

Murray, L., Fiori-Cowley, A. & Hooper, R. (1996a) The impact of postnatal depression and associated adversity on early mother–infant interactions and later infant outcome. *Child Development*, **67**, 2512–2526.

Murray, L., Hipwell, A. & Hooper, R. (1996b) The cognitive development of 5-year old children of postnatally depressed mothers. *Journal of Child Psychology and Psychiatry*, **37**, 927–935.

Nirmal, D., Thijs, I., Bethel, J., et al (2006) The incidence and outcome of concealed pregnancy among hospital deliveries in an 11 year population-based study in South Glamorgan. *Journal of Obstetrics and Gynaecology*, **26**, 118–121.

Nulman, I., Rovet, J., Stewart, D. E., et al (2002) Child development following exposure to tricyclic antidepressants or fluoxetine throughout fetal life: a prospective, controlled study. *American Journal of Psychiatry*, **159**, 1889–1895.

O'Connor, T. G. & Rutter, M. (2000) Attachment disorder behaviour following early severe deprivation: extension and longitudinal follow-up. English and Romanian Adoptees Study Team. *Journal of the American Academy of Child and Adolescent Psychiatry*, **39**, 703–712.

O'Connor, T. G., Rutter, M., Beckett, C., et al (2000) The effects of global severe privation on cognitive competence: extension and longitudinal follow-up. English and Romanian Adoptees Study Team. *Child Development*, **71**, 376–390.

O'Connor, T. G., Heron, J., Glover, V., *et al* (2002) Antenatal anxiety predicts child behavioural/emotional problems independently of postnatal depression. *Journal of the American Academy of Child and Adolescent Psychiatry*, **41**, 1470–1477.

O'Connor, T. G., Heron, J., Golding, J., *et al* (2003) Maternal antenatal anxiety and behavioural/emotional problems in children: a test of a programming hypothesis. *Journal of Child Psychology & Psychiatry*, **44**, 1025–1036.

Pajulo, M., Savonlathi, E. & Piha, J. (1999) Maternal substance abuse: Infant psychiatric interest: a review and hypothetical model of interaction. *American Journal of Drug and Alcohol Abuse*, **25**, 761–769.

Pallitto, C. C., Campbell, J. C. & O'Campo, P. (2005) Is intimate partner violence associated with unintended pregnancy? A review of the literature. *Trauma Violence and Abuse*, **6**, 217–35.

Park, R. J., Senior, R. & Stein, A. (2003) The offspring of mothers with eating disorders. *European Child and Adolescent Psychiatry*, **12(Suppl. 1)**, 110–119.

Phares, V. (1992) Where's poppa? The relative lack of attention to the role of fathers in child and adolescent psychopathology. *American Psychologist*, **47**, 656–674.

Phares, V., Fields, S., Kamboukos, D., *et al* (2005) Still looking for poppa: the continued lack of attention to the role of fathers in developmental psychopathology. *American Psychologist*, **60**, 735–736.

Pollock, P. H. & Percy, A. (1999). Maternal antenatal attachment style and potential abuse. *Child Abuse and Neglect*, **23**, 1345–1357.

Poobalan, A. S., Aucott, L. S., Ross, L., *et al* (2007) Effects of treating postnatal depression on mother–infant interaction and child development: systematic review. *British Journal of Psychiatry*, **191**, 378–386.

Quinlivan, J. A. & Condon, J. (2005) Anxiety and depression in fathers in teenage pregnancy. *Australian and New Zealand Journal of Psychiatry*, **39**, 915–920.

Ramchandani, P., Stein, A., Evans, J., *et al* (2005) Paternal depression in the postnatal period and child development: a prospective population study. *Lancet*, **365**, 2201–2205.

Raphael-Leff, J. (1985) Facilitators and regulators; vulnerability to postnatal disturbance. *Journal of Psychosomatic Obstetrics and Gynaecology*, **4**, 151–168.

Riordan, D., Appleby, L. & Faragher, B. (1999) Mother–infant interaction in post-partum women with schizophrenia and affective disorders. *Psychological Medicine*, **29**, 991–995.

Ross, L. E. (2005) Perinatal mental health in lesbian mothers: a review of potential risk and protective factors. *Women Health*, **41**, 113–128.

Rustico, M. A., Mastromatteo, C., Grigio, M., *et al* (2005) Two-dimensional *v.* two-plus four-dimensional ultrasound in pregnancy and the effect on maternal emotional status: a randomized study. *Ultrasound Obstetrics and Gynecology*, **25**, 468–472.

Rutter, M. (1999) Resilience concepts and findings: implications for family therapy. *Journal of Family Therapy*, **21**, 119–144.

Rutter, M., O'Connor, T. G. & The English and Romanian Adoptees (ERA) Study Team (2004) Are there biological programming effects for psychological development? Findings from a study of Romanian adoptees. *Developmental Psychology*, **40**, 81–94.

Sable, M. R. & Wilkinson, D. S. (2000) Impact of perceived stress, major life events and pregnancy attitudes on low birth weight. *Family Planning Perspectives*, **32**, 288–294.

Sanftner, J. L., Crowther, J. H., Crawford, P. A., *et al* (1996) Maternal influences (or lack thereof) on daughters' eating attitudes and behaviours. *Eating Disorders*, **4**, 147–159.

Savvidou, I., Bozikas, V. P., Hatzigeleki, S. *et al*, (2003) Narratives about their children by mothers hospitalized on a psychiatric unit. *Family Process*, **42**, 391–402.

Sears, R. R. (1943) *Survey of Objective Studies of Psychoanalytic Concepts*. Social Science Research Council.

Sedgman, B., McMahon, C., Cairns, D., *et al* (2006) The impact of two-dimensional versus three dimensional ultrasound exposure on maternal–fetal attachment and maternal health behaviour. *Ultrasound Obstetrics and Gynecology*, **27**, 245–251.

Sharps, P. W., Laughon, K. & Giangrande, S. K. (2007) Intimate partner violence and the childbearing year: maternal and infant health consequences. *Trauma Violence and Abuse*, **8**, 105–116.

Sidebotham, P., Heron, J. & ALSPAC Study Team, (2006) Child maltreatment in the 'children of the nineties': a cohort study of risk factors. *Child Abuse and Neglect*, **30**, 497–552.

Singer, L. T., Hawkins, S., Huang, J., *et al* (2001) Developmental outcomes and environmental correlates of very low birthweight, cocaine-exposed infants. *Early Human Development*, **64**, 91–103.

Singh, M. K., DelBello, M. P., Stanford, K. E., *et al* (2007) Psychopathology in children of bipolar patients. *Journal of Affective Disorders*, **102**, 131–136.

Slade, A., Sadler, L., De Dios-Kenn, C., *et al* (2005) Minding the Baby: a reflective parenting programme. *Psychoanalytic Study of the Child*, **60**, 74–100.

Social Exclusion Unit (1999) *Teenage Pregnancy: Report by the Social Exclusion Unit*. TSO (The Stationery Office).

Sohr-Preston, S. L. & Scaramella, L. V. (2006) Implications of timing of maternal depressive symptoms for early cognitive and language development. *Clinical Child and Family Psychology Review*, **9**, 65–83.

Spinelli, M. G. (2004) Maternal infanticide associated with mental illness: Prevention and the promise of saved lives. *American Journal of Psychiatry*, **161**, 1548–1557.

Spinelli, M. G. (2005) Infanticide: contrasting views. *Archives of Women's Mental Health*, **8**, 15–24.

Stanton, J. & Simpson, A. L. (2006) The aftermath: aspects of recovery described by perpetrators of maternal filicide committed in the context of severe mental illness. *Behavioural Sciences and the Law*, **24**, 103–112.

Stein, A., Woolley, H., Senior, R., *et al*, (2006) Treating disturbances in the relationship between mothers with bulimic eating disorders and their infants: a randomized, controlled trail of video feedback. *American Journal of Psychiatry*, **163**, 899–906.

Stern D. (2002) *The First Relationship: Mother and Infant*. Harvard University Press.

Stern, N. B. (1999) Motherhood: the emotional awakening. *Journal of Pediatric Healthcare*, **13**, S8–S12.

Suchman, N., Mayes, L. & Conti, J. (2004) Rethinking parenting interventions for drug dependent mothers: from behaviour management to fostering emotional bonds. *Journal of Substance Abuse Treatment*, **29**, 179–185.

Swain, J. E., Lorberbaum, J. P., Kose, S., *et al* (2007) Brain basis of early parent–infant interactions; psychology, physiology, and *in vivo* functional neuroimaging studies. *Journal of Child Psychology and Psychiatry*, **48**, 262–287.

Taggart, A. V., Short, S. D. & Barclay, L. (2000) 'She has made me feel human again': an evaluation of a volunteer home-based visiting project for mothers. *Health and Social Care in the Community*, **8**, 1–8.

Talge, N. M., Neal, C., Glover, V., *et al* (2007) Antenatal maternal stress and long-term effects on child neurodevelopment: how and why? *Journal of Child Psychology and Psychiatry*, **48**, 245–261.

Tan, L. H. & Quinlivan, J. A. (2006) Domestic violence, single parenthood and fathers in the setting of teenage pregnancy. *Journal of Adolescent Health*, **38**, 201–207.

Thomas, J. M., Chess, S., Birch, H. G. (1968) *Temperament and Behaviour Disorders in Children*. New York University Press.

Ukeje, I., Bendersky, M. & Lewis, M. (2001) Mother–infant interaction at 12 months in prenatally cocaine-exposed children. *American Journal of Drug and Alcohol Abuse*, **27**, 203–224.

Underdown, A., Barlow, J., Chung, V., *et al* (2006) Massage intervention for promoting mental and physical health in infants under six months. *Cochrane Database Systematic Reviews*, **18**, CD005038.

Van den Bergh, B. R., Mulder, E. J., Mennes, M., *et al* (2005) Antenatal maternal anxiety and stress and the neurobehavioural development of the fetus and child: links and possible mechanisms. A review. *Neuroscience and Biobehavioral Reviews*, **29**, 237–258.

Wadhwa, P. D., Sandman, C. A. & Gartie, T. J. (2001) The neurobiology of stress in human pregnancy. *Progress in Brain Research*, **133**, 131–142.

Wasserman, G. A., Liu, X., Pine, D. S., *et al* (2001) Contribution of maternal smoking during pregnancy and lead exposure to early child behavior problems. *Neurotoxicology and Teratology*, **23**, 13–21.

Waugh, E. & Bulik, C. M. (1999) Offspring of women with eating disorders. *International Journal of Eating Disorders*, **25**, 123–133.

Whitaker, R. C., Orzol, S. M. & Khan, R. S. (2006) Maternal mental health, substance use and domestic violence in the year after delivery and subsequent behaviour problems in children at age 3 years. *Archives of General Psychiatry*, **63**, 551–560.

Winnicott, D. W. (1970) The mother–infant experience of mutuality. In *Parenthood: Its Psychology and Psychopathology* (eds E. J. Anthony & T. Benedek), pp. 245–288. Little, Brown.

World Health Organization (1992). *International Classification of Diseases (10th edn) (ICD–10)*. WHO.

Zeanah, C. H., Boris, N. W. & Larrieu, J. A. (1997) Infant development and developmental risk: a review of the past 10 years. *Journal of the American Academy of Child and Adolescent Psychiatry*, **36**, 165–178.

CHAPTER 7

Screening and prevention

Researchers continue to observe that pregnant and postpartum women with mental disorders are not being identified and adequately treated (Kelly *et al*, 2001; Andersson *et al*, 2003; Coates *et al*, 2004; Smith *et al*, 2004; Thio *et al*, 2006) despite the fact they are routinely in contact with health professionals at this time. This chapter aims to address the issues concerning screening and prevention for both current and future disorders during pregnancy and the postpartum period, and point to best practice.

Definition of screening

The UK National Screening Committee has a very precise definition of screening (National Screening Committee, 2000):

> 'A public health service in which members of a defined population, who do not necessarily perceive that they are at risk of, or are already affected by a disease or its complications, are asked a question or offered a test to identify those individuals who are more likely to be helped than harmed by further tests or treatment to reduce the risk of disease or its complications.'

Another definition of screening is:

> 'The systematic application of a test or inquiry to identify individuals at risk of a specific disorder to benefit from further investigation or direct preventive among persons who have not sought medical attention on account of that disorder' (Peckham & Dezateux, 1998).

Screening was initially focused on conditions such as cancers, deafness in infants, risk factors for cardiovascular disease, and then more recently, psychological disorders. In 2002, the US Preventive Service Task Force recommended that clinical services screened adults for depression and several North American colleges and academies now advocate routinely asking patients about depression when taking a medical history.

Epidemiologists define case-finding as the search for additional disorders in those with medical problems and this fits most closely with the use of screening tools in pregnant and postpartum women.

There was considerable debate and consternation surrounding the National Screening Committee's initial recommendation that screening for postnatal depression was not justified and their website still states: 'Screening should not be offered. The evidence does not support the use of current screening tools or delivery' (National Screening Committee, 2006). After pressure from the Community Practitioners and Health Visitors Association this was modified to:

'... until more research is conducted into its potential for routine use in screening for postnatal depression, the National Screening Committee recommends that the Edinburgh Postnatal Depression Scale (EPDS) should not be used as a screening tool. It may, however, serve as a check list as part of a mood assessment for postnatal mothers, when it should only be used alongside professional judgement and a clinical interview' (National Screening Committee, 2006).

The National Screening Committee stated that the situation would be reviewed in late 2007, but the NICE guidelines published in February 2007 (National Institute for Health and Clinical Excellence, 2007) advocate asking two questions.

- During the past month, have you often been bothered by feeling down, depressed or hopeless?
- During the past month, have you often been bothered by having little interest or pleasure in doing things?

If there is a positive answer to both, the question 'Is this something you feel you need or want help with?' should be asked.

Although these questions have been validated in other healthcare settings (Whooley et al, 1997; McManus et al, 2005) there is, as yet, no evidence base to support their use in pregnant or postpartum women. A recent meta-analysis has found that requiring both questions to be endorsed results in substantial numbers of patients with depression being missed (Mitchell & Coyne, 2007) and a small study on teenage mothers found the anxiety sub-scale of the EPDS to be superior to the two above questions, with better sensitivity and negative predictive value (Kabir et al, 2007).

Screening instruments

Only three instruments have been developed specifically in order to screen for postnatal depression; the EPDS, the Postpartum Depression Screening Scale (PDSS) (Beck & Gable, 2000) and the Bromley Postnatal Depression Scale (Stein & van den Akker, 1992). Other self-report scales have been used in pregnant and postpartum populations but not all have been validated for this use. Boyd et al (2005) reviewed these and five other instruments in detail and critiqued their psychometric properties (reliability, sensitivity, specificity, positive predictive value and concurrent validity). They concluded that the EPDS is the most widely studied and has moderate psychometric soundness and also discussed some of the implications for clinicians and researchers.

The readability levels of the EPDS and PDSS have been assessed at US third and fourth grade respectively (Logsdon & Hutti, 2006) and it is stated that 95% of the UK adult population would be able to read the EPDS (Leverton, 2005). However, care should be taken not to assume literacy and anyone working with non-English-speaking women should consider whether a translation is available (see Cox & Holden, 2003; Henshaw & Elliott, 2005).

Edinburgh Postnatal Depression Scale

The first instrument developed specifically to screen for postnatal depression was the EPDS (Cox *et al*, 1987; Appendix III). This 10-item 'paper and pencil' has since been translated into numerous other languages and validated in many (Henshaw & Elliott, 2005), and remains the most widely used scale. It takes around 5 min to complete and is simple to score. Response categories are scored 0–3 according to the response, with items 3 and 5–10 being reverse scored, making the total score range of 0–30.

The original validation was done with Scottish women at 6 weeks postpartum. A cut-off score of 12/13 identified all the women with definite major depression and two of the three women with probable depression but there were false positives. A French study suggests that the EPDS is better at detecting women with anxious and anhedonic symptoms than those with psychomotor disability (Guedeney *et al*, 2000). Women from some cultures (e.g. Sylheti/Bengali) 'often prefer' to have the scale read to them than to complete it themselves (Fuggle *et al*, 2002).

The EPDS has been validated for use in pregnancy (Murray & Cox, 1990), some non-childbearing populations (Henshaw & Elliott, 2005) and fathers (Moran & O'Hara, 2006). However, in some non-Western settings, other instruments have been found to be superior, for example, the WHO Self-Reporting Questionnaire (Pollock *et al*, 2006). It has also been used with a simplified interview reference to an anchor event to emphasise timescales and a pictorial scale to assess severity in mothers with learning disabilities (Gaskin & James, 2006). One study of adolescent mothers reports that it may be possible to use three items from the anxiety sub-scale of the EPDS to make a preliminary diagnosis. (Kabir *et al*, 2007).

Matthey (2004) has calculated that a 4-point change indicates a clinical significance and this could be used in research trials. Some researchers and clinicians seem unaware that changing the format or cut-off score used can have a significant impact on the psychometrics of the scale. The variations found and the consequences for research and clinical practice are discussed in Matthey *et al* (2006).

The EPDS copyright is owned by the Royal College of Psychiatrists and the scale can only be reproduced provided this is published and includes the full reference.

Postpartum Depression Screening Scale

Cheryl Beck and Robert Gable developed the PDSS, a 35-item Likert-type self-report instrument which covers seven domains (Beck & Gable, 2000). There is also a short form (Beck & Gable, 2002) consisting of the first 7 items in the 35-item version.

The PDSS has been validated in Spanish and work is underway in several oher languages and communities. It has also been found to be reliable when administered over the telephone, which might be particularly useful in very remote areas (Mitchell *et al*, 2006).

Bromley Postnatal Depression Scale

This instrument consist of 10 items with open-ended and 'yes/no' questions plus a chart to identify when postnatal depression began. It assesses both current and past episodes of postnatal depression. There is no recommended cut-off score and only one published study of its psychometric properties has been undertaken (Stein & van den Akker, 1992).

General Health Questionnaire

Sharp (1988) carried out a validation study of the General Health Questionnaire (GHQ)–30 in early pregnancy and identified the optimum cut-off score of 5/6. However, Martin & Jomeen (2003), assessing the GHQ–12 in late pregnancy, full term and 28 days after delivery found that the scoring method had an impact both on the interpretation of data and on the prevalence of above-threshold 'cases'. They advised that further research should be undertaken to establish the optimum cut-off before the instrument is used in this population.

The GHQ has been found to have satisfactory sensitivity, specificity and positive predictive values in women who have had a miscarriage (Lok *et al*, 2004) and, although the EPDS performed slightly better, is a valid measure for screening for postnatal depression, anxiety and adjustment disorders (Navarro *et al*, 2007).

Hamilton Rating Scale for Depression

Scores on the HRSD in women in late pregnancy, 6 and 16 weeks postpartum were highly correlated with scores on measures that do not include somatic items, i.e. the Brief Symptom Inventory (Derogatis & Melisaratos, 1983) and the EPDS. Scores on somatic items did not correlate well with the total HRSD score in pregnancy, but did so at 6 weeks postpartum. However, scores on item 1 of the HRSD (depression) correlated less well with the total score at 6 weeks postpartum than during pregnancy. One explanation is that postpartum women may be less likely to articulate their difficulties as 'depression' and more likely to describe somatic complaints such as low energy or insomnia, and there is evidence to support this notion (Whitton *et al*, 1996).

Hospital Anxiety and Depression Scale

Factor analysis and internal reliability assessment of the Hospital Anxiety and Depression Scale (HADS) revealed that it does not reliably assess distinct domains of anxiety and depression in early pregnancy (Jomeen & Martin, 2004) or at 12 and 34 weeks (Karimova & Martin, 2003), and is therefore not a suitable screening tool for use in pregnant populations.

Beck Depression Inventory

Low scores on the BDI are determined mainly by somatic symptoms in pregnant women (Salamero *et al*, 1994), whereas higher scores are determined by depressive symptoms. Caution should, therefore, be exercised if using the BDI in this population and low scores should not be interpreted as indicating depressive symptomatology. A higher cut-off is advised when used with pregnant women than that usually employed in non-pregnant populations (Holcomb *et al*, 1996).

Other instruments and populations

A research diagnostic criteria-like algorithm based on items from the Self-Rating Depression Scale performed better than the scale itself in pregnant women (Kitamura *et al*, 1999).

Pictorial booklets entitled 'How Are You Feeling?' have been developed by the Community Practitioners and Health Visitors Association (Sobowale & Adams, 2005) to assist in the assessment of mental health, social and physical needs, and are available in Urdu, Bengali, Somali, Chinese, Arabic and English (useful for non-English speaking women with learning disabilities or those who are illiterate).

Downe *et al* (2007) reviewed the performance of the EPDS, the General Household Questionnaire, the Punjabi Postnatal Depression Scale and the Doop Chaon© (a visual tool) in screening for depressed mood after delivery in South Asian women living in the UK. They concluded that none of the tools met their quality criteria and qualitative data indicated that the women preferred face-to-face interviews to completing questionnaires.

There are several studies comparing the performance of one scale with others in pregnant and postpartum women. Interested readers are directed to Henshaw & Elliott (2005).

DeRosa & Logsdon (2006) highlight the poor psychometrics of the HRSD and BDI in adolescent mothers and point out that neither the EPDS nor the PDSS has been validated in this population.

Brockington *et al* (2001) have devised and validated a questionnaire to detect mother–infant bonding disorders, the Postpartum Bonding Instrument, which they propose using alongside the EPDS. It has been validated and translated into several languages. The authors suggest the instrument could also be used on a weekly basis to monitor change. Other instruments have also been devised to assess mother–infant interaction and bonding (see Chapter 3).

157

Acceptability

Screening with the EPDS appears to be acceptable to the majority of postpartum women (Buist *et al*, 2006; Gemmill *et al*, 2006) but not all would agree. In a study undertaken in Oxford, just over half of the women interviewed found screening with the EPDS less than acceptable (irrespective of whether or not they had depression). Particular issues were problems with how screening was carried out, for example the venue, the personal intrusion of it and stigma. Those interviewed had a clear preference for talking about how they felt, rather than filling out a questionnaire (Shakespeare *et al*, 2003). Similar findings are reported by Cubison & Munro (2005) regarding their 6-item scale which they erroneously called the EPDS. The women they interviewed had concerns about how the scale was administered (rushed, without any explanation, with others present and without any discussion about the score). Most were critical of the multiple choice type answers and some deliberately lied when answering it.

What are we screening for?

This is a crucial question. Is the intention to identify women with current mental disorder or those at risk of future disorder? This distinction will be borne in mind as we consider screening during pregnancy and in the postpartum period.

Pregnancy

Screening for current disorder

Up to a third of pregnant women are identified as suffering from a current psychiatric disorder (Kelly *et al*, 2001; Andersson *et al*, 2003; Kim *et al*, 2006), with depression followed by anxiety being the most common disorders. Both these conditions and others lead to poorer obstetric outcomes during pregnancy and at delivery (Andersson *et al*, 2004).

However, routine antenatal booking assessments do not identify all cases of psychiatric disorder in pregnant women. In a US antenatal care setting, 38% of women had a mental disorder but only 43% of these had their symptoms recorded, with less than a fifth having any mention in their records of a formal diagnosis. Just over a third had evidence of evaluation of their psychiatric problem in their maternity record but less than a quarter had their current treatment outlined (Kelly *et al*, 2001). Similarly, only 26% of pregnant women in public sector obstetric clinics with a mood or anxiety disorder and 12% of patients experiencing suicidal ideation had their problem recognised by their healthcare provider (Smith *et al*, 2004). Detection was more likely in this setting if the woman reported domestic violence. Low treatment rates of pregnant women with PTSD have also been reported (Loveland Cook *et al*, 2004).

However, ensuring that screening is universal can be problematic. A US programme, 'Identify, Screen, Intervene, Support' or 'ISIS', aimed to screen all pregnant women at 32 weeks of gestation with the EPDS, with high scorers being assessed further (including assessment of suicide risk) and referred on as appropriate to a brief psychosocial intervention for those with mild to moderate problems and to the psychiatric team if they had more severe or complex problems (Thoppil *et al*, 2005). They managed to screen 75% of patients.

There are no established biological markers for depression but Canadian investigators have observed that platelet serotonin levels correlate well with scores on the HRSD and propose that they might be a useful marker and guide to treatment response (Maurer-Spurej *et al*, 2007).

Screening for risk of postnatal depression

Austin & Lumley (2003) reviewed 16 studies that evaluated instruments used to screen women antenatally in order to identify those who are at risk of a postnatal depressive episode. Of the studies, 11 had devised scales specifically for this purpose, in 7 a study-specific instrument was combined with a standard self-report measure, 3 used a self-report measure alone and 3 used a diagnostic interview. They concluded that no instrument met criteria for routine population screening during pregnancy and postulated that this might have occurred because key risk predictors (personality, past history of abuse and depression, and severe blues) are not included in many of the instruments in question.

Austin *et al* (2005) then devised the Pregnancy Risk Questionnaire which identified risk factors and carried out a validation study. The questionnaire's sensitivity and specificity are better than previous scales but the positive predictive value remains limited.

In Canada, the Antenatal Psychosocial Health Assessment (ALPHA) was developed to screen women in relation to 15 risk factors and to identify those most at risk for a poorer psychosocial outcome. When compared against usual care in an RCT, more psychosocial concerns were identified by staff using the ALPHA, particularly those relating to family violence (Carroll *et al*, 2005). However, 65% of clinicians refused to take part in the trial, which raises questions about how easy more routine or widespread use would be.

The Postpartum Depression Predictors Inventory (PDPI), based on 13 risk factors has been developed, revised (the PDPI–R) and its psychometrics tested to an extent (Beck *et al*, 2006). It is designed to be the basis of an interview and is not a self-report scale. It performed well in pregnancy (validated against the EPDS), with a cut-off of 10.5 recommended, but has not been validated against a standardised interview.

Until more empirical data are available, systematic enquiry about past psychiatric history, the nature and severity of the illness and how it was treated are the way to assess the risk of depression after delivery. Dennis

& Ross (2006) observed that mothers with a psychiatric history were four times more likely to exhibit depressive symptoms at 8 weeks after delivery and that a history of previous postnatal depression and depression during the index pregnancy were also predictors, whereas family psychiatric history was not.

Screening for substance misuse and social problems

Screening for substance misuse is described in Chapter 5. An assessment should be made of any severe social problems including domestic violence following the guidance provided by the Department of Health (2005).

Screening for risk of severe mental illness

The high risk of recurrence after delivery in women with bipolar disorder, schizoaffective disorder or a history of puerperal psychosis or a severe depressive episode has been outlined in earlier chapters of this book. Failing to identify women at risk and failing to adequately manage that risk is a key point made in relation to maternal suicide and infanticide (Lewis & Drife, 2004).

It is crucial, therefore, that there should be a routine and systematic enquiry at antenatal booking about previous psychiatric history, its severity and the clinical presentation and the care received. Almost 10% of women who had a psychiatric admission before pregnancy will develop puerperal psychosis (Harlow *et al*, 2007). The risk increases with the number of hospitalisations, the closer they are in relation to pregnancy and the length of the most recent psychiatric hospitalisation.

General practitioners are advised to ensure that details regarding current and past psychiatric history are included in referral to antenatal booking and are advised not to use the term 'postnatal depression' or the acronym 'PND' in a generic way to describe all types of psychiatric disorder. However, 'Maternity Matters' (Department of Health, 2007) encourages women to refer themselves directly to midwives once they have confirmed they are pregnant, which gives rise to the risk of crucial aspects of the medical or psychiatric history not being communicated to those responsible for maternity care. Hence, the midwife undertaking a booking assessment must seek further details of the history from the woman's GP if she suspects there are or have been problems.

The precise details of previous illness, its severity and the treatment received should be obtained and recorded, and when a management plan has been decided upon, it must be communicated to the woman, all health professionals involved and inserted into all her records.

Role of midwives and obstetricians

The primary providers of antenatal care in the UK are midwives and they are ideally placed to enquire about mental disorder both at the booking interview and at subsequent visits. In 1999, 94% of in-maternity units in England and Wales reported that they asked about psychological problems at booking and a quarter undertook formal screening for depression during pregnancy (Tully *et al*, 2002). However, only 16% had offered any training to midwives to enable them to carry out this work and fewer than one in four had policies and guidelines regarding the management of women with depression let alone any other mental disorder. Results of a survey published in 2006 (Ross-Davie *et al*, 2006) indicate that although midwives have a positive attitude towards women with mental health problems and towards taking on a more developed role in mental health promotion, they also have many gaps in knowledge, including the signs and symptoms of serious illness and the risk of puerperal psychosis.

They feel less confident in managing women with depression or schizophrenia than those with rarer conditions such as HIV, cholestasis and symphisis pubis diastisis (Ross-Davie *et al*, 2006). Only 13% have had any post-registration training in mental health.

Like midwives, obstetricians should understand the risk of recurrence of serious mental illness in relation to childbirth, the timing and the likely nature of recurrences. They should be clear about what actions are needed during pregnancy and after delivery.

Postpartum

Similar to the situation in pregnancy, many women with postpartum depression or anxiety also go unrecognised (Thio *et al*, 2006.). Postnatal assessments are usually undertaken 4–6 weeks after delivery and certainly screening too early in the postpartum period, that is, less than 2 weeks, is likely to reduce the sensitivity of screening scales owing to the presence of blues symptoms (Lee *et al*, 2003).

Around 3–4 months after delivery is another opportunity to screen for depression whether by asking the two questions meantioned earlier (p. 155) or using a self-report questionnaire such as the EPDS to aid the clinical assessment. Using the EPDS in routine screening has been shown in several studies to increase the rate of diagnosed depression (Barnett *et al*, 1993; Hearn *et al*, 1998; Evins *et al*, 2000; Georgiopoulos *et al*, 2001).

However, the 3–5% of women who suffer from more severe postnatal depressive illnesses and those with psychotic disorders will present much earlier than 6 weeks after delivery. Two-thirds of women with postpartum-onset major depression dated the onset of their illness to a mean of 2.2 weeks (s.d. = 1.7) after delivery (Stowe *et al*, 2005). This means that health professionals should not dismiss early symptoms and assess maternal mental state much earlier than 6 weeks in any woman with a prior history of serious mood or psychotic disorder. A woman with a current or past serious mental illness should be asked about her mental health and symptoms at every postpartum contact.

Where should we screen?

Screening can take place in a variety of settings but the most frequently used in UK primary care are a woman's home or clinic. If others are present at home or the visit is unexpected it may be inconvenient and lack privacy. Administering a questionnaire in a busy clinic can lead to a woman feeling rushed and again privacy may be lacking. In one study, a clear preference was expressed for having the EPDS administered at home (Shakespeare *et al*, 2003). Clearly, there must be time and privacy to talk to the woman, explore any issues raised, and ask additional questions to clarify and answer her questions.

Child health settings

In the USA, babies are seen four to six times per year at well baby clinics and it has been suggested that this might afford the opportunity for paediatricians to assess maternal depression (Heneghan *et al*, 1998). However, without systematic screening, they do not appear to identify many of the mothers reporting depressive symptoms (Heneghan *et al*, 2000). Barriers appear to be the paediatrician's lack of education and training to diagnose and treat maternal depression and lack of time to take an adequate history (Olson *et al*, 2002; Wiley *et al*, 2004). There are also issues relating to whether or not they view it as their role. If they do, it is more likely that they will consider changing their practice towards identification of maternal depression. Improving communication skills via video feedback of assessment interviews can improve their ability to detect emotional disorders (Wissow *et al*, 1994).

Mothers are concerned about disclosure because of fear of judgement and the possibility of being referred to child protection services, and are more likely to disclose if they know their paediatrician well (Heneghan *et al*, 2004).

Role of health visitors

Health visitors in the UK are qualified nurses or midwives who have undergone further training in health promotion, child health and education. Every family with a child under the age of five has a named health visitor who can advise on everyday problems such as feeding, sleeping, behaviour problems and parenting in general, but who also assists with special needs, and may run immunisation programmes, child development checks and parenting classes.

Holden *et al* (1989) demonstrated in a small RCT that after brief training, health visitors could deliver an intervention based on Rogerian non-directive counselling which comprised eight 1-h 'listening visits' and that this was an effective intervention for mild to moderate non-psychotic unipolar postnatal depression. Health visitors in most areas now have had some form of training (although the quality and quantity of updates and supervision is very variable) and some form of screening and intervention is available in many parts of the UK.

Does screening lead to intervention?

Screening may not automatically lead to intervention for a variety of reasons. It is essential that there are clear care pathways so that professionals caring for pregnant or postpartum women know how to access assessment and treatment. The staff undertaking screening should have been trained and have sufficient ongoing supervision, consultation and contact with mental health professionals to enable them to access the pathways. Training will need to be updated and new entrants to the service trained. Workloads, vacancies and high turnover of staff are features of many services and failure in any of these areas can lead to women not receiving much needed treatment.

Shakespeare (2002) reports on the reasons why postpartum women in Oxford were not screened by health visitors (which occurred in a third to almost a half of the total sample). Around a quarter had cultural or language reasons, others had moved away. A total of 15% at 8 weeks and 13% at 8 months refused, others were unavailable, and for 26 and 30% no reason was given. Recording of EPDS scores was found to be haphazard with health visitors citing special circumstances such as staff shortages and workload issues as the reason for not recording them, but also being reluctant to label women as depressed which they felt could have negative consequences.

What do women think about screening?

Women themselves may be reluctant to disclose their problems or to access mental healthcare. In one study, most women in early pregnancy had not disclosed their emotional distress to their maternity care provider (Birndorf *et al*, 2001). However, they all expressed a willingness to see a mental health professional if they were referred. Robinson & Young (1982) report that 50% of postpartum mothers with depression identified by screening in an Australian baby health centre refused psychiatric referral. The main reason given was the stigma associated with psychiatric treatment, although women were happy to talk to clinic nursing staff. Even in a setting where screening is routine and has been explained to women, 16% of those with a high EPDS score ignored recommendations for follow-up (Buist *et al*, 2006). Some mothers fear admission to a psychiatric unit, being locked up or having their baby removed (Hall, 2006), and in some cultures partners and/or families will actively discourage a woman from disclosing her difficulties.

Netmums (2005) carried out an online survey of members, 63% of whom had been offered screening with the EPDS. Of these, 44% admitted lying to conceal their illness. The most common reason for this was feeling that if they admitted to having depression it meant admitting they were a failure, followed by not feeling comfortable confiding in the health visitor.

Women may lack knowledge or have misunderstandings about perinatal mental health problems and treatment as much of the information in the lay press or on websites is inaccurate and misleading (Martinez *et al*, 2000; Summers & Logsdon, 2005).

There are particular concerns that some of the most vulnerable women – those who are young, less well educated, poor attenders at appointments and whose infants have poorer outcomes – are being excluded from health visitor contact (Murray *et al*, 2003). Reasons for this may be mistrust of services and service providers, seeing health visitors as the 'baby police', feeling alienated from healthcare settings, lack of transport, relocation and multiple demands.

Prevention

Being familiar with the risk factors for postnatal depression and understanding the risk of recurrence after subsequent deliveries if a woman has had a postpartum episode together with the predictable timing of a likely episode of depression has led to numerous trials of preventive interventions. Some are delivered during pregnancy to women and others are delivered postpartum. Some are targeted at women with risk factors, others at women who have had a previous episode of depression or psychosis.

Depression

Several systematic reviews have now addressed the efficacy of a variety of interventions aimed at preventing postnatal depression (Dennis *et al*, 1999; Austin, 2003; Dennis, 2004; Dennis & Creedy, 2004; Dennis & Stewart, 2004; Bradley *et al*, 2005; Howard *et al*, 2005).

Antidepressants

Nortriptyline is not an effective prophylactic when given to women who have previously had postnatal depression (Wisner *et al*, 2001); however, sertraline led to significantly fewer recurrences when given to pregnant women without depression who had prior postnatal depression (Wisner *et al*, 2004).

Psychosocial and educational interventions

There is currently insufficient evidence to suggest that psychosocial or psychological interventions are effective in preventing postnatal depression (Dennis, 2004, 2005). However, it is possible that additional professional help postpartum might be beneficial. Antenatal group interventions have also largely proved unsuccessful (Austin, 2003) and are not recommended as being part of routine antenatal care (National Institute for Health and

Clinical Excellence, 2007). The NICE guideline does, however, recommend psychosocial interventions for women with subsyndromal symptoms in pregnancy, advising six sessions of interpersonal psychotherapy or CBT if they have a previous history of depression, or social support during pregnancy and postpartum if they do not.

Hormones

Progesterone and progestogens have been suggested as prophylaxis against recurrence of postnatal depression since Katharina Dalton's progesterone trial published in 1985 (Dalton, 1985) in which she claimed that it was an effective prophylactic. This is despite the fact that she used historical controls and the women were not randomised. Four years later she published a controlled trial, but again participants were not randomised (Dalton, 1989). Granger & Underwood (2001) reviewed the role of progesterone concluding that 'evidence to support its efficacy is lacking' and a Cochrane review states that progesterone does not have RCT data to support its use and notes that long-acting progestogens are associated with increased depressive symptoms (Dennis et al, 1999).

Sichel et al (1995) reported a small case series in which four women with a history of puerperal major depression were treated with high-dose oral oestrogen, none of whom experienced a recurrence. However, the risk of thrombosis associated with the postpartum period and oestrogen must be considered and heparinisation may be required.

Despite the positive association between thyroid antibody status and depression in postpartum women, thyroxine does not prevent the occurrence of postnatal depression (Harris et al, 2002).

Other interventions

Pregnant and recently delivered women often experience sleep disturbance and it has been proposed as a potential trigger for both postnatal depression and puerperal psychosis. A Canadian centre has piloted an intervention which they offer women who are considered at high risk for recurrence of depression postpartum (those with a personal or family history of depression or with subclinical symptoms during pregnancy). They are offered a hospital stay for five nights, during which mothers sleep in a single room, with their baby spending the night in the nursery. Breastfeeding mothers are encouraged to express milk during the day so that night feeds can be given by staff and hypnotics are used if required. A case-note review of the first 179 patients gave promising results (Steiner et al, 2003) but this has yet to be tested in an RCT.

There has also been interest in whether omega-3 fatty acids are a preventive intervention. Llorente et al (2003) gave docosahexaenoic acid supplementation or placebo to 138 breastfeeding mothers in an RCT. However, this did not confer any benefit on the rates of depressive symptoms or disorder. The following year, Marangell et al (2004) published a small open trial in which they gave omega-3 fatty acids to pregnant women (between 34 and 36 weeks) with a history of postpartum depression. However, four of the seven women became depressed and so prophylaxis with omega-3 fatty acids cannot be recommended (Freeman, 2006).

Calcium carbonate supplementation given as a prophylactic for pre-eclampsia in a double-blind placebo-controlled RCT led to significantly lower EPDS scores in the intervention group (Harrison-Hohner *et al*, 2001) but the participants were not selected on the basis of having a prior puerperal depressive episode and there remain no data to support this.

Puerperal psychosis

Disruption of the sleep–wake cycle, particularly reduced sleep and early waking, is associated with relapse of manic symptoms in non-puerperal populations (Wehr, 1989) and may well be a provoking factor in puerperal psychosis (Sharma, 2003). As far as is possible with a new infant, sleep loss and disruption should be minimised in vulnerable women. This could include support from a partner or family member in helping with night feeds (expressing milk during the day if breastfeeding).

Drugs

There are studies (but no RCTs) supporting the efficacy of lithium started in the immediate postpartum or in the last trimester for the prevention of puerperal psychosis (Stewart *et al*, 1991; Austin, 1992; Cohen *et al*, 1995). The last of these studies estimated the relative risk of relapse for those not taking mood stabilisers to be 8.6. However, maternal lithium levels must be checked regularly and care taken to avoid toxicity during delivery where fluid balance may be disrupted (by reducing the dose prior to delivery) during labour and in the postpartum when renal clearance (increased during pregnancy) returns to the pre-pregnant level.

A small naturalistic study (part of a larger study of bipolar disorder) examined whether olanzapine alone or in addition to antidepressants and/or mood stabilisers could prevent a puerperal psychotic episode (Sharma *et al*, 2006). Two (18.2%) of the women who took olanzapine experienced a postpartum episode (depression) as did eight (57.1%) women who did not take olanzapine (four depressive episodes, one mixed, one hypomania and two puerperal psychoses). It should be noted that the sample was of women with bipolar I and II disorder, not all of whom had had a previous puerperal psychotic episode, but it is of interest that olanzapine also appeared to prevent depressive episodes. Clearly this requires replication under controlled conditions.

Hormones

Both oestrogen and progesterone have been promoted as prophylactic agents for puerperal psychosis but with little success. Sichel *et al* (1995) gave seven women with histories of puerperal psychosis high-dose oral oestrogen immediately after delivery. The only woman to relapse postpartum had not been fully adherent with medication. However, transdermal oestradiol administered to 29 women with a diagnosis of bipolar disorder or schizoaffective disorder failed to reduce the rate of relapse (Kumar *et al*, 2003).

To date there is little evidence to support the use of oestrogen as prophylaxis for puerperal psychosis or recurrence of bipolar disorder postpartum and it should be remembered that there is an increased risk of thrombosis in the postpartum period and also with the use of oestrogens.

Conclusion

Mental disorders result in significant morbidity and mortality for pregnant and recently delivered women and can have lasting effects on their infants and families. As pregnant and postpartum women are in regular contact with health professionals this provides several opportunities for those suffering from or at risk of mental disorders to be detected and treated or for preventive strategies and monitoring to be put into place.

References

Andersson, L., Sundstrom-Poromaa, I., Bixo, M., *et al* (2003) Point prevalence of psychiatric disorders during the second trimester of pregnancy: a population-based study. *American Journal of Obstetrics and Gynecology*, **189**, 148–154.

Andersson, L., Sundstrom-Poromaa, I., Wulff, M., *et al* (2004) Implications of antenatal depression and anxiety for obstetric outcome. *Obstetrics and Gynecology*, **104**, 467–476.

Austin, M. P. (1992) Puerperal affective psychosis: is there a case for lithium prophylaxis? *British Journal of Psychiatry*, **161**, 692–694.

Austin, M. P. (2003) Targeted group antenatal prevention of postnatal depression: a review. *Acta Psychiatrica Scandinavica*, **107**, 244–250.

Austin, M. P. & Lumley, J. (2003) Antenatal screening for postnatal depression: a systematic review. *Acta Psychiatrica Scandinavica*, **107**, 10–17.

Austin, M. P., Hadzi-Pavlovic, D., Saint, K., *et al* (2005) Antenatal screening for the prediction of postnatal depression: validation of a psychosocial pregnancy risk questionnaire. *Acta Psychiatrica Scandinavica*, **112**, 310–317.

Barnett, B., Lockhart, K., Bernard, D., *et al* (1993) Mood disorders among mothers of infants admitted to a mothercraft hospital. *Journal of Paediatrics and Child Health*, **29**, 270–275.

Beck, C. T. & Gable, R. K. (2000) Postpartum depression screening scale: development and psychometric testing. *Nursing Research*, **49**, 272–282.

Beck, C. T. & Gable, R. K. (2002) *Postpartum Depression Scale Screening Manual*. Western Psychological Services.

Birndorf, C. A., Madden, A., Portera, L., *et al* (2001) Psychiatric symptoms, functional impairment, and receptivity toward mental health treatment among obstetrical patients. *International Journal of Psychiatry in Medicine*, **31**, 355–365.

Boyd, R. C., Le, H. N. & Somberg, R. (2005) Review of screening instruments for postpartum depression. *Archives of Women's Mental Health*, **8**, 141–153.

Bradley, E., Boath, E. & Henshaw, C. (2005) The prevention of postpartum depression: a narrative systematic review. *Psychosomatic Obstetrics and Gynecology*, **26**, 185–192.

Brockington, I., Oates, J., George, S., *et al* (2001) A screening questionnaire for mother–infant bonding disorders. *Archives of Women's Mental Health*, **3**, 133–140.

Buist, A., Condon, J., Brooks, J., *et al* (2006) Acceptability of routine screening for perinatal depression. *Journal of Affective Disorders*, **93**, 233–237.

Carroll, J. C., Reid, A. J., Biringer, A., *et al* (2005) Effectiveness of the Antenatal Psychosocial Health Assessment (ALPHA) form in detecting psychosocial concerns: a randomized controlled trial. *Canadian Medical Association Journal*, **173**, 253–259.

Coates, A. O., Schaefer, C. A. & Alexander, J. L. (2004) Detection of postpartum depression and anxiety in a large health plan. *Journal of Behavioral Health Services & Research*, **31**, 117–132.

Cohen, L., Sichel, D., Robertson, L., *et al* (1995) Postpartum prophylaxis for women with bipolar disorder. *American Journal of Psychiatry*, **152**, 1641–1645.

Cox, J. & Holden, J. (2003) Appendix 2: Translations of the Edinburgh Postnatal Depression Scale. In *Perinatal Mental Health: A Guide to the Edinburgh Postnatal Depression Scale*, pp. 71–110. Gaskell.

Cox, J. H., Holden, J. M. & Sagovsky, R. (1987) Detection of postnatal depression. Development of the 10-item Edinburgh Postnatal Depression Scale. *British Journal of Psychiatry*, **150**, 782–786.

Cubison, J. & Munro, J. (2005) Acceptability of using the EPDS as a screening tool. In *Screening for Perinatal Depression*, pp. 152–161. Jessica Kingsley.

Dalton, K. (1985) Progesterone prophylaxis used successfully in postnatal depression. *The Practitioner*, **229**, 507–508.

Dalton, K. (1989) Successful prophylactic progesterone for idiopathic postnatal depression. *International Journal of Prenatal and Perinatal Studies*, **1**, 323–327.

Dennis, C. L. (2004) Preventing postpartum depression part II: a critical review of nonbiological interventions. *Canadian Journal of Psychiatry*, **49**, 526–538.

Dennis, C. L. (2005) Psychosocial and psychological interventions for prevention of postpartum depression: systematic review. *BMJ*, **331**, 15–18.

Dennis, C. L. & Creedy, D. (2004) Psychosocial and psychological interventions for preventing postpartum depression. *Cochrane Database of Systematic Reviews*, **4**, CD001134.

Dennis, C. L. & Stewart, D. E. (2004) Treatment of postpartum depression, part 1: a critical review of biological interventions. *Journal of Clinical Psychiatry*, **65**, 1242–1251.

Dennis, C. L. & Ross, L. E. (2006) The clinical utility of maternal self-reported personal and familial psychiatric history in identifying women at risk for postpartum depression. *Acta Obstetricia Gynecologica Scandinavica*, **85**, 1179–1185.

Dennis, C. L., Ross, L. E. & Herxheimer, A. (1999) Oestrogens and progestins for preventing and treating postpartum depression. *Cochrane Database of Systematic Reviews*, **3**, CD001690.

Department of Health (2005) *Responding to Domestic Abuse: A Handbook for Health Professionals*. TSO (The Stationery Office).

Department of Health (2007) *Maternity Matters: Choice, Access and Continuity of Care in a Safe Service*. TSO (The Stationery Office).

Derogatis, L. R. & Melisaratos, N. (1983) The Brief Symptom Inventory: an introductory report. *Psychological Medicine*, **13**, 595–605.

DeRosa, N. & Logsdon, C. M. (2006) A comparison of screening instruments for depression in postpartum adolescents. *Journal of Child and Adolescent Psychiatry Nursing*, **19**, 13–20.

Downe, S. M., Butler, E. & Hinder, S. (2007) Screening tools for depressed mood after childbirth in UK-based South Asian women: a systematic review. *Journal of Advanced Nursing*, **57**, 565–583.

Evins, G. G., Theofrastous, J. P. & Galvin, S. L. (2000) Postpartum depression: a comparison of screening and routine clinical evaluation. *American Journal of Obstetrics and Gynecology*, **182**, 1080–1082.

Freeman, M. P. (2006) Omega-3 fatty acids and perinatal depression: a review of the literature and recommendations for future research. *Prostaglandins, Leukotrienes and Essential Fatty Acids*, **75**, 291–297.

Fuggle, P., Glover, L., Khan, F., *et al* (2002) Screening for postnatal depression in Bengali women: Preliminary observations from using a translated version of the Edinburgh Post-natal Depression Scale (EPDS). *Journal of Reproductive and Infant Psychology*, **20**, 71–82.

Gaskin, K. & James, H. (2006) Using the Edinburgh Postnatal Depression Scale with learning disabled mothers. *Community Practitioner*, **79**, 392–396.

Gemmill, A. W., Leigh, B., Ericksen, J., *et al* (2006) A survey of the clinical acceptability of screening for postnatal depression and non-depressed women. *BMC Public Health*, **6**, 211.

Georgiopoulos, A. M., Bryan, T. L., Wollan, T. L., *et al* (2001) Routine screening for postpartum depression. *Journal of Family Practice*, **50**, 117–122.

Granger, A. C. & Underwood, M. R. (2001) Review of the role of progesterone in the management of postnatal mood disorders. *Journal of Psychosomatic Obstetrics and Gynecology*, **22**, 49–55.

Guedeney, N., Fermanian, J., Guelfi, J. D., *et al* (2000) The Edinburgh Postnatal Depression Scale (EPDS) and the detection of major depressive disorders in early postpartum: some concerns about false negatives. *Journal of Affective Disorders*, **61**, 107–112.

Hall, P. (2006) Mothers' experiences of postnatal depression: an interpretative phenomenological analysis. *Community Practitioner*, **79**, 256–260.

Harlow, B. L., Vitonis, A. F., Sparen, P., *et al* (2007) Incidence of hospitalization for postpartum psychotic and bipolar episodes in women with and without prior prepregnancy or prenatal psychiatric hospitalizations. *Archives of General Psychiatry*, **64**, 42–48.

Harris, B., Oretti, R., Lazarus, J., *et al* (2002) Randomised trial of thyroxine to prevent postnatal depression in thyroid-antibody-positive women. *British Journal of Psychiatry*, **180**, 327–330.

Harrison-Hohner, J., Coste, S., Dorato, V., *et al* (2001) Prenatal calcium supplementation and postpartum depression: an ancillary study to a randomized trial of calcium for prevention of preeclampsia. *Archives of Women's Mental Health*, **3**, 141–146.

Hearn, G., Iliff, A., Jones, I., *et al* (1998) Postnatal depression in the community. *British Journal of General Practice*, **48**, 1064–1066.

Heneghan, A. M., Mercer, B. & DeLeone, N. (2004) Will mothers discuss parenting stress and depressive symptoms with their child's pediatrician? *Pediatrics*, **113**, 460–467.

Heneghan, A. M., Silver, E. J., Bauman, L. J., *et al* (1998) Depressive symptoms in inner-city mothers of young children: who is at risk? *Pediatrics*, **102**, 1394–1400.

Heneghan, A. M., Silver, E. J., Bauman, L. J., *et al* (2000) Do pediatricians recognize mothers with depressive symptoms? *Pediatrics*, **106**, 1367–1373.

Henshaw, C. & Elliott, S. (2005) Bibliography of translations and validation studies. In *Screening for Perinatal Depression*, pp. 205–211. Jessica Kingsley.

Holcomb, W. L., Stone, L. S., Lustman, P. J., *et al* (1996) Screening for depression in pregnancy: characteristics of the Beck Depression Inventory. *Obstetrics and Gynecology*, **88**, 1021–1025.

Holden, J. M., Sagovsky, R. & Cox, J. L. (1989) Counselling in a general practice setting: controlled study of health visitor intervention in treatment of postnatal depression. *BMJ*, **298**, 223–226.

Howard, L. M., Hoffbrand, S., Henshaw, C. *et al*, (2005) Antidepressant prevention of postnatal depression. *Cochrane Database of Systematic Reviews*, **2**, CD004363.

Jomeen, J. & Martin, C. (2004) Is the Hospital Anxiety and Depression Scale (HADS) a reliable screening tool in early pregnancy? *Psychology and Health*, **19**, 787–800.

Kabir, K., Sheeder, J., Kelly, L., *et al* (2007) identifying postpartum depression: 3 questions are as good as 10. *Journal of Pediatric and Adolescent Gynecology*, **20**, S135–S136.

Karimova, G. K. & Martin, C. R. (2003) A psychometric evaluation of the Hospital Anxiety and Depression Scale during pregnancy. *Psychology, Health and Medicine*, **8**, 89–103.

Kelly, R. H., Zatick, D. & Anders, T. F. (2001) The detection and treatment of psychiatric disorders and substance use among pregnant women cared for in obstetrics. *American Journal of Psychiatry*, **158**, 213–219.

Kim, H. G., Mandell, M., Crandall, C., *et al* (2006) Antenatal psychiatric illness and adequacy of prenatal care in an ethnically diverse inner-city obstetric population. *Archives of Women's Mental Health*, **9**, 103–107.

Kitamura, T., Sugawara, M., Shima, S., *et al* (1999) Temporal validity of self-rating questionnaires: improved validity of repeated use of Zung's Self-Rating Depression Scale among women during the perinatal period. *Journal of Psychosomatic Obstetrics and Gynaecology*, **20**, 112–117.

Kumar, C., McIvor, R. J., Davies, T., *et al* (2003) Estrogen administration does not reduce the rate of recurrence of affective psychosis after childbirth. *Journal of Clinical Psychiatry*, **64**, 112–118.

Lee, D. T. S., Yip, S. K., Chui, H. F. K., *et al* (2003) Postdelivery screening for postpartum depression. *Psychosomatic Medicine*, **65**, 357–361.

Leverton, T. (2005) Advantages and disadvantages of screening in clinical settings. In *Screening for Perinatal Depression* (eds C. Henshaw & S. Elliott), pp. 34–46. Jessica Kinglsey.

Lewis, G. & Drife, J. (2004) *Why Mothers Die 2000–2002. The Sixth Report of the Confidential Enquiries into Maternal Death in the United Kingdom*. RCOG Press.

Llorente, A. M., Jensen, C. L., Voigt, R. G., *et al* (2003) Effect of maternal docosahexaenoic acid supplementation on postpartum depression and information processing. *American Journal of Obstetrics and Gynecology*, **188**, 1348–1353.

Logsdon, M. C. & Hutti, M. H. (2006) Readability: an improtant issue impacting healthcare for women with postpartum depression. *American Journal of Maternal/Child Nursing*, **31**, 351–355.

Lok, I. H., Lee, D. T. S., Yip, S-K., *et al* (2004) Screening for post-miscarriage psychiatric morbidity. *American Journal of Obstetrics and Gynecology*, **191**, 546–550.

Loveland Cook, C. A., Flick, L. H., Homan, S. M., *et al* (2004) Posttraumatic stress disorder in pregnancy: prevalence, risk factors, and treatment. *Obstetrics and Gynecology*, **103**, 710–717.

Marangell, L. B., Martinez, J. M., Zboyan, H. A., *et al* (2004) Omega-3 fatty acids for the prevention of postpartum depression: negative data from a preliminary, open-label pilot study. *Depression and Anxiety*, **19**, 20–23.

Martin, C. R. & Jomeen, J. (2003) Is the 12-item General Health Questionnaire (GHQ–12) confounded by scoring method during pregnancy and following birth? *Journal of Reproductive and Infant Psychology*, **21**, 267–278.

Martinez, R., Johnston Robledo, I., Ulsh, H.M., *et al* (2000) Singing 'the baby blues': a content analysis of popular press articles about postpartum affective disturbances. *Women and Health*, **31**, 37–56.

Matthey, S. (2004) Calculating clinically significant change in postnatal depression studies using the Edinburgh Postnatal Depression Scale. *Journal of Affective Disorders*, **78**, 269–272.

Matthey, S., Henshaw, C., Elliott, S. A., *et al* (2006) Variability in use of cut-off scores and formats on the Edinburgh Postnatal Depression Scale – implications for research findings. *Archives of Women's Mental Health*, **9**, 309–315.

Maurer-Spurej, E., Pittendreigh, C. & Misri, S. (2007) Platelet serotonin levels support depression scores for women with postpartum depression. *Journal of Psychiatry and Neuroscience*, **32**, 23–29.

McManus, D., Pipkin, S. S. & Whooley, M. A. (2005) Screening for depression in patients with coronary heart disease (data from the Heart and Soul Study). *American Journal of Cardiology*, **96**, 1076–1081.

Mitchell, A. J. & Coyne, J. C. (2007) Do ultra-short screening instruments accurately detect depression in primary care? A pooled analysis and meta-analysis of 22 studies. *British Journal of General Practice*, **57**, 144–145.

Mitchell, A. M., Mittelstaedt, M. E. & Schott-Baer, D. (2006) Postpartum depression: the reliability of telephone screening. *American Maternal and Child Nurse*, **31**, 382–387.

Moran, T. E. & O'Hara, M. W. (2006) A partner-rating scale of postpartum depression: The Edinburgh Postnatal Depression Scale – Partner (EPDS–P). *Archives of Women's Mental Health*, **9**, 173–180.

Murray, D. & Cox, J. (1990) Screening for depression during pregnancy with the Edinburgh Postnatal Depression Scale (EPDS). *Journal of Reproductive and Infant Psychology*, **8**, 99–107.

Murray, L., Woolgar, M., Murray, J., *et al* (2003) Self-exclusion from health care in women at high risk from postpartum depression. *Journal of Public Health Medicine*, **25**, 131–137.

National Institute for Health and Clinical Excellence (2007) *Antenatal and Postnatal Mental Health. Clinical Management and Service Guidance*. NICE.

National Screening Committee (2000) *Second Report of the National Screening Committee*, pp. 27–28. Department of Health.

National Screening Committee (2006) National Screening Committee policy – postnatal depression screening. National Screening Committee, UK (http://www.library.nhs.uk/screening/ViewResource.aspx?resID=60978&tabID=288).

Navarro, P., Ascaso, C., Garcia-Esteve, L., *et al* (2007) Postnatal psychiatric morbidity: a validation study of the GHQ–12 and the EPDS as screening tools. *General Hospital Psychiatry*, **29**, 1–7.

Netmums (2005) Postnatal depression research. Netmums (http://www.netmums.com/h/n/PND/HOME//545//).

Olson, A. L., Kemper, K. J., Kelleher, K. J., *et al* (2002) Primary care pediatricians' roles and perceived responsibilities in the identification and management of maternal depression. *Pediatrics*, **110**, 1169–1176.

Peckham, C. & Dezateux, C. (1998) Issues underlying the evaluation of screening programmes. *British Medical Bulletin*, **54**, 767–778.

Pollock, J. I., Manaseki-Holland, S. & Patel, V. (2006) Detection of depression in women of child-bearing age in non-Western cultures: a comparison of the Edinburgh Postnatal Depression Scale and the Self-Reporting Questionnaire–20 in Mongolia. *Journal of Affective Disorders*, **92**, 267–271.

Robinson, S. & Young, J. (1982) Screening for depression and anxiety in the postnatal period: acceptance or rejection of a treatment offer. *Australian and New Zealand Journal of Psychiatry*, **16**, 47–51.

Ross-Davie, M., Elliott, S. A., Sarkar, A., *et al* (2006) A public health role in perinatal mental health: are midwives ready? *British Journal of Midwifery*, **14**, 330–334.

Salamero, M., Marcos, T., Gutierrez, F., *et al* (1994) Factorial study of the BDI in pregnant women. *Psychological Medicine*, **14**, 1031–1035.

Shakespeare, J. (2002) Health visitor screening for postnatal depression using the EPDS: a process study. *Community Practitioner*, **75**, 381–384.

Shakespeare, J., Blake, F. & Garcia, J. (2003) A qualitative study of the acceptability of routine screening of postnatal women using the Edinburgh Postnatal Depression Scale. *British Journal of General Practice*, **53**, 614–619.

Sharma, V. (2003) Role of sleep loss in the causation of puerperal psychosis. *Medical Hypotheses*, **61**, 477–481.

Sharma, V., Smith, A. & Mazmanian, D. (2006) Olanzapine in the prevention of postpartum psychosis and mood episodes in bipolar disorder. *Bipolar Disorders*, **8**, 400–404.

Sharp, D. J. (1988) Validation of the 3-item General Health Questionnaire in early pregnancy. *Psychological Medicine*, **18**, 503–507.

Sichel, D. A., Cohen, L. S., Robertson, L. M., *et al* (1995) Prophylactic estrogen in recurrent postpartum affective disorder. *Biological Psychiatry*, **38**, 814–818.

Smith, M. V., Rosenheck, R. A., Cavaleri, M. A., *et al* (2004) Screening for and detection of depression, panic disorder, and PTSD in public-sector obstetric clinics. *Psychiatric Services*, **55**, 407–414.

Sobowale, A. & Adams, C. (2005) Screening where there is no screening scale. In *Screening for Perinatal Depression* (eds C. Henshaw & S. Elliott), pp. 90–109. Jessica Kingsley.

Stein, G. & van den Akker, O. (1992) The retrospective diagnosis of postnatal depression by questionnaire. *Journal of Psychosomatic Research*, **36**, 67–75.

Steiner, M., Fairman, M. & Jansen, K. (2003) Can postpartum depression be prevented? *Archives of Women's Mental Health*, **6**, S106.

Stewart, D. E., Klompenhouwer, J. L., Kendell, R. E., *et al* (1991). Prophylactic lithium in puerperal psychosis. The experience of three centres. *British Journal of Psychiatry*, **158**, 393–397.

Stowe, Z. N., Hostetter, A. L. & Newport, D. J. (2005) The onset of postpartum depression: implications for clinical screening in obstetrical and primary care. *American Journal of Obstetrics and Gynecology*, **192**, 522–526.

Summers, A. L. & Logsdon, M. C. (2005) Web sites for postpartum depression: convenient, frustrating, incomplete, and misleading. *North American Journal of Maternal Child Nursing*, **30**, 88–94.

Thio, I. M., Oakley Browne, M. A., Coverdale, J. H., *et al* (2006) Postnatal depressive symptoms largely go untreated. *Social Psychiatry and Psychiatric Epidemiology*, **41**, 814–818.

Thoppil, J., Riutcel, T. L. & Nalesnik, S. W. (2005) Early intervention for perinatal depression. *American Journal of Obstetrics and Gynecology*, **192**, 1446–1448.

Tully, L., Garcia, J., Davidson, L., *et al* (2002) Role of midwives in depression screening. *British Journal of Midwifery*, **10**, 374–378.

US Preventive Service Task Force (2002) Screening for depression: recommendations and rationale. *Annals of Internal Medicine*, **136**, 760–764.

Wehr, T. A. (1989) Sleep loss: a preventable cause of mania and other excited states. *Journal of Clinical Psychiatry*, **50(Suppl.)**, 8–16.

Whitton, A., Warner, R. & Appleby, L. (1996) The pathway to care in post-natal depression: women's attitudes to postnatal depression and its treatment. *British Journal of General Practice*, **46**, 427–428.

Whooley, M. A., Avins, A. L., Miranda, J., *et al* (1997) Case-finding instruments for depression. Two questions are as good as many. *Journal of General Internal Medicine*, **12**, 439–445.

Wiley, C. C., Burke, G. S., Gill, P. A., *et al* (2004) Paediatricians' views of postpartum depression: a self-administered survey. *Archives of Women's Mental Health*, **7**, 231–236.

Wisner, K. L., Perel, J. M., Peindl, K. S., *et al* (2001) Prevention of recurrent postpartum depression: a randomized clinical trial. *Journal of Clinical Psychiatry*, **62**, 82–86.

Wisner, K. L., Perel, J. M., Peindl, K. S., *et al* (2004) Prevention of postpartum depression: a pilot randomized clinical trial. *American Journal of Psychiatry*, **161**, 1290–1292.

Wissow, L. S., Roter, D. L. & Wilson, M. E. H. (1994) Pediatrician interview style and mother's disclosure of psychosocial issues. *Pediatrics*, **93**, 289–295.

Further reading

Dennis, C. L. & Chung-Lee, L. (2006) Postpartum depression help-seeking barriers and maternal treatment preferences: a qualitative systematic review. *Birth*, **33**, 323–331.

Resources

For details of how to obtain the EPDS, the ALPHA scale, the PDSS and 'How Are You Feeling?' booklets, please see Appendices III and IV.

CHAPTER 8

Physical treatments during pregnancy

Given the substantial psychiatric morbidity during pregnancy described in Chapters 2 and 4, it is clear that many women will need drug treatment or other physical treatments during pregnancy either because non-pharmacological interventions have failed or because there is no alternative. However, only about a third of women with depression during pregnancy appear to receive any treatment (Flynn *et al*, 2006). A large population study in the Netherlands reported that 2% of pregnant women were taking antidepressants in the first trimester, most commonly fluoxetine and paroxetine (Ververs *et al*, 2006). Similar rates are found in Germany, but rates in the USA rose from 5.7% in 1999 to 13.4% in 2003 (Cooper *et al*, 2007) and were reported at almost 8% in 2004 and 2005 (Andrade *et al*, 2008). Women with severe mental illness are more likely to be taking more than one drug (mode=3) with more than a quarter taking six to ten drugs over the course of their pregnancy (Peindl *et al*, 2007).

There are a number of factors to be taken into consideration in the risk–benefit analysis, not least the impact of untreated psychiatric disorder on the foetus. The risks associated with untreated depression (adverse neonatal outcomes, maternal morbidity including suicidal ideas and attempts) were reviewed by Bonari *et al* (2004) who concluded:

> 'When making clinical decisions, clinicians should weigh the growing body of literature suggesting potential adverse effects of untreated depression during pregnancy against the literature that has failed to find risks with *in utero* antidepressant exposure.'

Readers should note that the evidence base in this area is changing rapidly and specialist drug information services should be contacted for an update before treating a pregnant woman. The following are general principles to be considered.

- Each case should have a careful risk–benefit assessment considering all aspects of maternal and foetal well-being.
- If the disorder is mild to moderate in severity, use a non-pharmacological intervention.

- Avoid first-trimester exposure if at all possible.
- Use the lowest effective dose for the shortest time.
- Tricyclics (amitriptyline, imipramine and nortriptyline) are the antidepressants of choice.
- If an SSRI is indicated, fluoxetine is the drug of choice.
- High-potency drugs (haloperidol, trifluoperazine) are the antipsychotics of choice.
- Avoid new depot medication; however, it is not usually necessary to discontinue depots if pregnancy occurs during established treatment but the woman should be warned about possible extrapyramidal side-effects in the infant.
- Avoid polypharmacy if at all possible, whether concurrently or sequentially.
- Consider whether medication should be tapered or withdrawn before delivery and when to reinstate afterwards after careful risk assessment.

Cohen *et al* (2006) demonstrated that 68% of women who discontinued antidepressants during pregnancy relapsed during pregnancy compared with 26% who maintained their medication, a fivefold increased risk. In addition, some childhood problems, for example internalising behaviours (depression, anxiety and withdrawal) in 4–5-year-old children are not associated with psychotropic medications being used during pregnancy but are linked to impaired maternal mood (Misri *et al*, 2006).

The potential risks of drugs include maternal and infant toxicity, side-effects or withdrawal symptoms and foetal teratogenicity both physical and behavioural. This must be balanced against the risk of not treating the mental disorder, which might result in adverse outcomes either as a direct consequence of the disorder or as a result of behaviours associated with the condition in question. For example, smoking or drug misuse, reduced self-care, poor attendance at antenatal appointments or deliberate self-harm are all associated with maternal mental illness.

In addition, pregnancy physiology may change drug pharmacokinetics (Table 8.1). The prescriber must be aware of this as changes to the dose or dosage schedule may be required and may need to be changed again at various stages during pregnancy and after delivery. For example, higher doses might be needed during pregnancy to achieve therapeutic serum levels if metabolism increases during pregnancy, but these may need to be reduced rapidly after delivery to avoid toxicity when pharmacokinetics rapidly return to the pre-pregnant state.

US Food and Drug Administration classification

The US Food and Drug Administration classifies drugs according to the risk they pose when given during pregnancy. Five categories range from A (controlled studies in humans show no risk) to D (positive evidence of risk;

Table 8.1   Pregnancy pharmacockinetics

Pregnancy physiology	Consequences
Increased absorption	Delayed gastric emptying
	Longer intestinal transit times
Reduced absorption	Reduced blood flow to legs in late pregnancy may reduce absorption of intramuscular drugs
Increased volume of distribution of psychotropics	Increased plasma volume
	Increased extracellular fluid
Serum lipids may compete for protein-binding sites and alter unbound drug concentrations	Increased body fat
Metabolism tissue delivery increased	Up to 50% increase in cardiac output but less of the output goes to the liver as it is diverted to the uterus
	Increased activity of CP450 and CYP3A4 but decreased CYP1A2 activity
Excretion can be increased	Increased renal blood flow
	Increased glomerular filtration rate
Increased constipation Lowered blood pressure exacerbating orthostatic hypotension	Side-effects might be worsened

See Jeffries & Bochner (1988).

human data show risk; benefits may outweigh risk) and X (contraindicated in pregnancy). Most tricyclics fall into category C (risk cannot be ruled out; human data lacking; animal studies positive or not done) and most of the SSRIs are in category B (no evidence of risk to humans; human data is reassuring; animal positive or positive or animal studies show no risk). The majority of antipsychotics are in category C, whereas mood stabilisers are in category D.

Routes of foetal exposure

Placental transfer

Psychotropics cross the placenta. Hostetter *et al* (2000*a*) reported three pregnant women treated with fluvoxamine, sertraline or venlafaxine. All three antidepressants and the metabolites of sertraline and venlafaxine were found in umbilical cord blood. A larger study examined umbilical cord blood samples in 38 women immediately after delivery. They had been taking citalopram, fluoxetine, paroxetine or sertraline. Both antidepressants and metabolites were detectable in 86.8% of umbilical cord samples with mean ratios of cord:maternal serum levels between 0.29 and 0.89. The lowest ratios were for sertraline and paroxetine. Maternal doses of sertraline and fluoxetine were correlated with umbilical cord blood sample concentrations

(Hendrick *et al*, 2003*a*). Rampono *et al* (2004) found the following cord:maternal concentration ratios: fluoxetine, 0.67; norfluoxetine, 0.72; sertraline, 0.63; desmethylsertraline, 0.63; paroxetine, 0.52; venlafaxine, 1.1; and O-desmethylvenlafaxine, 1.0.

Heikkinen *et al* (2002) found infant plasma levels of citalopram, desmethylcitalopram and didesmethylcitalopram which were 64%, 66% and 68% of maternal plasma concentrations respectively.

Amniotic fluid

Amniotic fluid reaches the foetus via several routes: inhalation into the respiratory tract, swallowing and possibly by transcutaneous absorption. The amount of amniotic fluid swallowed by the foetus increases as pregnancy progresses. Hostetter *et al* (2000*a*) found fluvoxamine and venlafaxine in the amniotic fluid but sertraline was below the level of detection of the assay. Metabolites of all three compounds were present. Loughhead *et al* (2006) examined the amniotic fluid of 27 women who were being treated with SSRIs and venlafaxine and undergoing amniocentesis for obstetric reasons. They found antidepressant concentrations were very variable with mean concentrations in amniotic fluid 11.6% of those in maternal serum. The highest ratios were for venlafaxine (172%) but the amniotic fluid:maternal serum ratio of metabolites was not consistent.

Risks to the foetus

In addition to routes of exposure, the clinician must consider the different types of potential risk to the foetus:

- intrauterine death
- risk of teratogenesis and organ malformation
- growth impairment
- risk of neonatal toxicity or withdrawal syndromes after delivery
- risk of long-term neurobehavioural sequelae.

The presence of other potential teratogens that might act in an additive or synergistic way must also be taken into account. These include non-prescribed drugs, herbal and homeopathic remedies, smoking and environmental toxins. A study examining the use of complementary therapies by pregnant women found that 87% reported using them (mega-vitamins, herbs, massage, aromatherapy and yoga) and viewed them as safe and effective (Gaffney & Smith, 2004). However, this should not be assumed.

Intrauterine death

Exposure to a teratogen before 2 weeks of gestation is likely to result in a non-viable 'blighted ovum'. Drugs taken later in pregnancy may cause miscarriage or stillbirth.

Teratogenesis and organ malformation

A drug is considered to be teratogenic if exposure during pregnancy raises the risk of congenital physical malformations over the baseline level of birth defects which is 2–4%. The period of maximum vulnerability is 3–12 weeks. The heart and great vessels are formed between 5 and 10 weeks after the last menstrual period, the lip and palate between 8 and 24 weeks, and the neural tube folds and closes around 5–6 weeks after. As around half of all conceptions in the UK are unplanned and most women do not learn of their pregnancy until around 6 weeks of gestation, exposure has often already happened when pregnancy is discovered.

Withdrawal syndromes and toxicity

Some drugs, having readily crossed the placenta, produce toxicity in the neonate as their immature metabolism may be unable to process the drug, leading to accumulation. Alternatively, there may be withdrawal symptoms in the infant following delivery as levels of the drug fall rapidly after birth.

Women's perceptions of drugs

Women taking antidepressants often discontinue them, fearing risk to their foetus. In one study, 87% of women taking antidepressants rated their risk of teratogenicity as greater than 1–3% (Bonari *et al*, 2004). Despite receiving reassuring information via counselling, 15% chose to stop taking them, saying that the first person they spoke to had advised discontinuation. The women sought information from multiple sources and there was often some time lapse between diagnosis and starting treatment that was not observed in the control groups on gastrointestinal or antibiotic drugs.

The manner in which the media report issues relating to drug exposure during pregnancy can give rise to great anxiety and lead to discontinuation of medication even when that has not been the core media message (Einarson *et al*, 2005). It is clear that perception of risk and decision-making are complex issues. Wisner *et al* (2000) describe a model that provides a structure for the decision-making process and give case examples in relation to depression.

Drugs

Tricyclic antidepressants

First-trimester exposure

Early reports suggested an association between tricyclics and limb reduction deformities. However, a systematic review of first-trimester exposure studies up to 1995 involving 414 women failed to indicate an association between exposure to tricyclics and increased rates of congenital malformations, concluding that they are relatively safe (Altshuler *et al*, 1996).

McElhatton *et al* (1996) examined outcomes in 689 women of whom 330 had taken tricyclics during pregnancy. The incidence of congenital malformations, spontaneous abortions and late foetal deaths was within the expected range for the general population. Long-term therapy (usually in association with other drugs) was associated with neonatal withdrawal symptoms. There was no increase in the rate of congenital malformations in the prospective study carried out by Ericson *et al* (1999) in which 390 women were taking tricyclics (the majority clomipramine). Simon *et al* (2002) also found no association between tricyclic exposure and malformations or adverse perinatal outcomes in 209 infants.

More recently, a Swedish study (Källen & Otterblad Olausson, 2006) examined the rate of congenital cardiac defects in the infants of 6896 women who had taken antidepressants during pregnancy. Nineteen per cent had taken tricyclics. They found an increased risk of ventricular or atrial septal defects with clomipramine (OR=2.11).

Obstetric and neonatal outcomes

Källen (2004) found an increased risk of preterm birth (OR=1.96), low birth weight (OR=1.98), respiratory distress (OR=2.21), a low APGAR score (OR=2.33), neonatal convulsions (OR=1.90) and hypoglycaemia (OR 1.62), particularly after tricyclic exposure. Davis *et al* (2007) reported an increase in preterm delivery risk, respiratory distress, endocrine and metabolic disorders, and temperature regulation problems.

One study revealed a rate of miscarriage in those exposed to tricyclics when compared with controls (Pastuzak *et al*, 1993) and a more recent meta-analysis of cohort studies from 1966 to 2003 found a miscarriage rate of 12.4% in women taking antidepressants (all classes), a relative risk of 1.45. However, depression itself might have contributed to this increase (Hemels *et al*, 2005).

Dose requirements appear to increase during the second half of pregnancy to 1.3–2 times the non-pregnant dose (Wisner *et al*, 1993). This increased clearance rapidly returns to normal levels by the end of the second postpartum week. Nortriptyline serum levels have been shown to rise in the early postpartum weeks despite stable dosing. This is due to an apparent refractoriness in its processing which continues until 6–8 weeks after delivery (Wisner *et al*, 1997). Cholestasis has been reported in association with dothiepin (Milkiewicz *et al*, 2003).

Neonatal withdrawal symptoms have been observed when tricyclics have been used in the third trimester and it is often suggested that a gradual taper and discontinuation before delivery is undertaken. However, women who require tricyclics in late pregnancy are likely to be those most at risk of recurrence or worsening of symptoms postpartum, so discontinuation may not be the most appropriate strategy (Altshuler *et al*, 1996) and each individual case requires careful assessment before deciding on tapering. There are also case reports of symptoms (respiratory distress, hypotonia and jitteriness) correlating with serum drug levels, suggesting toxicity (e.g. Schimmell *et al*, 1991).

Long-term neurodevelopmental outcomes

Follow-up studies of exposed infants at 5–86 months of age revealed no effect of tricyclics on global IQ, language development or behaviour (Nulman *et al*, 1997, 2002).

Selective serotonin reuptake inhibitors

Pharmacokinetics

A study tracking fluoxetine and norfluoxetine during pregnancy and after delivery observed low trough samples during pregnancy on doses from 20 to 40 mg/day and mean norfluoxetine/fluoxetine ratios in late pregnancy 2.4 times higher than at 2 months after delivery. This may be partly due to increased demethylation by cytochrome P450 2D6 (CYP2D6) and could mean that the dose has to be increased to achieve therapeutic benefit (Heikkinen *et al*, 2003). Sit *et al* (2008) report similar findings for citalopram, escitalopram and sertraline. Hostetter *et al* (2000*b*) followed 34 women on SSRIs throughout pregnancy. Two-thirds required dose increases to maintain euthymia and the increases tended to occur in the early part of the third trimester. Doses at delivery were around 1.86 times higher than the initial dose. Kim *et al* (2006) observed that umbilical vein fluoxetine and norfluoxetine concentrations at birth were 65% and 72% of maternal concentrations respectively.

First-trimester exposure

In 2000, a meta-analysis of first-trimester exposure to fluoxetine covering studies published between 1988 and 1996 and involving 367 women, concluded that there was no evidence that fluoxetine caused an increase in the rate of congenital malformations (Addis & Koren, 2000). Subsequent to this, Kulin *et al* (1998) reported no increased incidence of malformations in the infants of 267 women exposed to fluvoxamine, paroxetine or sertraline, and Ericson *et al* (1999) also found no increase in malformations in over 500 women, of whom 375 were taking citalopram.

Only 1 out of 108 infants was born with major malformations from a cohort of mothers with first-trimester exposure to citalopram (Sivojelezova *et al*, 2005). Simon *et al* (2002) also found no association between SSRIs and congenital malformations, as did Hendrick *et al* (2003*b*). In the series reported by Yaris *et al* (2005), 74 women were taking SSRIs (some with other drugs). One woman taking fluoxetine had a miscarriage. Alwan *et al* (2005) report an increased rate of craniosynostosis (OR=1.8) and omphalocele in infants exposed to SSRIs (OR=3.0), but a meta-analysis by Einarson & Einarson (2005) again concluded that SSRIs do not increase the rate of malformations. This was also confirmed by a Finnish population study which concluded that other than an increased risk of admission to a neonatal unit with third-trimester exposure (OR=1.6), SSRIs did not increase the risk of malformations, preterm birth, small-for-gestational-age or low-birth-weight infants (Malm *et al*, 2005). A Danish population-based study, however, did find an increased risk of malformations with an adjusted relative risk of 1.34 for exposure any time during early pregnancy and 1.84 for exposure during the second and third months. The association was not specific to any particular malformation (Wogelius *et al*, 2006).

Källen & Otterblad Olausson (2006) found an increased risk of cardiac malformations with paroxetine (OR=2.22), as did Diav-Citrin *et al* (2005*a*). Alwan *et al* (2005) found that paroxetine accounted for 36% of the SSRI exposures in omphalocele cases (OR=6.30). Hence, the manufacturer revised the pregnancy sub-section of the product information in October 2005 and advised prescribing paroxetine to a pregnant woman only 'if the potential benefit outweighs the potential risk' (Dollow, 2006). Louik *et al* (2007) observed an association between sertraline and omphalocele (OR=5.7) and septal defects (OR=2.0), and between right ventricular outflow tract obstruction and paroxetine exposure.

Two meta-analyses have now been conducted. The first (Rahimi *et al*, 2006) included studies conducted between 1990 and 2005 and concluded that there was no increase in congenital malformations but the risk of spontaneous abortion was significantly increased. Bar-Oz *et al* (2007) included studies published between 1985 and 2006, concluding that paroxetine was associated with a significant increase in cardiac malformations (OR=4.11) but could not rule out a detection bias.

Some of the conflicting evidence in these studies might relate to the fact that there does appear to be a dose–response relationship between paroxetine and malformations with OR=2.23 for a major malformation and OR=3.07 for a cardiac malformation if the dose was above 25 mg/day during the first trimester (Bérard *et al*, 2007). Odds ratios also appear to be higher for polytherapy involving paroxetine compared with paroxetine monotherapy (Cole *et al*, 2007). The most recent study to compare rates of cardiac defects following first-trimester exposure to paroxetine (>3000 infants) with an unexposed cohort found the rate of cardiac congenital malformations to be similar to the population incidence (Einarson *et al*, 2008), and another study identified that exposure to both SSRIs and benzodiazepines is associated with congenital heart defects, whereas SSRI monotherapy was only associated with atrial septal defects (Oberlander *et al*, 2008*a*).

The duration of exposure to antidepressants does not appear to be associated with an increased risk of major congenital malformations (Ramos *et al*, 2008).

Obstetric and neonatal complications

Cholestasis has been reported in association with both citalopram and paroxetine (Milkiewicz *et al*, 2003). There is a case report of an infant with necrotising enterocolitis associated with exposure to escitalopram during pregnancy and breastfeeding (Potts *et al*, 2007). Chambers *et al* (1996) reported that infants exposed to fluoxetine in the third trimester had a higher incidence of preterm delivery (as did Davis *et al*, 2007), admission to neonatal units, poor neonatal adaptation and lower birth rate. Simon *et al* (2002) also reported an increase in preterm delivery following exposure to SSRIs and lower APGAR scores in third-trimester exposure. It is unclear whether this deceleration of weight gain is due to the antidepressant or depression. Bodnar *et al* (2006) describe a case in which poor maternal weight gain was associated with sertraline treatment commencing at 22 weeks gestation and outline the methods used to counteract this. However, there does not appear to be an increased risk of postpartum haemorrhage (Salkeld *et al*, 2008).

Chambers *et al* (2006) found an increased risk of persistent pulmonary hypertension in newborns of mothers exposed to SSRIs after 20 weeks gestation compared with the rate in matched controls. This condition has a mortality rate of 10–20%. The relative risk was 6 but the absolute risk only 0.5%. Other antidepressants had lower risks compared with controls. The mechanism is not known.

In contrast, Cohen *et al* (2000) found no difference in gestational age, APGAR scores, or the timing of hospital-to-home discharge in infants born to mothers with late rather than early exposure to fluoxetine. Paroxetine use during the third trimester was associated with neonatal distress in a prospective controlled study (Costei *et al*, 2002). Suri *et al* (2004) found no adverse obstetric outcomes in 64 women with depression taking fluoxetine. Hendrick *et al* (2003*b*) also found no increase in neonatal complications but noted that the three women treated with high doses of fluoxetine (40–80 mg/day) had low-birth-weight infants. Zeskind & Stephens (2004) reported more activity and tremulousness, fewer changes in behavioural state and more rapid-eye-movement sleep. Lattimore *et al* (2005) pooled the above-mentioned studies in a meta-analysis and observed the following ORs: prematurity, 1.85; low birth weight, 3.64; neonatal unit admission, 3.30; and poor neonatal adaptation, 4.08.

Animal studies have shown transient decreases in uterine artery blood flow, foetal oxygen pressure, oxygen saturation and foetal PH, plus foetal carbon dioxide pressure increases with fluoxetine (Morrison *et al*, 2002). If repeated, this might provide one mechanism for poor outcomes.

Wen *et al* (2006) in a large population cohort reported low birth weight, preterm birth, foetal death, infant death, seizures and use of mechanical ventilation in infants exposed to paroxetine during pregnancy. There are case reports of neonatal subdural, intraventricular and subarachnoid haemorrhage associated with maternal SSRI use. Selective serotonin reuptake inhibition of platelet serotonin leading to decreased platelet aggregation is thought to be responsible, although it is not clear that SSRIs increase the rate of intracranial haemorrhage above the expected rate. Later in the same year, a large population study found exposure to SSRIs during pregnancy was associated with an increased risk of low birth weight and respiratory distress even when the severity of maternal depression was taken into account (Oberlander *et al*, 2006), and a prospective study identified that antidepressants (the majority of which were SSRIs) rather than antenatal depressive symptoms predicted lower gestational age and preterm delivery (Suri *et al*, 2007).

Case reports, case series and cohort studies have been reporting a neonatal behavioural syndrome associated with SSRI exposure in late pregnancy for several years. Moses-Kolko *et al* (2005) reviewed the literature and discussed the clinical implications. They concluded that the risk of a neonatal behavioural syndrome was 3.0 when compared with early gestational or no exposure, the risk of admission to a neonatal unit was 2.6 and of respiratory difficulty 2.3. The most commonly reported drugs involved were paroxetine and fluoxetine. The most common symptoms are (in decreasing order of frequency) irritability, hypertonia, jitteriness, difficulty feeding, tremor, agitation, seizures, tachypnoea and posturing. More rarely, seizures and electroencephalography abnormalities have been reported. It is not clear whether these phenomena are due to discontinuation syndrome or serotonin toxicity, although Knoppert *et al* (2006) report a case in which symptoms were correlated with high serum levels of paroxetine, suggesting the latter. Laine *et al* (2003) reported that neonates exposed to SSRIs had more serotonergic symptoms and that the severity of these symptoms was related to cord blood 5-hydroxyindoleacetic acid levels, and there is a case in which a neonate with two defective CYP2D6 alleles who was exposed to paroxetine in late pregnancy and experienced particularly severe adverse effects is described (Laine *et al*, 2004).

Nordeng & Spigset (2005) have also reviewed neonatal withdrawal syndrome and summarise the data relating to each individual drug. Oberlander *et al* (2004) observed that infants exposed to paroxetine alone or in combination with clonazepam were more likely to experience poor adaptation (respiratory distress) but noted higher maternal and infant plasma levels in the combined therapy group and an increased risk of neonatal symptoms than in the single therapy group, highlighting the need to consider all exposures and avoid polypharmacy if at all possible.

The syndrome is usually mild and self-limiting (e.g. a median duration of 3 days; Ferreira *et al*, 2007) and onsets within hours or days of birth. A French study observed the median onset as 1 day after delivery (Cissoko *et al*, 2005). A recent controlled study of full-term infants estimated the prevalence at 30% of those exposed to SSRIs *in utero* (Levinson-Castiel *et al*, 2006) and length of exposure rather than timing appears to be important (Oberlander *et al*, 2008*b*). Infants with serotonin transporter *SLC6A4* promoter genotype are more likely to experience respiratory distress and other adverse outcomes with SSRI exposure (Oberlander *et al*, 2008*c*)

Management is usually supportive care in a neonatal unit. More severe cases might need respiratory support, ventilation and fluid replacement or anticonvulsant therapy. Bot *et al* (2006) suggested a 3-day observation period for infants born to mothers who used SSRIs in the last trimester. Chlorpromazine has been used in cases of withdrawal from paroxetine (*n*=3) and fluoxetine (*n*=1) (Nordeng *et al*, 2001).

In order to prevent the neonatal behavioural syndrome it is suggested that SSRIs should be tapered off (or stopped in the case of fluoxetine) around 2 weeks before the expected date of delivery and resumed afterwards. The timing of delivery is hard to predict and there is a risk with tapering of precipitating an antenatal recurrence and/or increasing the risk of a postpartum depressive episode. There must be, therefore, a full risk–benefit analysis in vulnerable women. It should be noted that there are at present no data to indicate that tapering and discontinuing SSRIs prevents the neonatal syndrome. Sanz *et al* (2005) advise not to prescribe paroxetine to pregnant women and if this is not possible to use the lowest effective dose. Certainly, an infant delivered to a woman taking an SSRI must be closely monitored for adverse events and any that occur must be reported to the Medicines and Healthcare Products Regulatory Agency (see p. 201).

Long-term neurodevelopmental outcomes

Nulman *et al* (1997, 2002) reported no impact of *in utero* exposure to fluoxetine on outcomes such as global IQ, language development or behaviour. However, lower APGAR scores and lower scores on Bayley Psychomotor Development Index and the motor quality factor of the Bayley Behavioural Rating Scale have been found in non-exposed children compared with infants exposed to SSRIs (Casper *et al*, 2003). An attenuated response to heel prick pain has also been shown in infants with prenatal SSRI exposure compared with unexposed infants (Oberlander *et al*, 2005). Animal research has shown that early exposure to SSRIs produces selective behavioural changes in adult rats, including increased locomotor activity and decreased sexual behaviour (Macaig *et al*, 2005). This implies that early exposure to SSRIs disrupts the normal maturation of the serotonin system and could alter serotonin-dependent neuronal processes. It is not known whether these effects are also seen in humans but it is certainly possible that pregnancy exposure to SSRIs may have longer-term consequences. One small study has shown that exposure to SSRIs during foetal life led to reduced 5-HT uptake in infants (Anderson *et al*, 2004).

Conclusion

It does appear that there is a small increased risk of congenital malformations (particularly cardiac with paroxetine) with first-trimester exposure to SSRIs. There is also increasing evidence that there is an association with pregnancy exposure and withdrawal symptoms, and possibly a small reduction in gestational age. Hence, paroxetine is best avoided if possible, although if a woman becomes pregnant while taking it, a full risk–benefit analysis must be undertaken before switching or stopping medication.

Other antidepressants

Venlafaxine

Venlafaxine does not appear to increase the rate of congenital malformations above the base rate (Einarson *et al*, 2001; Yaris *et al*, 2004; Einarson & Einarson, 2005) and there does not appear to be any increased risk of obstetric complications. However, Einarson *et al* (2001) found a non-significant trend towards a higher rate of miscarriage in exposed pregnancies. There are reports of a withdrawal syndrome including restlessness, jitteriness, irritability, tremor, convulsions, hypotonia, hyperreflexia, diarrhoea, hypoglycaemia and poor feeding (e.g. Pakalapati *et al*, 2006). In one case, improvement was achieved by giving the infant 1 mg venlafaxine. The symptoms had ceased by the eighth day postpartum (de Moor *et al*, 2003). Yaris *et al* (2004) followed up, for 12 months, infants of 10 women who had taken venlafaxine and observed no congentital malformations or developmental delay. Klier *et al* (2007) report reduced bioavailability of venlafaxine across the three trimesters.

Mirtazapine

Mirtazapine is a piperazino-azepine with a tetracyclic structure and is not related to any other antidepressant. There are 169 published pregnancy exposures to mirtazapine at the time of writing.

The first study was of a woman who used mirtazapine only in the first month of pregnancy with a successful outcome (Simhandl *et al*, 1998). Two cases reported in 2002 by Kesim & Yaris resulted in one uneventful delivery and healthy infant, but the second infant was delivered at 39 weeks by Caesarean section for premature rupture of membranes and experienced neonatal hyperbilirubinaemia but did not require phototherapy. Yaris *et al* (2004) reported eight women who took mirtazapine during pregnancy. There were no adverse outcomes in seven, but one woman (who also took alprazolam, diazepam and nefazodone) miscarried.

Out of 13 554 women in a prescription event-monitoring study of mirtazapine, 41 became pregnant. Of these, 8 experienced miscarriages, 8 had the pregnancy terminated and 24 had live births of which 4 were preterm. One of these infants had a patent ductus arteriosus. The outcome of another pregnancy was not known (Biswas *et al*, 2003). Three papers report the use of mirtazapine in the treatment of hyperemesis gravidarum in a total of 11 women, 1 woman with a twin pregnancy (Saks, 2001; Rohde *et al*, 2003; Guclu *et al*, 2005). Djulus *et al* (2006) carried out a prospective study with two comparison groups: disease-matched pregnant women diagnosed with depression taking other antidepressants and pregnant women exposed to non-teratogens. There were 77 live births, 1 stillbirth, 20 miscarriages, 6 therapeutic abortions and 2 major malformations in the mirtazapine group. The mean birth weight was 3335 g (s.d. = 654) and the mean gestational age at delivery was 38.9

weeks (s.d.=2.5). Most (95%) of the women took mirtazapine in the first trimester, but only 25% of the women took it throughout pregnancy. The rate of miscarriage was higher in both antidepressant groups (19% in the mirtazapine group and 17% in the other antidepressant group) than in the non-teratogen group (11%), but none of the differences were statistically significant. The rate of preterm births was also higher in the mirtazapine group (10%) and in the other antidepressant group (7%) than in the non-teratogen group (2%). The difference was statistically significant between the mirtazapine group and the non-teratogen group ($P=0.04$). The most recent report is that of monozygotic twins whose mother was treated with mirtazapine throughout pregnancy and who presented with recurrent hypothermia unattributable to other causes (Sokolover *et al*, 2008).

Nefazodone

The limited data available ($n=89$, Einarson *et al*, 2003; $n=2$, Yaris *et al*, 2004; $n=2$, Yaris *et al*, 2005) have shown no increase in the rates of malformations or complications. This drug has been discontinued in the UK but may still be available elsewhere.

Buproprion

A controlled study following up 136 women taking buproprion for depression after smoking cessation found no increase in congenital malformations and a miscarriage rate similar to that of other antidepressants (Chan *et al*, 2005). One review notes that the manufacturer has a register containing over 400 prospectively monitored pregnancies with a possible increase in the rate of malformations, mostly cardiac, and that there are other case studies yet to be published (Anonymous, 2005).

Trazodone

In the 58 cases of trazodone exposure reported by Einarson *et al* (2003) there was no increase in the rate of congenital malformations.

Monoamine oxidase inhibitors

There are animal studies reporting an association between monoamine oxidase inhibitors (MAOIs) and foetal growth retardation (Poulson & Robson, 1964), and results from a small case series of women treated with phenelzine and tranylcypromine during pregnancy found a higher rate of abnormalities than would be expected (Heinonen, *et al*, 1977). In addition, the diet has to be adhered to and the possibility of hypertensive crisis during pregnancy or labour indicate that they should be avoided if at all possible, particularly if an operative delivery is likely, as MAOIs interact with several anaesthetic agents. Gracious & Wisner (1997) report the successful treatment of a woman with depression with phenelzine throughout pregnancy and delivery.

Moclobemide

There is one case report of an uneventful pregnancy and delivery of a healthy infant in a women exposed to moclobemide during pregnancy (Rybakowski, 2001), and of seven women exposed to the drug in a report by Yaris *et al* (2005). One of these women took moclobemide in conjunction with amitriptyline and had a preterm delivery.

Reboxetine

Hackett *et al* (2006*a*) reported outcomes for four women who took reboxetine during pregnancy. One infant out of the four had developmental problems unrelated to reboxetine, the others met normal developmental milestones and there were no adverse events.

Duloxetine

There are no published data on the safety of duloxetine in pregnancy.

St John's wort

Several animal studies report no toxicity or impact on development of mice or rats exposed to St John's wort during prenatal life (Cada *et al*, 2001; Rayburn *et al*, 2001*a*, 2001*b*; Borges *et al*, 2005) but an uncontrolled study reported hepatic and renal damage in rats exposed during pregnancy and breastfeeding (Gregoretti *et al*, 2004). It would seem prudent, therefore, to avoid St John's wort exposure during pregnancy until sufficient controlled human data exist to be certain there are no increased risks. Dougoua *et al* (2006), on systematically reviewing the evidence, concluded that 'caution is warranted until further research is conducted' and pointed out that when used concomitantly with other medications metabolised by CYP450 their serum levels may be reduced. Einarson *et al* (2000) note that although doctors are very reluctant to recommend St John's wort to pregnant patients, 49% of women surveyed taking naturopathic medicine felt comfortable doing so. Pregnant women should therefore be asked routinely whether or not they are taking any herbal remedies.

Anxiolytics and hypnotics

Benzodiazepines

Dolovitch *et al* (1998) carried out a systematic review and meta-analysis of 23 studies examining major malformations and, in particular, oral clefts in infants exposed to benzodiazepines during the first trimester. They found that pooled data from cohort studies revealed no association between foetal exposure to benzodiazepines and major malformations or oral clefts. However, when they pooled data from case–control studies, there appeared to be an increased risk of major malformations or oral cleft. Only pregnancies resulting in live or stillbirths were included in the review and not those that were terminated. Pregnancies may have been terminated because of first-trimester exposure, in which case this review would underestimate the risk.

However, Khan *et al* (1999) undertook a logistic regression, which revealed that the case–control studies exaggerated the OR for the risk of exposure by 55% and concluded that there is no association. Since then, a large population-based case–control study involving 22 865 women taking benzodiazepines and 38 151 controls again found no excess of congenital malformations (Eros *et al*, 2002). McElhatton (1994) compiled a comprehensive review of benzodiazepines in relation to pregnancy and lactation. However, a recent analysis of the French Central-East registry of congenital malformation data 1976–1997 found no increased rate of malformations with benzodiazepine use as a group but when analysed by individual drug, lorazepam was found to be associated with anal atresia with an OR of 6.2 (Bonnot *et al*, 2003).

If a pregnant woman is exposed to benzodiazepines, an ultrasound scan at 20 weeks should be performed to detect any oral or palatal clefts and other anomalies.

Benzodiazepines are thought to be responsible for two major neonatal complications if prescribed in the last trimester of pregnancy. The first of these is neonatal withdrawal in which hypertonia, hyperreflexia, feeding difficulties, restlessness, irritability, with abnormal sleep patterns, poor suckling, bradycardia, apnoea and an increased incidence of low APGAR scores have been reported, particularly where benzodiazepines have been given during labour.

The second is floppy infant syndrome. This includes tremors, hyperactivity, hypothermia, lethargy and feeding problems. Infants do not appear to have long-lasting sequelae of either syndrome and usually recover in a few weeks. A French study of benzodiazepine use in the last month of pregnancy found 51% of infants developed adverse reactions. Hypotonia was reported in 42% and neonatal withdrawal in 20%, with tremulousness the most common symptom (Swortfiguer *et al*, 2005).

Advice is, therefore, to keep to the lowest possible dose and shortest possible time, and to avoid if possible or decrease the dose in late pregnancy and before delivery to reduce the risk of neonatal withdrawal and floppy infant syndrome.

Benzodiazepine receptor agonists

There are very few human data evaluating the safety of zopiclone, zolpidem and zaleplon in pregnancy. The Toronto Motherisk Program have reported 40 cases of first-trimester exposure to zopiclone finding no increase in congenital malformations or complications compared with a control group (Diav-Citrin *et al*, 1999). There are reports of hepatotoxicity associated with zolpidem in adults (Karsenti *et al*, 1999) and a structurally similar drug was withdrawn as a result. There should, therefore, be raised awareness of the possibility of hepatotoxicity if a pregnant woman is exposed to zolpidem.

The initial management of a pregnant woman with sleep problems should be advice regarding sleep hygiene such as bedtime routine, avoiding caffeine and reducing activity before sleep, and only if this fails or the problem is severe and chronic should low-dose chlorpromazine or amitriptyline be used.

Buspirone

There are no human data in the literature regarding the safety of buspirone in pregnancy.

Antipsychotics

Typical antipsychotics have been in use for over 40 years and the use of atypicals is increasing; yet a Cochrane review failed to find any trial data comparing any antipsychotics with any other with respect to maternal or foetal/infant outcomes (Webb *et al*, 2004). Hence, there is a very limited evidence base on which to advise practitioners.

Typical antipsychotics

Phenothiazines

Altshuler *et al* (1996) undertook a meta-analysis of the effects of first-trimester low-potency phenothiazines on pregnancy outcomes. The pooled results of the five English language studies between 1966 and 1995 (many of the women studied had hyperemesis gravidarum) resulted in an OR ratio for congenital malformation of 1.21 – a small but significant risk. However, phenothiazines do not appear to be related to any specific abnormality.

A records review carried out by the French National Institute of Health examined 12 764 births (Godet & Marie-Cardine, 1999). The rate of congenital malformations was 1.6% in the whole population and 3.5% in those infants exposed to phenothiazines. Although this was a significant difference, the study did not control for maternal age, so it may not necessarily be a drug effect. The same paper reported no increase in the rate of malformations in children born to 199 mothers with schizophrenia (2.5%) when all medications were grouped together; however, when considered separately, the risk was higher with haloperidol and lowest with phenothiazines. There was an increased incidence of prematurity in the whole sample of 12.3% compared with 5.6% in the general population (Godet & Marie-Cardine, 1991).

There are reports of cholestatic liver disease and ductopaenia associated with pregnancy use of chlorpromazine (e.g. Moradpour *et al*, 1994; Chlumska *et al*, 2001), neonatal fever and cyanotic spells (Ben-Amitai & Merlob, 1991) and extrapyramidal symptoms in exposed infants (e.g. Levy & Wisniewski, 1974). One infant who was exposed to chlorpromazine and lithium is reported to have had 'neurologic depression' for the first 9 days of life (Nielson *et al*, 1983). The use of depot medication may result in more persistent adverse events. For example, an infant exposed to both chlorpromazine and fluphenazine decanoate experienced neurological symptoms for 9 months (O'Connor *et al*, 1981).

Two studies found normal cognitive and emotional development in a total of 118 children exposed to chlorpromazine during foetal life (Kris *et al*, 1965; Stika *et al*, 1990).

Butyrophenones

Haloperidol is reported to have a placental passage ratio of 65.5% (Newport *et al*, 2007). Early case reports suggested an association between first-trimester exposure to haloperidol and limb deformities. However, controlled studies of antipsychotics used for pregnancy emesis found no increase in abnormalities, and more recently a multicentre prospective controlled study comparing the outcomes in 219 women exposed to haloperidol (*n*=188) or penfluridol (*n*=27) found no difference in the rate of congenital anomalies between the exposed group and controls (Diav-Citrin *et al*, 2005*b*). There was an increased rate of preterm birth and lower birth weights in the exposed group. There were two cases of limb defects in the haloperidol/penfluridol group and the authors could not rule out an association because of the sample size. They advise that any pregnancy exposed to butyrophenones in the first trimester should have a Level II ultrasound performed with emphasis on the limbs.

Other reported adverse events related to maternal haloperidol include severe hypothermia in an infant who was also exposed to benztropine (Mohan *et al*, 2000) and dyskinetic symptoms (Collins & Comer, 2003). There is a case report of thrombocytosis persisting for 3 months in the infant of a woman treated with haloperidol, biperiden, promethazine hydrochloride, nitrazepam and chlorpromazine (Nako *et al*, 2001).

A woman who, at 34 weeks gestation, took an overdose of 300 mg haloperidol (Hansen *et al*, 1997) became unresponsive and experienced an extrapyramidal reaction but recovered within 48 h. On admission there was no foetal movement or 'breathing' and the heart rate was non-reactive. The foetal biophysical profile returned to normal 5 days after admission. Pregnancy-induced hypertension and oligohydramnios were detected at 39 weeks, labour was induced and a healthy infant delivered.

One study followed up the children (until age seven) of mothers who took a variety of typical antipsychotics (Platt *et al*, 1988). Children aged seven who had been exposed for more than 2 months *in utero* were 3 cm taller than controls but shorter at 4 months of age.

Diphenylbutylpiperadines

Published data are limited to one case report of a woman with Tourette syndrome and obsessive–compulsive disorder who took pimozide and fluoxetine during pregnancy until pimozide was withdrawn 2 weeks prior to delivery. A healthy male infant was born (Bjarnason *et al*, 2006).

189

Atypical antipsychotics

Placental passage rates for atypical antipsychotics appear to be highest for olanzapine, followed by haloperidol, risperidone and quetiapine (Newport *et al*, 2007). A recent small study observed a significantly higher incidence of large-for-gestational-age infants when exposed to atypical antipsychotics ($n=25$) compared with typical antipsychotics ($n=45$) and a control group exposed to non-teratogens ($n=38$) (Newham *et al*, 2008).

Olanzapine

Most of the data are in relation to olanzapine and clozapine. Olanzapine is reported to have the highest placental passage ratio (compared with haloperidol, risperidone and quetiapine) at 72.1% (Newport *et al*, 2007). Goldstein *et al* (2000) reported all the known cases of exposure to olanzapine up to October 1998. Of the prospectively identified pregnancies ($n=37$), 14 were aborted (with no foetal anomaly detected), 13% of the remainder ended in miscarriage (the expected rate in controls is 15%) and there were no malformations in the remaining 20. There was one stillbirth at 37 weeks gestation in a case complicated by drug misuse, hepatitis and gestational diabetes. The authors also identified retrospectively reported cases ($n=11$). The two anomalies found in this group (Down syndrome and unilateral renal atresia) were not attributed to olanzapine. A further paper extended the available information on prospectively identified cases to 96 cases of exposure to olanzapine (Ernst & Goldberg, 2002). The rate of major malformations in the olanzapine-exposed group was 8.3%.

Since then there have been several case reports of successful outcomes with healthy infants where mothers have taken olanzapine and others where problems have occurred (e.g. hypertension, gestational diabetes and pre-eclampsia) but it is not known whether olanzapine was a contributor (Littrell *et al*, 2000). In 2005, McKenna *et al* reported 151 pregnancy outcomes in women exposed to atypicals ($n=60$ olanzapine; $n=49$ risperidone; $n=36$ quetiapine; $n=6$ clozapine) and pregnant controls who were not. The only outcome that was statistically significantly different between the two groups was an increased risk of low birth weight (10% *v.* 2%) in the exposed group. There was no difference in the rates of malformations, miscarriage, gestational age, stillbirth or neonatal distress. Others have reported increased rates of low birth weight and neonatal unit admission with olanzapine (Newport *et al*, 2007) and there have been case reports of a large-for-gestational-age infant with Erb's palsy (Friedman & Rosenthal (2003), developmental dysplasia of the hip (Spyropoulos *et al*, 2006), meningocoele and ankyloblepharon (Arora & Prahaj, 2006), and atrioventricular canal defect and club foot (Yeshayahu, 2007). One case report of a woman who took an overdose of 112.5 mg olanzapine at 16 weeks gestation and continued to take it along with oxazepam reported no adverse events (Dervaux *et al*, 2007).

Quetiapine

There are five case reports in the literature documenting pregnancy exposure to quetiapine with successful outcomes in four (Tényi *et al*, 2002; Taylor *et al*, 2003; Yaris *et al*, 2004; Çabuk *et al*, 2007) and neonatal jitteriness (but normal development until 1 year of age) in the fifth (Klier *et al*, 2007). McKenna *et al* (2005) reported 36 women exposed to quetiapine with no reports of congenital malformations. A post-marketing surveillance study reported six pregnancies, five with first-trimester-only exposure (Twaites *et al*, 2007). There were no malformations in the five live births. Newport *et al* (2007) report a placental passage ratio in 21 women taking quetiapine of 24.1%, siginifically lower than that for haloperidol and risperidone, and Klier *et al* (2007) observed reduced bioavailability of quetiapine across the three trimesters of pregnancy.

Risperidone

Nine pregnancies exposed to risperidone were reported in a post-marketing study of over 7000 patients (Mackay *et al*, 1998). These resulted in seven live births, two terminations of pregnancy and no congenital abnormalities.

There is a report of exaggerated hypotension during a spinal anaesthetic for Caesarean section in a woman who was taking risperidone which has α_1-adrenergic antagonistic properties (Williams & Hepner, 2004). There is a case report of an uncomplicated pregnancy and successful delivery where the mother was taking risperidone long term (Ratnayake & Libretto, 2002), while McKenna *et al* (2005) studied 49 women with no reported malformations. The most recently published and largest post-marketing study identified 713 pregnancies exposed to risperidone (Coppola *et al*, 2007). Of 68 prospectively reported exposures with known outcomes there were malformations in 3.8% and spontaneous abortions in 16.9%, similar to general population rates. Twelve of the retrospectively reported pregnancies involved malformations and there were 37 with perinatal syndromes, including 21 with possible withdrawal syndrome. Risperidone has been reported to have a placental passage ratio of 49.2% (Newport *et al*, 2007).

There are two case reports of women managed on long-acting injectable risperidone throughout pregnancy with no maternal or infant adverse events (Dabbert & Heinze, 2006; Kim *et al*, 2007).

Amisulpride

There are no human data in the literature relating to amisulpride and pregnancy.

Aripiprazole

There are three case reports of pregnancy exposure to aripiprazole. In one, the pregnancy was uneventful but foetal tachycardia necessitated a Caesarean section at full term. The mother experienced failed lactation but her infant was healthy and developed normally over the 6-month follow-up period (Mendhekar *et al*, 2006*a*), as did the infant of a woman who took 15 mg/day from week 29 of gestation (Mendhekar *et al*, 2006*b*). Another woman experienced pregnancy-induced hypertension at 39 weeks but delivered a healthy infant (Mervak *et al*, 2008).

Zotepine and ziprasidone

There are no published human data relating to zotepine or ziprasidone in pregnancy.

Clozapine

In the 1990s there were several reports of successful pregnancies exposed to clozapine with no suggestion of an increase in congenital anomalies and a report of four women successfully treated whose infants were followed up to 6–10 years (Gáti *et al*, 2001). However, there have been various problems reported including: gestational diabetes (Waldman & Safferman, 1993; Dickson & Hogg, 1998); an infant with floppy infant syndrome born to a mother on clozapine and lorazepam (di Michele *et al*, 1996); a seizure in an 8-day-old infant (Stoner *et al*, 1997); a still birth (Mendhekar *et al*, 2003); and reduced foetal heart rate variability (Yogev *et al*, 2002). There is a report of foetal serum clozapine levels greater than those in maternal serum which the authors suggest may be due to the higher concentration of albumin in foetal blood (Barnas *et al*, 1994). A woman attempting suicide when 9 months pregnant took an overdose of clozapine, resulting in the neonatal death of her infant (Klys *et al*, 2007).

Nguyen & Lalonde (2003) reviewed six cases published in the literature and summarised data from almost 200 cases known to Novartis. The authors concluded that no specific risk could be attributed to clozapine but noted that foetal plasma levels could be higher than maternal levels and that there were case reports of neonatal hypotonia and of convulsions. They advised that use of clozapine in pregnancy must be limited to cases where the benefits clearly outweigh potential risks.

Obstetric anaesthetists have described a case in which they chose to use general anaesthesia for an emergency Caesarean section in a woman who was obese who had taken clozapine throughout pregnancy (Doherty *et al*, 2006). This was chosen because of the risk of profound hypotension following neuraxial blockade which can be resistant to vasopressors. They provide a comprehensive account of the issues related to pre-, peri- and post-operative deliveries involving clozapine exposure, including the increased risk of thromboembolism, intestinal paralysis and need to monitor temperature in post-operative parturient women. Psychiatrists assessing such women or caring for them in mother and baby units will find this paper a useful resource.

Koren *et al* (2002) identified obesity and a low intake of folate in women with schizophrenia taking atypical antipsychotics. This puts them at higher risk of having infants with neural tube defects.

Anticholinergics

There are few data relating to anticholinergic drugs and pregnancy but they should only be used for extrapyramidal side-effects in the short-term and only if absolutely necessary. Preferably the dose of the drug should be reduced.

Mood stabilisers

Lithium

Lithium crosses the placenta and a recent study found a mean mother–infant lithium ratio of 1.05 (Newport *et al*, 2005). Early data in the 1970s from case registers based on voluntary submissions suggested that there was an increased incidence of cardiac malformations, particularly Ebstein's anomaly, in infants exposed to lithium in the first trimester. The risk was estimated at 400 times the expected rate in the general population (Nora *et al*, 1974). Cohen *et al* (1994) reviewed the evidence including controlled epidemiological studies and reported risk ratios of between 1.5 and 3.0 for all congenital malformations and 1.2 and 7.7 for cardiac malformations. The risk for Ebstein's anomaly rises from 1 in 20 000 in the general population to 1 in 1000. The window of risk for cardiac malformations is between 4 and 9 weeks. If a woman has been exposed during this time, a Level II ultrasound and a foetal echocardiogram between 16 and 18 weeks are advised to assess cardiac development. A follow-up study of 60 women exposed in the second and third trimester did not detect any malformations (Schou, 1974), and a more recent trial of 20 pregnancies in 14 women also reported no problems other than induction of labour to shorten time off lithium (Kramer *et al*, 2003).

Assuming the pregnancy is continued, a decision whether or not to carry on with lithium has to be made. If lithium is continued throughout pregnancy, the lowest dose to achieve therapeutic levels should be used. This might mean a dose increase as pregnancy progresses owing to increased clearance via the increased glomerular filtration rate (30–50% in the second half of pregnancy). Levels should be checked more frequently: twice weekly in the second trimester, weekly in the third; urea, electrolytes and thyroid function should also be checked. Divided doses are said to reduce peak levels, so twice-daily dosage can be considered. If this is the case, levels should be monitored just before the next dose.

If lithium is to be discontinued, this should be done gradually as rapid discontinuation can trigger relapse. This same advice applies to women who are contemplating pregnancy and wish to stop treatment before attempting to conceive. Dependent on the severity of illness and likelihood of recurrence, lithium may be restarted during the second trimester.

Tapering and discontinuation of lithium 3–4 weeks before delivery is suggested to avoid foetal toxicity and maternal toxicity during labour. There are numerous reports (for reviews see Pinelli *et al*, 2002 and Kozma, 2005) of neonatal problems including poor respiratory effort and cyanosis, cardiac rhythm disturbances, nephrogenic diabetes insipidus, thyroid dysfunction, goitre, hypoglycaemia, hypotonia and lethargy, hyperbilirubinaemia and large-for-gestational-age infants. Newport *et al* (2005) confirmed in a controlled study that lower APGAR scores, longer hospital stays and higher rates of CNS and neuromuscular complications were observed in infants with higher lithium concentrations at delivery. They demonstrated that withholding lithium for 48 h before delivery reduced maternal concentrations by 0.28 meq/l. This might be a strategy for women in whom it is too risky to discontinue for a longer period. Lithium should be reinstated after delivery at a lower dose (renal clearance falls to non-pregnant levels dramatically postpartum).

If a woman is taking lithium she should deliver in hospital and close monitoring is required by the obstetric team during delivery to maintain fluid balance and avoid toxicity.

Carbamazepine

Animal studies and the majority of human studies indicate that carbamazepine is teratogenic. Neural tube defects appear in 0.5–1% of infants, which is five to ten times the rate of the general population, cardiovascular anomalies occur in 1.5–2%, cleft lip and palate occur five times more than in controls, and skeletal and brain malformations have been observed. A meta-analysis of 1255 pregnancies revealed an overall rate of major malformations of 6.7% (OR=3.0) (Matalon *et al*, 2002). The studies of neurodevelopmental outcomes in children exposed to carbamazepine are inconsistent (Ornoy, 2006). A recent case study highlights the fact that skin eruptions of varying degrees of severity occur in 3% of people taking carbamazepine. Angioedema is a potentially life-threatening complication which is more common in women and has a peak incidence in the third decade of life (Elias *et al*, 2006). Anticonvulsants taken during pregnancy (of which carbamazepine was the most commonly used drug) increase the risk of pre-eclampsia, haemorrhage after vaginal delivery and respiratory distress (Pilo *et al*, 2006).

Clearance varies during pregnancy and serum levels may decrease, so serum levels during pregnancy are recommended with dosage adjustment as indicated. Foetal serum levels are 50–80% of maternal serum levels. Carbamazepine is associated with vitamin K deficiency, which can impair clotting, so supplementation with this vitamin is recommended.

Sodium valproate

Sodium valproate (also known as divalproex semisodium and valproic acid) has been used in the treatment of epilepsy for many years and soon after its introduction an increase in the rate of neural tube defects was observed. Also, other congenital malformations have been noted (e.g. cranial facial defects, foetal valproate syndrome (brachycephaly, high forehead, shallow orbits, ocular hypertelorism, small nose and mouth, low-set posteriorly rotated ears, long overlapping fingers and toes, and hyperconvex fingernails), fingernail hypoplasia, cardiac defects) and the use of valproate as a mood stabiliser has increased.

Koren *et al* (2006) carried out a meta-analysis of studies published between 1978 and 2005. The relative risk for any malformation when monotherapy is compared with other anticonvulsants is 2.59, and 3.16 when compared with untreated patients with epilepsy and 3.77 when compared with the general population. The relative risk increased if valproate was given with other anticonvulsants. The risk increased at a dose of 600 mg/day and the largest risk appeared when doses were >1000 mg/day, a finding replicated by Vajda *et al* (2006) using Australian Pregnancy Register data with doses above 1100 mg/day. There are reports of lowered verbal IQs in children exposed to valproate but these data could not be entered into the meta-analysis. A study in which valproate was the second most commonly prescribed anticonvulsant reported an increased risk for adverse delivery events (Pilo *et al*, 2006).

Women of childbearing age should be warned about these risks, adequate contraception ensured and folate 5 mg/day is advised as this may afford some protection against neural tube defects. Animal and human studies have shown variable results and a recent population-based case–control study suggested that the risk may be reduced but not eliminated (Kjaer *et al*, 2008). If there is first-trimester exposure, then detailed ultrasound at 16–18 weeks and alpha-foetoprotein assay is advised. Clearance during pregnancy is variable.

Other reported problems are a risk of haemorrhage caused by impaired vitamin K-dependent clotting factors and the risk of transient neonatal hepatic dysfunction.

Lamotrigine

Lamotrigine clearance is increased by up to 300% in the last trimester of pregnancy and reverts quickly after delivery. There also seems to be considerable individual variation in pharmacokinetic changes during pregnancy underlining the need to closely monitor serum levels (Petrenaite *et al*, 2005).

Rates of congenital malformations reported range from 0 to 7% (Vajda *et al*, 2003; Cunnington *et al*, 2005; Morrow *et al*, 2006). Initial prospective studies seemed to indicate that doses of lamotrigine of 200 mg/day or below have minimal teratogenic effect. One study has found that doses above this level are associated with a higher risk of malformations (5.4%), higher still if given with valproate (Morrow *et al*, 2006), but Cunnington *et al* (2007) report no effect of dose on the rate of malformations.

There are also emerging concerns about a possible increased risk of oral clefts (Holmes *et al*, 2006) when lamotrigine monotherapy is used in the first trimester. This led to the manufacturer issuing guidance stating that it should only be used in pregnancy if the benefits of treatment outweigh possible risks to the foetus. All these data are drawn from populations with epilepsy and, as yet, there are extremely limited data in psychiatric populations. Gentile (2006) recommends lamotrigine as the mood stabiliser of choice during pregnancy but also warns that combining it with sodium valproate markedly increases the risk of teratogenicity.

If lamotrigine is to be continued after pregnancy, it should be noted that its interaction with combined oral contraceptives can render them less effective.

Gabapentin

Animal studies at dosages higher than those used in humans have shown skeletal development and renal problems. Öhman et al (2005) reported six women with epilepsy or pain disorders who took gabapentin throughout pregnancy. One had a preterm infant at 32 weeks; all deliveries were uneventful but one infant experienced short-lived hypotonia and cyanosis. A study of 39 women with 48 pregnancy outcomes (97% had first-trimester exposures) found a higher rate of preterm births (22.9%) when all births including six twin deliveries were counted and 9.1% when they were excluded. The malformation rate was 6.8% (Montouris, 2003). One of the women in this study had a bipolar disorder.

Clinicians should bear in mind two things.

1. Anticonvulsants should only be prescribed to women of childbearing age if the benefits outweigh the disadvantages and the prescriber must ensure that reliable contraception is in place. Current evidence suggests that this practice is far from universal (Wieck et al, 2007).
2. The incidence of teratogenesis increases significantly with all anticonvulsants in polytherapy, particularly if valproate is involved.

Calcium channel blockers

Calcium channel blockers have been used in obstetrics as antihypertensives, antiarrythmics and tocolytics for some time. A prospective analysis of 78 women exposed to calcium channel blockers (41% verapamil, 44% nifedipine) found no increase in the rate of congenital malformations or neonatal problems (Magee et al, 1996). A meta-analysis of 75 tocolytic studies (Berkman et al, 2003) reported that calcium channel blockers are rated as low risk for short-term neonatal harm. They are now beginning to emerge as mood stabilisers but the safety data are extremely limited in this population.

- Goodnick (1993) reported the treatment of three women with bipolar who became symptomatic during pregnancy.
- The use of verapamil in a sequential series of women with bipolar (some pregnant) is discussed by Wisner et al (2002).
- There is a case report of nimodipine use during pregnancy (Yingling et al, 2002).

Stimulants

It was found that in infants of mothers taking methylphenidate at doses ranging from 35 to 80 mg/day for ADHD the infant's dose was estimated at

0.2% and 0.7% of the maternal weight-adjusted dose (Hackett *et al*, 2005, 2006*b*). Another paper reports a woman 11 months postpartum taking oral immediate-release methylphenidate 5 mg in the morning and 10 mg at noon. The authors estimated that a fully breastfed infant would receive a dose of 0.16% of the maternal weight-adjusted dose (Spigset *et al*, 2007). Cases where infant plasma levels have been taken have found the drug to be undetectable. Of eight infants whose mothers were taking either dextroamphetamine or methylphenidate, seven had no methylphenidate-related adverse reactions and development was age-appropriate (Hackett *et al*, 2005).

A 1973 newsletter report (Ayd, 1973) contains a personal communication from the drug company, which reported that of 103 breastfeeding mothers treated with dextroamphetamine (dose not specified) for depression, no infant showed evidence of stimulation or insomnia.

Rapid tranquillisation of the pregnant woman

If a pregnant woman requires rapid tranquillisation she should be managed according to the NICE guidelines on the short-term management of disturbed and violent behaviour (National Institute for Health and Clinical Excellence, 2005). Most National Health Service (NHS) trusts have rapid tranquillisation policies based on these. However, there are some additional factors to consider.

- Restraint procedures should take pregnancy into account and not use any that might compromise the foetus.
- The woman should not be placed in seclusion after rapid tranquillisation.
- Antipsychotics or benzodiazepines with a short half life are the preferred medication and both should be given at the minimum effective dose. If a benzodiazepine is used in late pregnancy, the risks of floppy infant syndrome must be considered.
- Should a woman require rapid tranquillisation close to term, in labour or soon after delivery, paediatric and anaesthetic opinions are advised.

Non-drug interventions

Electroconvulsinve therapy

There are several successful case reports of ECT being an effective treatment for depression during pregnancy (Repke & Berger, 1984; Wise *et al*, 1984; Yellowlees & Page, 1990; Livingston *et al*, 1994; Echevarria Moreno *et al*, 1998; Gilot *et al*, 1999; Forray & Ostroff, 2007) and mania (Finnerty *et al*, 1996). It may be the treatment of choice if the patient has severe depression or psychosis as it minimises medication exposure and avoids the use of polypharmacy, which may be needed and for which there are few safety data.

However, although some of the cases reported had positive outcomes for the mother and foetus, others report complications. One foetus developed ascites at 34 weeks and died 9 days after delivery following surgery (Gilot *et al*, 1999). There is a report of foetal heart decelerations when ECT was used (DeBattista *et al*, 2003) and one young woman had a miscarriage after her third treatment (Echevarria Moreno *et al*, 1998). Uterine contractions, reduced foetal heart variability and contraction-related late cardiac decelerations indicating a compromised foetus were reported by Bhatia *et al* (1999). The other case reported in this paper was without complications. Uterine contractions and bleeding suggesting placental abruption occurred after each treatment in another report (Sherer *et al*, 1991); there is also a report of premature labour (Polster & Wisner, 1999) and status epilepticus (Balki *et al*, 2006). With any general anaesthetic there is the risk of hypoxia.

Miller (1994) reviewed 300 case reports between 1942 and 1991, finding 28 with reported complications, most of which did not apparently have a causal relationship with ECT. She concluded that ECT is safe during pregnancy provided precautions are taken and full informed consent is given.

The following advice is gleaned from the literature.

- Obstetric assessment including pelvic examination is advised prior to each treatment.
- Assessment of uterine contractions or vaginal bleeding after treatment is recommended.
- Foetal heart monitoring is recommended by most.
- Place the patient in a slightly left lateral position to minimise aortocaval compression.
- As patients beyond the first trimester are at increased risk of regurgitation of gastric contents, anaesthetic assessment is required regarding the use of anticholinergics and whether intubation is advised.
- Pregnancy is accompanied by mild hyperventilation. Respiratory alkalosis caused by excessive hyperventilation which is sometimes used to reduce the seizure threshold should be avoided as it can reduce oxygen transfer from maternal to foetal haemoglobin.

Transcranial magnetic stimulation

There are case reports of pregnant women treated successfully with transcranial magnetic stimulation with no adverse events (Nahas *et al*, 1999; Klirova *et al*, 2008).

Vagus nerve stimulation

Vagus nerve stimulation is receiving interest as a possible intervention for treatment-resistant depression. There is one case report of a woman with unipolar depression who became pregnant during a pilot study of vagus nerve stimulation. She continued to receive the intervention along with citalopram and bupropion throughout her pregnancy and normal delivery. She experienced a short-lived episode of depression lasting 11 days after delivery, which resolved spontaneously and her daughter was a healthy full-term infant (Husain *et al*, 2005).

Bright light therapy

Bright light therapy is also being explored as a possible treatment for pregnant women with depression. Oren *et al* (2002) carried out an open trial of bright light therapy in an A-B-A design for 3–5 weeks in 16 pregnant patients with major depression. After 3 weeks of treatment, mean depression ratings improved by 49% and benefits were seen through 5 weeks of treatment with no evidence of adverse effects of light therapy on pregnancy.

Epperson *et al* (2004) randomly assigned 10 pregnant women with major depressive disorder to a 5-week trial with either a 7000 lux (active) or 500 lux (placebo) light box. At the end of the RCT the women had the option of continuing in a 5-week extension phase. Results of the RCT were not significant but after a further 5 weeks, the presence of active *v.* placebo light produced a clear treatment effect with an effect size (0.43) similar to that seen in antidepressant drug trials. This was associated with phase advances of the melatonin rhythm.

Omega-3 fatty acids

Su *et al* (2001) report treating a woman with omega-3 fatty acids who had long-standing schizophrenia and became pregnant. She experienced a reduction in both positive and negative symptoms and there were no adverse effects.

Aromatherapy and massage

Massage and aromatherapy using essential oils has been suggested as an intervention for anxiety in pregnant women and one that might be more acceptable than drugs. However, animal studies have shown some essential oils to be responsible for intrauterine growth retardation and congenital anomalies and there is a lack of both efficacy and safety data in human pregnancy (Bastard & Tiran, 2006).

Reporting adverse events in pregnant women

Any adverse or suspected adverse event in relation to a drug or herbal medicine must be reported to the Medicines and Healthcare Products Regulatory Agency via the Yellow Card Scheme. Both healthcare professionals and patients can complete electronic Yellow Card reports via www.yellowcard. gov.uk: Yellow Cards can be obtained from any pharmacy and can also be found in copies of the *British National Formulary*, the *Nurse Prescribers'*

Formulary, the *Monthly Index of Medical Specialties (MIMS) Companion*, and from the Association of the British Pharmaceutical Industry (ABPI) Compendium of Data Sheets and Summaries of Product Characteristics. There is also a freephone Yellow Card hotline (0808 100 3352). Do not worry about duplicating a report. Even if you think someone else might have reported the event, report it anyway.

The National Teratology Information Service (NTIS)

The National Teratology Information Service (http://www.nyrdtc.nhs.uk/Services/teratology/teratology.html) provides a 24-h service on all aspects of toxicity of drugs and chemicals in pregnancy throughout the UK. All enquiries are confidential.

Contact details

Regional Drug & Therapeutics Centre,
Wolfson Unit,
Claremont Place,
Newcastle upon Tyne NE2 4HH

General enquiries: 0191 232 1525
Urgent enquiries: 0191 282 5944
Poisoning and chemical exposures in pregnancy out of hours: 0844 892 0111

Motherisk

Motherisk (www.motherisk.org) is a Canadian website run by the Hospital for Sick Children in Toronto, giving advice and providing resources for patients and professionals regarding pregnancy exposures.

Helpline numbers

Alcohol and substance: +1-877-327-4636
Nausea and vomiting: +1-800-436-8477
HIV and HIV treatment: +1-888-246-5840
Motherisk's home line: +1-416-813-6780

References

Addis, A. & Koren, G. (2000) Safety of fluoxetine during the first trimester of pregnancy: a meta-analytical review of epidemiological studies. *Psychological Medicine*, **30**, 89–94.

Altshuler, L. L, Cohen, L., Szuba, M. P., *et al* (1996) Pharmacologic management of psychiatric illness during pregnancy: dilemmas and guidelines. *American Journal of Psychiatry*, **153**, 592–606.

Alwan, S., Reefhuis, J., Rasmussen, S., *et al* (2005) Maternal use of selective serotonin reuptake inhibitors and risk for birth defects. *Birth Defects Research (Part A): Clinical and Molecular Teratology*, **73**, 291.

Anderson, G. M., Czarkowski, K., Ravski, N., *et al* (2004) Platelet serotonin in newborns and infants: ontogeny, heritability and effect of *in utero* exposure to selective serotonin reuptake inhibitors. *Pediatric Research*, **56**, 418–422.

Andrade, S. E., Raebel, M. A., Brown, J., *et al* (2008) Use of antidepressant medications during pregnancy: a multisite study. *American Journal of Obstetrics and Gynecology*, **198**, 194.e1–194.e5.

Anonymous (2005) Bupropion (amfebutamone): caution during pregnancy. *Prescrire International*, **14**, 225.

Arora, M. & Prahaj, S. K. (2006) Meningocele and ankyloblepharon following *in utero* exposure to olanzapine. *European Psychiatry*, **21**, 345–346.

Ayd, F. J. (1973) Excretion of psychotropic drugs in human breast milk. *International Drug Therapy Newsletter*, **8**, 33–40.

Balki, M., Castro, C., & Ananthanarayan, C. (2006) Status epilepticus after electroconvulsive therapy in a pregnant patient. *International Journal of Obstetric Anesthesia*, **15**, 325–328.

Bar-Oz, B., Einarson, A., Boskovic, R., *et al* (2007) Paroxetine and congenital malformations: meta-analysis and consideration of potential confounding factors. *Clinical Therapeutics*, **29**, 918–926.

Barnas, C., Bergant, A., Hummer, M., *et al* (1994) Clozapine concentrations in maternal and fetal plasma, amniotic fluid, and breast milk. *American Journal of Psychiatry*, **151**, 945.

Bastard, J. & Tiran, D. (2006) Aromatherapy and massage for antenatal anxiety: its effect on the fetus. *Complementary Therapies in Clinical Practice*, **12**, 48–54.

Ben-Amitai, D. & Merlob, P. (1991) Neonatal fever and cyanotic spells from maternal chlorpromazine. *DICP: The Annals of Pharmacotherapy*, **25**, 1009–1010.

Bérard, A., Ramos, É., Rey, É., *et al* (2007) First trimester exposure to paroxetine and risk of cardiac malformations in infants: the importance of dosage. *Birth Defects Research Part B: Developmental and Reproductive Toxicology*, **80**, 12–17.

Berkman, N. D., Thorp, J. M., Lohr, K. N., *et al* (2003) Tocolytic treatment for the management of preterm labour: a review of the evidence. *American Journal of Obstetrics and Gynecology*, **188**, 1648–1659.

Bhatia, S. C., Baldwin, S. A. & Bhatia, S. K (1999) Electroconvulsive therapy during the third trimester of pregnancy. *Journal of ECT*, **15**, 270–274.

Biswas, P. N., Wilton, L. V. & Shakir, S. A. (2003) The pharmacovigilance of mirtazepine: results of a prescription event monitoring study on 13,554 patients in England. *Journal of Psychopharmacology*, **17**, 121–126.

Bjarnason, N. H., Rode, L. & Kim, D. (2006) Fetal exposure to pimozide: a case report. *Journal of Reproductive Medicine*, **51**, 443–444.

Bodnar, L. M., Sunder, K. R. & Wisner, K. L. (2006) Treatment with selective serotonin reuptake inhibitors during pregnancy: deceleration of weight gain because of depression or drug? *American Journal of Psychiatry*, **163**, 986–991.

Bonari, L., Pinto, N., Ahn, E., *et al* (2004) Perinatal risks of untreated depression during pregnancy. *Canadian Journal of Psychiatry*, **49**, 726–735.

Bonnot, O., Vollset, S.-E., Godet, P-F., *et al* (2003) Exposition *in utero* au lorazepam et atresia anale: signal épidémiologique. *Encéphale*, **29**, 553–559.

Borges, L. V., do Carmo Cancino, J. C., Peters, V. M., *et al* (2005) Development of pregnancy in rats treated with *Hypericum perforatum*. *Phytotherapy Research*, **19**, 885–887.

Bot, P. B., Semmekrot, B. A. & van der Stappen, J. (2006) Neonatal effects of exposure to selective serotonin reuptake inhibitors during pregnancy. *Archives of Diseases of Childhood, Fetal and Neonatal Edition*, **91**, F153.

Çabuk, D., Sayn, A., Derinöz, O., *et al* (2007) Quetiapine use for the treatment of manic episode during pregnancy. *Archives of Women's Mental Health*, **10**, 235–236.

Cada, A. M., Hansen, D. K., LaBorde, J. B., *et al* (2001) Minimal effects from developmental exposure to St. John's wort (*Hypericum perforatum*) in Sprague-Dawley rats. *Nutritional Neuroscience*, **4**, 135–141.

Casper, R. C., Fleisher, B. E., Lee-Ancajas, J. C., *et al* (2003) Follow-up of children of depressed mothers exposed or not exposed to antidepressant drugs during pregnancy. *Journal of Pediatrics*, **142**, 402–408.

Chambers, C., Johnson, K., Dick, L., *et al* (1996) Birth outcomes in pregnant women taking fluoxetine. *New England Journal of Medicine*, **335**, 1010–1015.

Chambers, C. D., Hernandez-Diaz, S., Van Marter, L. J., *et al* (2006) Selective serotonin-reuptake inhibitors and risk of persistent pulmonary hypertension of the newborn. *New England Journal of Medicine*, **354**, 579–587.

Chan, B., Koren, G., Fayez, I., *et al* (2005) Pregnancy outcome of women exposed to buproprion during pregnancy: a prospective comparative study. *American Journal of Obstetrics and Gynecology*, **192**, 932–936.

Chlumska, A., Curik, R., Boudova, L., *et al* (2001) Chlorpromazine-induced cholestatic liver disease with ductopenia. *Ceskoslovenska Patologie*, **37**,118–122.

Cissoko, H., Swortfiguer, B., Giraudeau, B., *et al* (2005) Exposition aux antidépresseurs inhibiteurs de la recapture de la sérotonine (IRS) en fin de grossesse: retentissement neonatal. *Archives de Pédiatrie*, **12**, 1081–1084.

Cohen, L. F., Jefferson, J. M., Johnson, J. W., *et al* (1994) A reevaluation of risk of *in utero* exposure to lithium. *JAMA*, **271**, 146–150.

Cohen, L. S., Heller, V. L., Bailey, J. W., *et al* (2000) Birth outcomes following prenatal exposure to fluoxetine. *Biological Psychiatry*, **48**, 996–1000.

Cohen, L. S., Altshuler, L. L., Harlow, B. L., *et al* (2006) Relapse of major depression during pregnancy in women who maintain or discontinue antidepressant treatment. *JAMA*, **295**, 499–507.

Cole, J. A., Ephross, S. A., Cosmatos, I. S., *et al* (2007) Paroxetine in the first trimester and the prevalence of congenital malformations. *Pharmacoepidemiology and Drug Safety*, **16**, 1075–1085.

Collins, K. & Comer, J. (2003) Maternal haloperidol therapy associated with dyskinesia in a newborn. *American Journal of Health-System Pharmacy*, **60**, 2253–2255.

Cooper, W. O., Willy, M. E., Pont, S. J., *et al* (2007) Increasing use of antidepressants in pregnancy. *American Journal of Obstetrics and Gynecology*, **196**, 544.e1–544.e5.

Coppola, D., Russo, L-J., Kwarta, Jr, F. R. (2007) Evaluating the postmarketing experience of risperidone use during pregnancy: pregnancy and neonatal exposures. *Drug Safety*, **30**, 247–264.

Costei, A. M., Kozer, E., Ho, T., *et al* (2002) Perinatal outcome following third trimester exposure to paroxetine. *Archives of Pediatrics and Adolescent Medicine*, **156**, 1129–1132.

Cunnington, M., Tennis, P. & International Lamotrigine Pregnancy Registry Scientific Advisory Committee (2005) Lamotrigine and the risk of malformations in pregnancy. *Neurology*, **64**, 955–960.

Cunnington, M., Ferber, S., Quartey, G., *et al* (2007) Effect of dose on the frequency of major birth defects following fetal exposure to lamotrigine monotherapy in an international observational study. *Epilepsia*, **48**, 1207–1210.

Dabbert, D. & Heinze, M. (2006) Follow-up of a pregnancy with risperidone microspheres. *Pharmacopsychiatry*, **39**, 235.

Davis, R. L., Rubanowice, D., McPhillips, H., *et al* (2007) Risks of congenital malformations and perinatal events among infants exposed to antidepressant medications during pregnancy. *Pharmacoepidemiology & Drug Safety*, **16**, 1086–1094.

de Moor, R. A., Mourad, L., ter Haar, J., *et al* (2003) Withdrawal symptoms in a neonate following exposure to venlafaxine during pregnancy. *Nederlands Tijdschrift voor Geneeskunde*, **147**, 1370–1372.

DeBattista, C., Cochran, M., Barry, J. J., *et al* (2003) Fetal heart rate decelerations during ECT-induced seizures: is it important? *Acta Anaesthesiologica Scandinavica*, **47**, 101–103.

Dervaux, A., Ichou, P., Pierron, G., *et al* (2007) Olanzapine exposure during pregnancy. *Australian and New Zealand Journal of Psychiatry*, **41**, 706.

di Michele, V., Ramenghi, L.A. & Sabatino, G. (1996) Clozapine and lorazepam administration in pregnancy. *European Psychiatry*, **11**, 214.

Diav-Citrin, O., Okotore, B., Lucarelli, K., *et al* (1999) Pregnancy outcome following first-trimester exposure to zopiclone: a prospective controlled cohort study. *American Journal of Perinatology*, **16**, 157–160.

Diav-Citrin, O., Schechtman, S., Winbaum, D., *et al* (2005*a*) Paroxetine and fluoxetine in pregnancy: a mulitcenter, prospective controlled study. *Reproductive Toxicology*, **20**, 459.

Diav-Citrin, O., Schechtman, S., Ornoy, S., *et al* (2005*b*) Safety of haloperidol in pregnancy: a multicentre, prospective, controlled study. *Journal of Clinical Psychiatry*, **66**, 317–322.

Dickson, R. A. & Hogg, L. (1998) Pregnancy of a patient treated with clozapine. *Psychiatric Services*, **49**, 1081–1083.

Djulus, J., Koren, G., Einarson, T. R., *et al* (2006) Exposure to mirtazapine during pregnancy: a prospective, comparative study of birth outcomes. *Journal of Clinical Psychiatry*, **67**, 1280–1284.

Doherty, J., Bell, P. F. & King, D. J. (2006) Implications for anaesthesia in a patient established on clozapine. *International Journal of Obstetric Anesthesia*, **15**, 59–62.

Dollow, S. (2006) Important safety information (letter). GlaxoSmithKline.

Dolovich, L. R., Addis, A., Vaillancourt, J. M. R., *et al* (1998) Benzodiazepine use in pregnancy and major malformations or oral cleft: meta-analysis of cohort and case–control studies. *BMJ*, **317**, 839–843.

Dougoua, J. J., Mills, E., Perri, D., *et al* (2006) Safety and efficacy of St John's Wort (hypericum) during pregnancy and lactation. *Canadian Journal of Clinical Pharmacology*, **13**, e268–e276.

Echevarria Moreno, M., Martin Munoz, J., Sanchez Valderrabanos, J., *et al* (1998) Electroconvulsive therapy in the first trimester of pregnancy. *Journal of ECT*, **14**, 251–254.

Einarson, T. R. & Einarson, A. (2005) Newer antidepressants in pregnancy and rates of major malformations: a meta-analysis of prospective comparative studies. *Pharmacoepidemiology and Drug Safety*, **14**, 823–827.

Einarson, A., Lawrimore, T., Brand, P., *et al* (2000) Attitudes and practices of physicians and naturopaths toward herbal products, including use during pregnancy and lactation. *Canadian Journal of Clinical Pharmacology*, **7**, 45–49.

Einarson, A., Fatoye, B., Sarkar, M., *et al* (2001) Pregnancy outcome following gestational exposure to venlafaxine: a multicenter prospective controlled study. *American Journal of Psychiatry*, **158**, 1728–1730.

Einarson, A., Bonari, L., Voyer-Lavigne, S., *et al* (2003) A multicentre prospective controlled study to determine the safety of trazodone and nefazodone use during pregnancy. *Canadian Journal of Psychiatry*, **48**, 106–110.

Einarson, A., Schachtschneider, A. K., Halil, R., *et al* (2005) SSRIs and other antidepressant use during pregnancy and potential neonatal adverse effects: impact of a public health advisory and subsequent reports in the news media. *BMC Pregnancy and Childbirth*, **5**, 11.

Einarson, A., Pistelli, A., Desantis, M., *et al* (2008) Evaluation of the risk of congenital cardiovascular defects associated with use of paroxetine during pregnancy. *American Journal of Psychiatry*, **165**, 749–752.

Elias, A., Madhusoodana, S., Pudukkadan, D., *et al* (2006) Angioedema and maculopular eruptions associated with carbamazepine administration. *CNS Spectrums*, **11**, 352–354.

Epperson, C. N., Terman, M., Terman, J. S., *et al* (2004) Randomized clinical trial of bright light therapy for antepartum depression: preliminary findings. *Journal of Clinical Psychiatry*, **65**, 421–425.

Ericson, A., Kallen, B. & Wilhon, B. (1999) Delivery outcome after the use of antidepressants in early pregnancy. *European Journal of Clinical Pharmacology*, **55**, 503–508.

Ernst, C. L. & Goldberg, J. F. (2002) The reproductive safety profile of mood stabilizers, atypical antipsychotics, and broad-spectrum psychotropics. *Journal of Clinical Psychiatry*, **63**(Suppl. 4), 42–55.

Eros, E., Czeizel, A. E., Rockenbauer, M., *et al* (2002) A population-based case–control teratologic study of nitrazepam, medazepam, tofisopam, alprazolum and clonazepam treatment during pregnancy. *European Journal of Obstetrics and Gynecology and Reproductive Biology*, **10**, 147–154.

Ferreira, E., Carceller, A. M., Agogue, C., *et al* (2007) Effects of selective serotonin reuptake inhibitors and venlafaxine during pregnancy in term and preterm neonates. *Pediatrics*, **119**, 52–59.

Finnerty, M., Levin, Z. & Miller, L. (1996) Acute manic episodes in pregnancy. *American Journal of Psychiatry*, **153**, 261–263.

Flynn, H. A., Blow, F. C. & Marcus, S. M. (2006) Rates and predictors of depression treatment among pregnant women in hospital-affiliated obstetrics practices. *General Hospital Psychiatry*, **28**, 289–295.

Forray, A. & Ostroff, R. B. (2007) The use of electroconvulsive therapy in postpartum affective disorders. *Journal of ECT*, **23**, 188–193.

Friedman, S. H. & Rosenthal, M. B. (2003) Treatment of perinatal delusional disorder: a case report. *International Journal of Psychiatry in Medicine*, **33**, 391–394.

Gaffney, L. & Smith, C. (2004) The views of pregnant women towards the use of complementary therapies and medicines. *Birth Issues*, **13**, 43–50.

Gáti, A., Trixler, M. & Tényi, T. (2001) Pregnancy and atypical antipsychotics. *European Neuropsychopharmacology*, **11**, S247.

Gentile, S. (2006) Prophylactic treatment of bipolar disorder in pregnancy and breastfeeding: focus on emerging mood stabilizers. *Bipolar Disorder*, **8**, 207–220.

Gilot, B., Gonzalez, D., Bournazeau, J. A., *et al* (1999) Case report: electroconvulsive therapy during pregnancy. *Encéphale*, **25**, 590–594.

Godet, P. F. & Marie-Cardine, M. (1991) Neuroleptiques, schizophrenie et grossesse: étude epidemiologique et teratologique. *Encéphale*, **17**, 543–547.

Goldstein, D. J., Corbin, L. A. & Fung, M. C. (2000) Olanzapine-exposed pregnancies and lactation: early experience. *Journal of Clinical Psychopharmacology*, **20**, 399–403.

Goodnick, P. J. (1993) Verapamil prophylaxis in pregnant women with bipolar disorder. *American Journal of Psychiatry*, **150**, 10.

Gracious, B. L. & Wisner, K. L. (1997) Phenelzine use throughout pregnancy and the puerperium: case report, review of the literature, and management recommendations. *Depression and Anxiety*, **6**, 124–128.

Gregoretti, B., Stebel, M., Candussio, L., *et al* (2004) Toxicity of *Hypericum perforatum* (St. John's wort) administered during pregnancy and lactation in rats. *Toxicology and Applied Pharmacology*, **200**, 201–205.

Guclu, S., Gol, M., Dogan, E., *et al* (2005) Mirtazepine use in resistant hyperemesis gravidarum: report of three cases and review of the literature. *Archives of Gynecology and Obstetrics*, **272**, 298–300.

Hackett, L. P., Ilett, K. F., Kristensen, J. H., *et al* (2005) Infant dose and safety of breastfeeding for dexamphetamine and methylphenidate in mothers with attention deficit hyperactivity disorder. *Therapeutic Drug Monitoring*, **27**, 220–221.

Hackett, L. P., Ilett, K. F., Rampono, J., *et al* (2006a) Transfer of reboxetine into breastmilk, its plasma concentrations and lack of adverse events in the breastfed infant. *European Journal of Clinical Pharmacology*, **62**, 633–638.

Hackett, L. P., Kristensen J. H., Hale, T. W., *et al* (2006b) Methylphenidate and breastfeeding. *Annals of Pharmacotherapy*, **40**, 1890–1891.

Hansen, L. M., Megerian, G. & Donnenfeld, A. E. (1997) Haloperidol overdose during pregnancy. *Obstetrics and Gynecology*, **90**, 659–661.

Heikkinen, T., Ekblad, U., Kero, P., *et al* (2002) Citalopram in pregnancy and lactation. *Clinical Pharmacology and Therapeutics*, **72**, 184–191.

Heikkinen, T., Ekblad, U., Palo, P., *et al* (2003) Pharmacokinetcs of fluoxetine and norfluoxetine in pregnancy and lactation. *Clinical Pharmacology and Therapeutics*, **73**, 330–336.

Heinonen, O. P., Slone, D. & Shapiro, S. (1977) *Birth Defects and Drugs in Pregnancy.* Publishing Services Group.

Hemels, M. E. H., Einarson, A., Koren, G., *et al* (2005) Antidepressant use during pregnancy and the rates of spontaneous abortions: a meta-analysis. *Annals of Pharmacotherapy,* **39,** 803–809.

Hendrick, V., Stowe, Z. N., Altshuler, L. L., *et al* (2003*a*) Placental passage of antidepressant medications. *American Journal of Psychiatry,* **160,** 993–996.

Hendrick, V., Smith, L., Suri, R., *et al* (2003*b*) Birth outcomes after prenatal exposure to antidepressant medication. *American Journal of Obstetrics and Gynecology,* **188,** 812–815.

Holmes, L. B., Wyszynski, D. F., Baldwin, E. J., *et al* (2006) Increased risk for non-syndromic cleft palate among infants exposed to lamotrigine during pregnancy. *Birth Defects Research Part A: Clinical and Molecular Teratology,* **76,** 96–104.

Hostetter, A., Ritchie, J. C. & Stowe, Z. N. (2000*a*) Amniotic fluid and umbilical cord blood concentrations of antidepressants in three women. *Biological Psychiatry,* **48,** 1032–1034.

Hostetter, A., Stowe, Z. N., Strader, J. R., Jr., *et al* (2000*b*) Dose of selective serotonin uptake inhibitors across pregnancy: clinical implications. *Depression and Anxiety,* **11,** 51–57.

Husain, M. H., Stegman, D. & Trevino, K. (2005) Pregnancy and delivery while receiving vagus nerve stimulation for the treatment of major depression: a case report. *Annals of General Psychiatry,* **4,** 16.

Jeffries, W. S. & Bochner, F. (1988) The effect of pregnancy on drug pharmacokinetics. *Medical Journal of Australia,* **149,** 675–677.

Källen, B. (2004) Neonate characteristics after maternal use of antidepressants in late pregnancy. *Archives of Pediatric and Adolescent Medicine,* **158,** 312–316.

Källen, B. & Otterblad Olausson, P. (2006) Antidepressant drugs during pregnancy and infant congenital heart defect. *Reproductive Toxicology,* **21,** 221–222.

Karsenti, D., Blanc, P., Bacq, Y., *et al* (1999) Hepatotoxicity associated with zolpidem treatment. *BMJ,* **318,** 1179.

Kesim, M. & Yaris, F. (2002) Mirtazepine use in two pregnant women: is it safe? *Teratology,* **66,** 204.

Khan, K. S., Wykes, C. & Gee, H. (1999) Quality of studies must influence inferences made from meta-analyses. *BMJ,* **319,** 918.

Kim, J., Riggs, K. W., Misri, S., *et al* (2006) Stereoselective disposition of fluoxetine and norfluoxetine during pregnancy and breast-feeding. *British Journal of Clinical Pharmacology,* **61,** 155–163.

Kim, S-W., Kim, K-M., Kim, J-M., *et al* (2007) Use of long-acting injectable risperidone before and throughout pregnancy in schizophrenia. *Progress in Neuro-Psychopharmacology and Biological Psychiatry,* **31,** 543–545.

Kjaer, D., Horvath-Puho, E., Christensen, J., *et al* (2008) Antiepileptic drug use, folic acid supplementation, and congenital abnormalities: a population-based case–control study. *British Journal of Obstetrics and Gynaecology,* **115,** 98–103.

Klier, C. M., Mossaheb, N., Saria, A., *et al* (2007) Pharmacokinetics and elimination of quetiapine, venlafaxine and trazodone during pregnancy and postpartum. *Journal of Clinical Psychopharmacology,* **27,** 720–722.

Klirova, M., Novak, T., Kopecek, M., *et al* (2008) Repetitive transcranial magnetic stimulation (rTMS) in major depressive episode during pregnancy. *Neuroendocrinology Letters,* **29,** 69–70.

Klys, M., Rojek, S. & Rzepecka-Wozniak, E. (2007) Neonatal death following clozapine self-poisoning in late pregnancy: an unusual case report. *Forensic Science International,* **171,** e5–e10.

Knoppert, D. C., Nimkar, R., Principi, T., *et al* (2006) Paroxetine toxicity in a newborn after in utero exposure: clinical symptoms correlate with serum levels. *Therapeutic Drug Monitoring,* **28,** 5–7.

Koren, G., Cohn, T., Chitayat, D., et al (2002) Use of atypical antipsychotics during pregnancy and the risk of neural tube defects in infants. *American Journal of Psychiatry*, **159**, 136–137.

Koren, G., Nava-Ocampo, A. A., Moretti, M. E., et al (2006) Major malformations with valproic acid. *Canadian Family Physician*, **52**, 441–447.

Kozma, C. (2005) Neonatal toxicity and transient neurodevelopmental deficits following prenatal exposure to lithium: another clinical reports and review of the literature. *American Journal of Medical Genetics*, **132A**, 441–444.

Kramer, A., Knoppert-Van der Klein, E. A. M., Van Kamp, I. L., et al (2003) Bipolar and pregnant? No problem! A clinical evaluation of lithium use during pregnancy. *European Neuropsychopharmacology*, **13**, S246.

Kris, E. B. (1965) Children of mothers maintained on pharmacotherapy during pregnancy and postpartum. *Current Therapeutic Research–Clinical and Experimental*, **7**, 785–789.

Kulin, N. A., Pastuszak, A., Sage, S. R., et al (1998) Pregnancy outcome following maternal use of the new selective serotonin reuptake inhibitors: a prospective controlled multicenter study. *JAMA*, **279**, 609–610.

Laine, K., Kytola, J. & Bertilsson, L. (2004) Severe adverse effects in a newborn with two defective CYP2D6 alleles after exposure to paroxetine during late pregnancy. *Therapeutic Drug Monitoring*, **26**, 685–687.

Laine, K., Heikkinen, T., Ekblad, U., et al (2003) Effects of exposure to selective serotonin reuptake inhibitors during pregnancy on serotonergic symptoms in newborns and cord blood monoamine and prolactin concentrations. *Archives of General Psychiatry*, **60**, 720–726.

Lattimore, K. A., Donn, S. M., Kaciroti, N., et al (2005) Selective serotonin reuptake inhibitor (SSRI) use during pregnancy and effects on the fetus and newborn: a meta-analysis. *Journal of Perinatology*, **25**, 595–604.

Levinson-Castiel, R., Merlob, P., Linder, N., et al (2006) Neonatal abstinence syndrome after in utero exposure to selective serotonin reuptake inhibitors in term infants. *Archives of Pediatric and Adolescent Medicine*, **160**, 173–176.

Levy, W. & Wisniewski, K. (1974) Chlorpromazine causing extrapyramidal dysfunction in newborn infant of psychotic mother. *New York State Journal of Medicine*, **74**, 684–685.

Littrell, K. H., Johnson, C. G., Peabody, C. D., et al (2000) Antipsychotics during pregnancy. *American Journal of Psychiatry*, **157**, 1342.

Livingston, J. C., Johnstone, W. M. Jr. & Hadi, H. A. (1994) Electroconvulsive therapy in a twin pregnancy: a case report. *American Journal of Perinatology*, **11**, 116–118.

Loughhead, A. M., Fisher, A. D., Newport, D. J., et al (2006a) Antidepressants in amniotic fluid: another route of fetal exposure. *American Journal of Psychiatry*, **163**, 145.

Louik, C., Lin, A. E., Werler, M. M., et al (2007) First-trimester use of selective serotonin-reuptake inhibitors and the risk of birth defects. *New England Journal of Medicine*, **356**, 2675–2683.

Macaig, D., Simpson, K., Coppinger, D., et al (2005) Neonatal antidepressant exposure has lasting effects on behavior and serotonin circuitry. *Neuropsychopharmacology*, **31**, 47–57.

Mackay, F. J., Wilton, L. V., Pearce, G. L. et al (1998) The safety of risperidone: a post-marketing study on 7684 patients. *Human Psychopharmacology and Clinical Experience Journal*, **13**, 413–418.

Magee, L., Schick, B., Donnenfeld, A., et al (1996) The safety of calcium channel blockers in human pregnancy: a prospective, multicenter cohort study. *American Journal of Obstetrics and Gynecology*, **174**, 823–828.

Malm, H., Klaukka, T. & Neuvonen, P. J. (2005) Risks associated with selective serotonin reuptake inhibitors in pregnancy. *Obstetrics and Gynaecology*, **106**, 1289–1296.

Matalon, S., Schechtman, S., Goldzweig, G., et al (2002) The teratogenic effect of carbamazepine: a meta-analysis of 1255 exposures. *Reproductive Toxicology*, **16**, 9–11.

McElhatton, P. R. (1994) The effects of benzodiazepine use during pregnancy and lactation. *Reproductive Toxicology*, **8**, 461–475.

McElhatton, P. R., Garbis, H. M., Elefant, E., *et al* (1996) The outcome of pregnancy in 689 women exposed to therapeutic doses of antidepressants. A collaborative study of the European Network of Teratology Information Services (ENTIS). *Reproductive Toxicology,* **10,** 285–294.

McKenna, K., Koren, G., Tetelbaum, M., *et al* (2005) Pregnancy outcome of women using atypical antipsychotic drugs: a prospective comparative study. *Journal of Clinical Psychiatry,* **66,** 444–449.

Mendhekar, D. N., Sharma, J. B., Srivastava, P. K., *et al* (2003) Clozapine and pregnancy. *Journal of Clinical Psychiatry,* **64,** 850.

Mendhekar, D., Sunder, K. R. & Andrade, C. (2006a) Aripiprazole in a pregnant schizoaffective woman. *Bipolar Disorders,* **8,** 299–300.

Mendhekar, D., Sharma, J. & Srilakshmi, P. (2006b) Use of aripiprazole during late pregnancy in a woman with psychotic illness. *Annals Pharmacotherapy,* **40,** 575.

Mervak, B., Collins, J. & Valenstein, M. (2008) Case report of aripiprazole usage during pregnancy. *Archives of Women's Mental Health,* **11,** 249–250.

Milkiewicz, P., Chilton, A. P., Hubscher, S. G., *et al* (2003) Antidepressant induced cholestasis: hepatocellular redistribution of multidrug resistant protein (MRP2). *Gut,* **52,** 300–303.

Miller, L. J. (1994) Use of electroconvulsive therapy during pregnancy. *Hospital and Community Psychiatry,* **45,** 444–450.

Misri, S., Corral, M., Wardrop, A. A., *et al* (2006) Quetiapine augmentation in lactation. A series of case reports. *Journal of Clinical Psychopharmacology,* **26,** 508–511.

Mohan, M. S., Patole, S. K. & Whitehall, J. S. (2000) Severe hypothermia in a neonate following antenatal exposure to haloperidol. *Journal of Paediatrics and Child Health,* **36,** 412–413.

Montouris, G. (2003) Gabapentin exposure in human pregnancy: results from the Gabapentin Pregnancy Registry. *Epilepsy and Behavior,* **4,** 310–317.

Moradpour, D., Altorfer, J., Greminger, P., *et al* (1994) Chlorpromazine-induced vanishing bile duct syndrome leading to biliary cirrhosis. *Hepatology,* **20,** 1437–1471.

Morrison, J. L., Chien, C., Riggs, K. W., *et al* (2002) Effect of maternal fluoxetine administration on uterine blood flow, fetal blood gas status, and growth. *Pediatric Research,* **51,** 433–442.

Morrow, J., Russell, A., Guthrie, E. *et al* (2006) Malformation risks of antiepileptic drugs in pregnancy: a prospective study from the UK Epilepsy and Pregnancy Register. *Journal of Neurology, Neurosurgery and Psychiatry,* **77,** 193–198.

Moses-Kolko, E. L., Bogen, D., Perel, J., *et al* (2005) Neonatal signs after late in utero exposure to serotonin reuptake inhibitors: literature review and implications for clinical applications. *JAMA,* **293,** 2372–2383.

Nahas, Z., Bohning, D. E., Molloy, M. A., *et al* (1999) Safety and feasibility of repetitive transcranial magnetic stimulation in the treatment of anxious depression in pregnancy: a case report. *Journal of Clinical Psychiatry,* **60,** 50–52.

Nako, Y., Tachibana, A., Fujiu, T., *et al* (2001) Neonatal thrombocytosis resulting from the maternal use of non-narcotic antischizophrenic drugs during pregnancy. *Archives of Disease in Childhood–Fetal and Neonatal Edition,* **84,** F198–F200.

National Institute for Health and Clinical Excellence (2005) *Violence: The Short-Term Management of Disturbed/Violent Behaviour in Psychiatric In-patient and Emergency Departments.* Royal College of Nursing (http://www.nice.org.uk/nicemedia/pdf/cg025fullguideline.pdf).

Newham, J. J., Thomas, S. H., MacRitchie, K., *et al* (2008) Birth weight of infants after maternal exposure to typical and atypical antipsychotics: prospective comparison study. *British Journal of Psychiatry,* **192,** 333–337.

Newport, D. J., Viguera, A. C., Beach, A. J., *et al* (2005) Lithium placental passage and obstetrical outcome: implications for clinical management during late pregnancy. *American Journal of Psychiatry,* **162,** 2162–2170.

Newport, D. J., Calamaras, M. R., DeVane, C. L., *et al* (2007) Atypical antipsychotic administration during late pregnancy: placental passage and obstetrical outcomes. *American Journal of Psychiatry,* **164,** 1214–1220.

Nguyen, H-N. & Lalonde, P. (2003) Clozapine et grossesse. *Encéphale*, **29**, 119–124.

Nielsen, H. C., Wiriyathian, S., Rosenfeld, R., *et al* (1983) Chlorpromazine excretion by the neonate following chronic *in utero* exposure. *Pediatric Pharmacology*, **3**, 1–5.

Nora, J. J., Nora, A. H. & Toews, W. H. (1974) Lithium, Ebstein's anomaly and other congenital heart defects. *Lancet*, **2**, 594–595.

Nordeng, H. & Spigset, O. (2005) Treatment with selective serotonin reuptake inhibitors in the third trimester of pregnancy. *Drug Safety*, **28**, 565–581.

Nordeng, H., Lindemann, R., Perminov, K. V., *et al* (2001) Neonatal withdrawal syndrome after *in utero* exposure to selective serotonin reuptake inhibitors. *Acta Paediatrica*, **90**, 288–291.

Nulman, I., Rovet, J., Stewart, D. E., *et al* (1997) Neurodevelopment of children exposed *in utero* to antidepressant drugs. *New England Journal of Medicine*, **336**, 258–263.

Nulman, I., Rovet, J., Stewart, D. E., *et al* (2002) Child development following exposure to tricyclic antidepressants or fluoxetine throughout fetal life: a prospective, controlled study. *American Journal of Psychiatry*, **159**, 1889–1895.

Oberlander, T. F., Misri, S., Fitzgerald, C. E., *et al* (2004) Pharmacologic factors associated with transient neonatal symptoms following prenatal psychotropic medication exposure. *Journal of Clinical Psychiatry*, **65**, 230–237.

Oberlander, T. F., Grunau, R. E., Fitzgerald, C., *et al* (2005) Pain reactivity in 2-month-old infants after prenatal and postnatal serotonin reuptake inhibitor medication exposure. *Pediatrics*, **115**, 411–425.

Oberlander, T. F., Warburton, W., Misri, S., *et al* (2006) Neonatal outcomes after prenatal exposure to selective serotonin reuptake inhibitor antidepressants and maternal depression using population-based linked health data. *Archives of General Psychiatry*, **63**, 898–906.

Oberlander, T. F., Warburton, W., Misri, S., *et al* (2008a) Major congenital malformations following prenatal exposure to serotonin reuptake inhibitor and benzodiazepines using population-based health data. *Birth Defects Research B. Developmental & Reproductive Technology*, **83**, 68–76.

Oberlander, T. F., Warburton, W., Misri, S., *et al* (2008b) Effects of timing and duration of gestational exposure to serotonin reuptake inhibitor antidepressants: population-based study. *British Journal of Psychiatry*, **192**, 338–343.

Oberlander, T. F., Bonaguro, R. J., Misri, S., *et al* (2008c) Infant serotonin transporter (SLC6A4) promoter genotype is associated with adverse neonatal outcomes after prenatal exposure to serotonin reuptake inhibitor medications. *Molecular Psychiatry*, **13**, 65–73.

O'Connor, M., Johnson, G. H. & James, D. I. (1981) Intrauterine effect of phenothiazines. *Medical Journal of Australia*, **1**, 416–417.

Öhman, I., Vitols, S. & Tomson, T. (2005) Pharmacokinetics of gabapentin during delivery, in the neonatal period, and lactation: does a fetal accumulation occur during pregnancy? *Epilepsia*, **10**, 1621–1624.

Oren, D. A., Wisner, K. L., Spinelli, M., *et al* (2002) An open trial of morning light therapy for treatment of antepartum depression. *American Journal of Psychiatry*, **159**, 666–669.

Ornoy, A. (2006) Neuroteratogens in man: an overview with special emphasis on the teratogenicity of antiepileptic drugs in pregnancy. *Reproductive Toxicology*, **22**, 214–226.

Pakalapati, R. K., Bolisetty, S., Austin, M-P., *et al* (2006) Neonatal seizures from in utero venlafaxine exposure. *Journal of Pediatrics and Child Health*, **42**, 737–738.

Pastuzak, A., Schick-Boschetto, B., Zuber, C., *et al* (1993) Pregnancy outcome following first-trimester exposure to fluoxetine (Prozac). *JAMA*, **269**, 2246–2248.

Peindl, K. S., Masand, P., Mannelli, P., *et al* (2007) Polypharmacy in pregnant women with major psychiatric illness: a pilot study. *Journal of Psychiatric Practice*, **13**, 385–391.

Petrenaite, V., Sabers, A. & Hansen-Schwartz, J. (2005) Individual changes in lamotrigine plasma concentrations during pregnancy. *Epilepsy Research*, **65**, 185–188.

Pilo, C., Wilde, K. & Windbladh, B. (2006) pregnancy, delivery and neonatal complications after treatment with anticonvulsants. *Acta Obstetricia Gynecologica Scandinavica*, **85**, 643–646.

Pinelli, J. M., Symington, A. J., Cunningham, K. A., *et al* (2002) Case report and review of the perinatal implications of maternal lithium use. *American Journal of Obstetrics & Gynecology*, **187**, 245–249.

Platt, J. E., Friedhoff, A. J., Broman, S. H., *et al* (1988) Effects of prenatal exposure to neuroleptic drugs on children's growth. *Neuropsychopharmacology*, **1**, 205–212.

Polster, D. S. & Wisner, K. L. (1999) ECT-induced premature labor: a case report. *Journal of Clinical Psychiatry*, **60**, 53–54.

Potts, A. L., Young, K. L., Carter, B. S., *et al* (2007) Necrotizing enterocolitis associated with *in utero* and breast milk exposure to the selective serotonin reuptake inhibitor, escitalopram. *Journal of Perinatology*, **27**, 120–122.

Poulson, E. & Robson, J. M. (1964) Effects of phenelzine and some related compounds on pregnancy. *Journal of Endocrinology*, **30**, 205–215.

Rahimi, R., Nikfar, S. & Abdollahi, M. (2006) Pregnancy outcomes following exposure to serotonin reuptake inhibitors: a meta-analysis of clinical trials. *Reproductive Toxicology*, **22**, 571–575.

Ramos, E., St-Andre, M., Rey, E., *et al* (2008) Duration of antidepressant use during pregnancy and risk of major congenital malformations. *British Journal of Psychiatry*, **192**, 344–350.

Rampono, J., Proud, S., Hackett, P. L., *et al* (2004) A pilot study of newer antidepressant concentrations in cord and maternal serum and possible affects in the neonate. *International Journal of Neuropsychopharmacology*, **7**, 329–334.

Ratnayake, T. & Libretto, S. E. (2002) No complications with risperidone treatment before and throughout pregnancy and during the nursing period. *Journal of Clinical Psychiatry*, **63**, 76–77.

Rayburn, W. F., Christensen, H. D., Gonzalez, C. L., *et al* (2001*a*) Effect of antenatal exposure to Saint John's wort (Hypericum) on neurobehavior of developing mice. *American Journal of Obstetrics and Gynecology*, **183**, 1225–1231.

Rayburn, W. F., Gonzalez, C. L., Christensen, H. D., *et al* (2001*b*) Impact of hypericum (St-Johns-wort) given prenatally on cognition of mice offspring. *Neurotoxicology and Teratology*, **23**, 629–637.

Repke, J. T. & Berger, N. G. (1984) Electroconvulsive therapy in pregnancy. *Obstetrics and Gynecology*, **63**, S39–S41.

Rohde, A., Dembinski, J. & Dorn, C. (2003) Mirtazepine (Remergil) for treatment resistant hyperemesis gravidarum: rescue of a twin pregnancy. *Archives of Gynecology and Obstetrics*, **268**, 219–221.

Rybakowski, J. K. (2001) Moclobemide in pregnancy. *Pharmacopsychiatry*, **34**, 82–83.

Saks, B. R. (2001) Mirtazepine, treatment of depression, anxiety, and hyperemesis gravidarum in the pregnant patient. A report of seven cases. *Archives of Women's Mental Health*, **3**, 165–170.

Salkeld, E., Ferris, L. E. & Juurlink, D. N. (2008) The risk of postpartum hemorrhage with selective serotonin reuptake inhibitors and other antidepressants. *Journal of Clinical Psychopharmacology*, **28**, 230–234.

Sanz, E. J., De Las Cuevas, C., Kiuru, A., *et al* (2005) Selective serotonin reuptake inhibitors in pregnant women and neonatal withdrawal syndrome: a database analysis. *Lancet*, **365**, 482–487.

Schimmell, M. S., Katz, E. Z., Shaag, Y., *et al* (1991) Toxic neonatal effects following maternal clomipramine therapy. *Clinical Toxicology*, **29**, 479–484.

Schou, M. (1974) What happened to all the lithium babies? A follow up study of children born without malformations. *Acta Psychiatrica Scandinavica*, **54**, 193–197.

Sherer, D. M., D'Amico, M. L., Warshal, D. P., *et al* (1991) Recurrent mild abruptio placentae occurring immediately after repeated electroconvulsive therapy in pregnancy. *American Journal of Obstetrics and Gynecology*, **165**, 652–653.

Simhandl, C., Zhoglami, A. & Pinder, R. (1998) Pregnancy during use of mirtazepine. *European Neuropsychopharmacology*, **8**, S146.

Simon, G. E., Cunningham, M. L. & Davis, R. L. (2002) Outcomes of prenatal antidepressant exposure. *American Journal of Psychiatry*, **159**, 2055–2061.

Sit, D. K., Perel, J. M., Helsel, J. C., *et al* (2008) Changes in antidepressant metabolism and dosing across pregnancy and early postpartum. *Journal of Clinical Psychiatry*, **69**, 652–658.

Sivojelezova, A., Shuhaiber, S., Sarkissian, L., *et al* (2005) Citalopram use in pregnancy: Prospective comparative evaluation of pregnancy and fetal outcome. *American Journal of Obstetrics and Gynecology*, **193**, 2004–2009.

Sokolover, N., Merlob, P. & Klinger, G. (2008) Neonatal recurrent prolonged hypothermia associated with maternal mirtazepine treatment during pregnancy. *Canadian Journal of Clinical Pharmacology*, **15**, e188–e190.

Spigset, O., Brede, W. R. & Zahlsen, K. (2007) Excretion of methylphenidate in breast milk. *American Journal of Psychiatry*, **164**, 348.

Spyropoulos, A. C., Zervas, I. M. & Soldatos, C. R. (2006) Hip dysplasia following a case of olanzapine during pregnancy. *Archives of Women's Mental Health*, **9**, 219–222.

Stika, L., Elisova, K., Honzakova, L., *et al* (1990) Effects of drug administration in pregnancy on children's school behaviour. *Pharmaceutisch Weekblad – Scientific Edition*, **12**, 252–255.

Stoner, S. C., Sommi, R. W., Marken, P., *et al* (1997) Clozapine use in two full term pregnancies. *Journal of Clinical Psychiatry*, **58**, 364–365.

Su, K. P., Shen, W. W. & Huang, S. Y. (2001) Omega-3 fatty acids as a psychotherapeutic agent for a pregnant schizophrenic patient. *European Neuropsychopharmacology*, **11**, 295–299.

Suri, R., Altshuler, L., Hendrick, V., *et al* (2004) The impact of depression and fluoxetine on obstetrical outcome. *Archives of Women's Mental Health*, **7**, 193–200.

Suri, R., Altshuler, L., Hellemann, G., *et al* (2007) Effects of antenatal depression and antidepressant treatment on gestational age at birth and risk of preterm birth. *American Journal of Psychiatry*, **164**, 1206–1213.

Swortfiguer, D., Cissoko, H., Giraudeau, B., *et al* (2005) Retentissement neonatal de l'exposition aux benzodiazepines en fin de grossesse [Neonatal consequences of benzodiazepines used during the last month of pregnancy]. *Archives de Pédiatrie*, **12**, 1327–1331.

Taylor, T. M., O'Toole, M. S., Ohlsen, R. I., *et al* (2003) Safety of quetiapine during pregnancy. *American Journal of Psychiatry*, **160**, 588.

Tényi, T., Trixler, M. & Keresztes, Z. (2002) Quetiapine and pregnancy. *American Journal of Psychiatry*, **159**, 674.

Twaites, B. R., Wilton, L. V. & Shakir, S. A. W. (2007) The safety of quetiapine: results of a post-marketing surveillance study on 1728 patients in England. *Journal of Psychopharmacology*, **21**, 392–399.

Vajda, F. J., O'Brien, T. J., Hitchcock, A., *et al* (2003) The Australian registry of anti-epileptic drugs in pregnancy: experience after 30 months. *Journal of Clinical Neuroscience*, **10**, 543–549.

Vajda, F. J. E., Hitchcock, A., Graham, J., *et al* (2006) Foetal malformations and seizure control: 52 months data of the Australian Pregnancy Registry. *European Journal of Neurology*, **13**, 645–654.

Ververs, T., Kaasenbrood, H., Visser, G., *et al* (2006) Prevalence and patterns of antidepressant use during pregnancy. *European Journal of Clinical Pharmacology*, **62**, 863–870.

Waldman, M. & Safferman, A. (1993) Pregnancy and clozapine. *American Journal of Psychiatry*, **150**, 168–169.

Webb, R. T. Howard, L., Abel, K. M. (2004) Antipsychotic drugs for non-affective psychotic illnesses during pregnancy and postpartum. *Cochrane Database of Systematic Reviews*, **2**, CD004411.

Wen, S. W., Yang, Q., Garner, P., *et al* (2006) Selective serotonin reuptake inhibitors and adverse pregnancy outcomes. *American Journal of Obstetrics and Gynecology*, **194**, 961–966.

Wieck, A., Rao, S., Sein, K., *et al* (2007) A survey of antiepileptic prescribing to women of childbearing potential in psychiatry. *Archives of Women's Mental Health*, **10**, 83–85.

Williams, J. H. & Hepner, D. L. (2004) Risperidone and exaggerated hypotension during a spinal anesthetic. *Anesthetics and Analgesia*, **98**, 240–241.

Wise, M. G., Ward, S. C., Townsend-Parchman, W., *et al* (1984) Case report of ECT during high-risk pregnancy. *American Journal of Psychiatry*, **141**, 99–101.

Wisner, K. L., Perel, J. M. & Wheeler, S. B. (1993) Tricyclic dose requirements across pregnancy. *American Journal of Psychiatry*, **150**, 1541–1542.

Wisner, K. L., Perel, J. M., Peindl, K. S., *et al* (1997) Effects of the postpartum period on nortriptyline pharmacokinetics. *Psychopharmacology Bulletin*, **33**, 243–248.

Wisner, K. L., Zarin, D. A., Holmboe, E. S., *et al* (2000) Risk–benefit decision making for treatment of depression during pregnancy. *American Journal of Psychiatry*, **157**, 1933–1940.

Wisner, K. L., Peindl, K. S., Perel, J. M., *et al* (2002) Verapamil treatment for women with bipolar disorder. *Biological Psychiatry*, **51**, 745–752.

Wogelius, P., Nørgaard, M., Gislum, M., *et al* (2006) Maternal use of selective serotonin reuptake inhibitors and risk of CMs. *Epidemiology*, **17**, 701–704.

Yaris, F., Kadioglu, M., Kesim, M., *et al* (2004) Newer antidepressants in pregnancy: prospective outcome of a case series. *Reproductive Toxicology*, **19**, 235–238.

Yaris, F., Ulku, C., Kesim, M., *et al* (2005) Psychotropic drugs in pregnancy: a case–control study. *Progress in Neuro-Psychopharmacology and Biological Psychiatry*, **29**, 333–338.

Yellowlees, P. M. & Page, T. (1990) Safe use of electroconvulsive therapy in pregnancy. *Medical Journal of Australia*, **153**, 679–680.

Yeshayahu, Y. (2007) The use of olanzapine in pregnancy and congenital cardiac and musculoskeletal abnormalities. *American Journal of Psychiatry*, **164**, 1759–1760.

Yingling, D. R., Utter, G., Vengalil, S., *et al* (2002) Calcium channel blocker, nimodipine, for the treatment of bipolar disorder during pregnancy. *American Journal of Obstetrics and Gynecology*, **187**, 1711–1712.

Yogev, Y., Ben-Haroush, A. & Kaplan, B. (2002) Maternal clozapine treatment and decreased fetal heart rate variability. *International Journal of Gynaecology and Obstetrics*, **79**, 259–260.

Zeskind P. S. & Stephens, L. E. (2004) Maternal selective serotonin reuptake inhibitor use during pregnancy and newborn behaviour. *Pediatrics*, **113**, 368–375.

Further reading

American College of Obstetricians and Gynecologists (2008) ACOG Practice Bulletin: Clinical management guidelines for obstetrician–gynecologists number 92, April 2008. Use of psychiatric medications during pregnancy and lactation. *Obstetrics & Gynecology*, **111**, 1001–1020.

Costa, L. G., Steardo, L. & Cuomo, V. (2004) Structural effects and neurofunctional sequelae of developmental exposure to psychotherapeutic drugs: experimental and clinical aspects. *Pharmacological Reviews*, **56**, 103–147.

Lattimore, K. A., Donn, S. M., Kaciroti, N., *et al* (2005) Selective serotonin reuptake inhibitor (SSRI) use during pregnancy and effects on the fetus and newborn. *Journal of Perinatology*, **25**, 595–604.

Pollard, I. (2007) Neuropharmacology of drugs and alcohol in mother and fetus. *Seminars in Fetal and Neonatal Medicine*, **12**, 106–113.

Psychopharmacology for perinatal psychiatry

Consensus views from a round table discussion at a joint meeting of the Section of Perinatal Psychiatry and the Psychopharmacology Special Interest Group on 'Psychotropic prescribing in pregnancy, striving to "first do no harm"', held on 22 November 2007, Royal College of Obstetricians and Gynaecologists, London (http://pgxpsy.blogspot.com).

General principles for the prescribing of psychotropic drugs during pregnancy can be found in the Royal College of Psychiatrists' 2007 College Report (CR142) *Use of Licensed Medicines for Unlicensed Applications in Psychiatric Practice.*

CHAPTER 9

Physical treatments and breastfeeding

It is without doubt that breastfeeding has enormous health benefits both for infants and their mothers. Bottle-fed infants are more prone to infections, allergies, being overweight at school entry, and more likely to develop type 1 insulin-dependent diabetes and childhood cancers. Mothers who do not breastfeed are at increased risk of obesity, osteoporosis, and ovarian and breast cancer in later life. Breastfeeding can promote mother–infant interaction and increase maternal self-esteem. It is in this context and the recommendations from health organisations that breastfeeding must be promoted, that the treatment of mothers with mental illness sits.

There is a rapidly expanding evidence base, so clinicians should ensure that they contact a specialist drug information service before prescribing to ensure that they have the most up-to-date information.

Factors influencing infant exposure

Most drugs do pass into breast milk and the amount is influenced by several factors (Box 9.1).

There are additional factors that influence the amount the infant receives and these are summarised in Box 9.2.

General guidelines

- Sick or preterm infants are more vulnerable than healthy full-term infants, so exercise additional caution.
- If possible, use drugs with a short half-life so that there is the possibility of timing feeds when maternal serum levels are lowest, i.e. just before the next dose. Another option is to express milk when serum levels are highest and discard that sample. However, these should not be hard and fast rules as it may not be possible with a hungry demand-fed infant and can be one obstacle too much for a mother with depression.
- If maternal sleep deprivation is a problem, express milk if possible (before next dose) and arrange for someone else to undertake night

---

Box 9.1 Factors affecting drug concentration in breast milk

- Maternal plasma level: dependent upon dose, timing and route of administration, maternal metabolism and excretion
- Drug half-life
- Lipid solubility: breast milk is fatty and therefore concentrates lipophilic drugs including psychotropics
- Protein binding: free drugs transfer into breast milk
- Time since delivery: in early postpartum there are larger gaps between alveolar cells in the breast, increasing the amount of drug that passes from maternal blood. After 4 days this reduces
- Fat content of milk: lipophilic drugs will show increased transfer in hind milk rather than fore milk

---

feeds or consider whether supplementing with formula is a suitable option.

- Monitor the feeding, activity level, sleep and conscious level of any breastfed infant whose mother is taking psychotropics.
- Be sensitive to the feelings of any mother who has to stop breastfeeding or is unable to/does not want to. It is all too easy to engender guilt and self-blame.

Antidepressants

When considering potential risks to an infant from exposure to an antidepressant via breast milk, the risks must be balanced against the considerable body of existing knowledge we have about the adverse impact of untreated maternal depression on infant development (e.g. Murray & Cooper, 1997; Murray *et al*, 1999; Hipwell, *et al*, 2005).

Tricyclics

Yoshida & Kumar (1996) reviewed the available literature on tricyclics and breastfeeding in 1996. Many of these studies were of single cases only; the largest cohort was 15 and the total number of mother–infant pairs 44. There appeared to be considerable inter-individual variation of the level of tricyclics and their metabolites in plasma and milk samples in women taking the same dose.

There are some reports of amitriptyline concentrations being higher in milk than maternal serum. Levels of tricyclics were undetectable in most infants but there were low levels of 10-hydroxynortriptyline in two babies aged 3 and 8 weeks (Wisner & Perel, 1991). There are two cases of apparent toxicity. One occurred in an infant exposed to doxepin who became pale, sweaty and drowsy with depressed respiration and who

---

Box 9.2 Factors affecting infant plasma drug levels

- Amount of drug ingested: dependent upon whether exclusively breastfed or not, whether fore or hind milk ingested and timing since last maternal dose. Infants usually require 150 ml/kg/day of milk
- Infant metabolism: neonates have a reduced capacity to metabolise drugs for at least the first 2 weeks and this could be extended if the infant is preterm or ill
- Infant excretion: the neonatal kidney is less efficient than that of an adult and the glomerular filtration rate does not become equivalent to that of an adult until 2–5 months
- CNS exposure: the blood–brain barrier is immature in neonates

---

recovered on cessation of breastfeeding (Matheson *et al*, 1985). In the other case, reported in 1999 (Frey *et al*), the 9-day-old infant became hypotonic, with poor feeding and vomiting. His mother had taken doxepin during late pregnancy and while breastfeeding. Otherwise, there were no adverse events associated with tricyclics.

The only group to follow-up exposed infants is Buist & Janson (1995), who assessed at 3–5 years of age the children of 30 women who had breastfed while taking dothiepin, and the children of 36 women without depression. There were no differences in cognitive scores between the two groups, although marital conflict and child behaviour were most pronounced in the dothiepin group. This of course, could be related to depressive illness.

Following the 1996 review, Yoshida *et al* (1997*a*) studied 10 breastfeeding mothers who were taking tricyclics and compared outcomes in both mothers and infants with 15 mothers taking trycyclics and their bottle-fed infants. Maternal plasma levels had a linear relationship with oral dose and closely reflected the concentrations in milk. The daily dose ingested by the infants was around 1% of the maternal dose/kg and very small amounts of tricyclics were detected in infant plasma and urine. There were no acute toxic effects seen in the breastfed infants and no evidence of developmental delay when compared with the bottle-fed babies.

In summary, tricyclics have been widely prescribed and with the exception of doxepin appear to be relatively safe in breastfeeding, with levels of infant serum either low or undetectable. However, they are toxic in overdose and this may be a risk to the mother or other small children in the household who may accidentally ingest them. The main side-effects are sedation, and anticholinergic and postural hypotension that could all be problematic for new mothers. The drug with the lowest toxicity in overdose is lofepramine and tricyclics that appear in low levels in breast milk are nortriptyline and imipramine.

Selective serotonin reuptake inhibitors

Fluoxetine

Fluoxetine is the SSRI with most published data on its use in breastfeeding mothers. Doses of 20–40 mg (Heikkinen *et al*, 2002*a*) and 20 mg or less (Hendrick *et al*, 2001*a*) during pregnancy produce relatively low trough fluoxetine–norfluoxetine concentrations. The first of these studies observed that at delivery, infants had umbilical vein levels 65% and 72% respectively of maternal levels, and the estimated infant exposures were 2.4% of maternal dose at 2 weeks of age and 3.8% at 2 months.

There are three single case reports of exposure to fluoxetine via breastfeeding from the early 1990s (Isenberg, 1990; Burch & Wells, 1992; Lester *et al*, 1993). The dose in each case was 20 mg. There were no adverse events in the first two cases but the infant in the third experienced colic, vomiting and watery stools. In 1996, Taddio *et al* reported 10 women nursing 11 infants. The average daily dose of fluoxetine and its metabolite received by the infant was 6.5%. This was considered safe, as it is less than 10% of the maternal dose. No adverse events were reported during the short period of observation. However, Brent & Wisner (1998) reported a 3-week-old infant, breastfed by a mother taking fluoxetine, carbamazepine and buspirone, who experienced 60–90 s episodes in which her eyes rolled back, her limbs stretched out and she became limp. These did not recur but at 4 months of age she began having episodes in which she became limp and unresponsive for a few seconds several times per week. Investigations revealed nothing and she displayed no further symptoms at 1 year of age.

Since then, there has been a report of a full-term infant who was born to a mother who had taken 40 mg fluoxetine throughout pregnancy. During breastfeeding the infant became sleepy, hypotonic, difficult to rouse, pyrexial, fed poorly and began to moan with an expiratory grunt (Hale *et al*, 2001). She had been normal at birth and the symptoms remitted on cessation of breastfeeding. No infectious or metabolic cause was found for her symptoms. It is assumed that having been exposed to fluoxetine *in utero*, and in addition via breast milk, she had higher plasma levels. Exposure to long half-life drugs via breast milk could lead to accumulation and toxicity in neonates unable to metabolise them efficiently. Kristensen *et al* (1999) have demonstrated that neonates exposed to fluoxetine during pregnancy and via breast milk had higher concentrations of fluoxetine and norfluoxetine. Stereoselective disposition of fluoxetine and its metabolite in the mother, fetus, breast milk and infant lead to greater exposure of the infant to the biologically active entantiomer S-norfluoxetine (Kim *et al*, 2006).

Epperson *et al* (2003) studied the effect of fluoxetine in breast milk on platelet serotonin in 11 infants and observed that all but one experienced little or no decline, suggesting that there were minimal effects on peripheral and central serotonin transporter blockade. In another infant, levels dropped substantially and were associated with a measurable fluoxetine level. Yoshida *et al* (1998*a*) tracked the development of four infants exposed to fluoxetine *in utero* until the age of 12–13 months using the Bayley scales and found no evidence of delay.

Chambers *et al* (1999) observed an excess of breastfed infants who weighed less than two standard deviations below the mean when their mothers were taking fluoxetine. However, Hendrick *et al* (2003) reported that breastfed infants of mothers with depression who were taking antidepressants (citalopram, fluoxetine, fluvoxamine, paroxetine, sertraline or venlafaxine) did not gain any more weight than 6-month-old infants from normative populations.

Taking all the above into consideration, fluoxetine should be avoided while breastfeeding if at all possible, especially if the infant is very young, preterm or sick, or who may have an immature or impaired metabolism. If it is unavoidable, keep to the lowest possible therapeutic dose and monitor the infant's well-being very closely. If high doses, for example 60 mg, must be used (e.g. in the treatment of bulimia), then the mother should be advised not to breastfeed.

The advantages and disadvantages of various sampling analysis methods are discussed in Suri *et al* (2002).

Paroxetine

The highest concentrations of mean estimated dose of paroxetine found in infants has been reported at 0.7–2.9% (Öhman et al, 1999), 1.13% (Begg et al, 1999) and 1.1% (Misri et al, 2000) of the maternal dose, occurring 4–7 h after ingestion. This last study found infant plasma levels below the assay's ability to detect them and the second found levels undetectable in all but one infant whose level was unquantifiable. Paroxetine is certainly present in breast milk (Stowe *et al*, 2000) but again this study found undetectable amounts in infant sera and observed no adverse events.

Merlob *et al* (2004) did not find any effect of paroxetine on infant weight at 6 and 12 months and observed no adverse events other than one infant being reported as irritable. Developmental milestones in those infants exposed were normal. Given the low amounts of paroxetine found in infant plasma, the lack of adverse events and the fact that it has no active metabolites, paroxetine is one choice for breastfeeding mothers.

Sertraline

Sertraline has a weak metabolite and has been detected in breast milk but only low or undetectable levels have been observed in infant plasma (Altshuler *et al*, 1995; Mammen *et al*, 1997; Stowe *et al*, 1997; Kristensen *et al*, 1998; Epperson *et al*, 2001; Perel *et al*, 2003; Stowe *et al*, 2003). Breast milk levels peak between 1 and 9 h post-ingestion, with lowest levels occurring 1 h before the next dose.

Mean estimates of infant exposure range from 0.54 to 0.90% for sertraline and 0.49 to 1.32% of the maternal dose for N-desmethylsertraline. Epperson *et al* (2001) demonstrated unaltered platelet serotonin uptake in infants of nursing mothers, suggesting that peripheral or central serotonin transport is unaffected by exposure to sertraline via breast milk. No adverse events have been reported other than withdrawal symptoms in an infant who was breastfed after its mother had taken 200 mg sertraline daily throughout pregnancy (Kent & Laidlaw, 1995). Hendrick *et al* (2001*b*) compared concentration of sertraline, paroxetine and fluvoxamine in breastfeeding women. Sertraline was detected in the serum of 24% of exposed infants but the levels were low and there were no adverse events reported. The likelihood of a detectable infant serum level was increased if the mother's dose was 100 mg or above. Overall, there are now more than 100 cases reported with no adverse events identified.

Citalopram

Spigset *et al* (1997) demonstrated in two women a relative dose of 1.8% of the weight-adjusted maternal dose, which is less than those reported for fluoxetine but higher than paroxetine and sertraline. Rampono *et al* (2000) studied seven women and found infant doses of 3.7% for citalopram and 1.4% for desmethylcitalopram. There were no adverse events. Lepola *et al*, 2000) studied seven women and found an infant dose of 0.03%. Two case reports have reported an infant dose of 5.4% (Schmidt *et al*, 2000) and 4.8% (Jensen *et al*, 1997). The latter study found levels in milk higher than maternal serum, and the mother in Schmidt *et al*'s study, having received 2–3 nights of citalopram treatment, reported that her infant slept uneasily.

Heikkinen *et al* (2002*b*) monitored 11 women and 10 matched controls. They found infant doses of 0.3% at 2 weeks and 0.2% at 2 months. All infants were followed up for 1 year and there were no differences in weight or development between the exposed infants and the controls. In a prospective cohort study, Lee *et al* (2004) assessed 31 breastfeeding women taking citalopram, 12 women with depression taking citalopram and 31 healthy women matched by age and parity. They found no differences between the groups in the rate of adverse events and no events related to citalopram; however, seven women with depression in the control groups were taking other SSRIs.

Escitalopram

Ilett *et al* (2005) reported on five lactating mothers taking escitalopram and their infants. Relative infant doses in milk were 4.5% (s.d.=1.8) for escitalopram and 1.7% (s.d.=0.7) for desmethylescitalopram. Both were undetectable in infant plasma in two infants that were sampled. Castberg & Spigset (2006) published a case report of a breastfeeding woman treated with escitalopram alone and then in combination with valproate. The relative doses of escitalopram in the infant were 5.1% when used alone and 7.7% when valproate was added. No adverse events were observed in either report.

Duloxetine

An open-label study observed the pharmacokinetics of 40 mg duloxetine in six nursing mothers (Lobo *et al*, 2008). The mean milk:plasma ratio was 0.25 and the infant dose estimated at 0.14% of the maternal dose.

Fluvoxamine

Early single-case reports estimated the milk:plasma ratio for fluvoxamine as 0.29 (Wright *et al*, 1991; Yoshida *et al*, 1997b). A later case study found a higher milk:plasma ratio (1.32) and a mean infant dose of 1.58% of the maternal dose (Hägg *et al*, 2000). Piontek *et al* (2001) studied two mother–infant pairs and found infant serum levels that were too low to quantify, as did Kristensen *et al* (2002) and Hendrick *et al* (2001b). Mean infant doses were 1.38% and 0.8% respectively. Fluvoxamine has no active metabolites. The only adverse event potentially related to fluvoxamine was jaundice which resolved spontaneously despite continuation of the drug and breastfeeding.

Venlafaxine

There are now published data on over 20 breastfed infants who have been exposed to venlafaxine. A small case-series of three mothers and their infants observed that the mean dose infants received was 7.6% of the maternal weight-adjusted dose (Ilett *et al*, 1998). There were no adverse effects. Hendrick *et al* (2001c) studied two mother–infant pairs. No venlafaxine was detectable in infant serum but low levels of the metabolite O-desmethylvenlafaxine were found; however, there were no adverse effects. In 2002, Ilett *et al* studied six women and their infants. Mean maternal plasma values for venlafaxine and O-desmethylvenlafaxine were 2.5 and 2.74, which led to mean relative infant doses of 3.2% for venlafaxine and 3.2% for O-desmethylvenlafaxine. There were no adverse events observed in the seven infants.

An infant whose mother had been taking venlafaxine 375 mg daily during pregnancy presented with symptoms of lethargy, poor sucking ability, and dehydration at 2 days of age. After being allowed to breastfeed, the symptoms subsided over 1 week and the authors concluded that the symptoms were probably withdrawal symptoms that were reduced by the venlafaxine in the breastmilk (Koren *et al*, 2006).

Monoamine oxidase inhibitors

Pons *et al* (1990) studied the pharmacokinetics of moclobemide and its metabolites in six lactating women. Concentrations in milk were highest 3 h after the dose and absent after 12 h. On average the concentration in milk was 72% of the serum concentration. An infant would receive an estimated 1% of the maternal dose.

There are no published safety data relating to phenelzine, tranylcypromine or isocarboxazid, so these drugs should be avoided in breastfeeding mothers.

Mirtazapine

Maternal levels of mirtazapine in breast milk remain low if the dose remains below 120 mg/day: exclusively breastfed infants receive 0.6–2.8% (average 1.5%) of the maternal dose of mirtazapine and 0.4% (range 0.1–0.7%) of its metabolite desmethylmirtazapine (Aichhorn *et al*, 2004; Klier *et al*, 2007; Kristensen *et al*, 2007).

Trazodone

Peak levels of trazodone in milk occur around 2 h after the dose and it is estimated that an exclusively breastfed infant would receive 0.65% of the maternal weight-adjusted dose (Verbeeck *et al*, 1986). However, the active metabolite was not measured. The infant of a mother who took trazodone 200 mg daily for 12 weeks starting at 4 weeks postpartum was followed up at 12 months of age when no adverse effects on growth and development were found (Misri & Sivertz, 1991). Another woman took trazodone 75 mg in addition to venlafaxine 75 mg/day and quetiapine 75 mg/day before conception, during pregnancy and during breastfeeding. Her breastfed infant's development was tested at 12 months and was within normal limits (Misri *et al*, 2006).

Nefazodone

Infant intake of nefazodone and its active metabolite hydroxynefazodone are estimated at 6.2% and 2% respectively (Dodd *et al*, 1999). There is one report of a premature (36-weeks adjusted gestational age) infant becoming drowsy and lethargic, not feeding well and being unable to maintain normal body temperature when her mother was taking 300 mg nefazodone daily (Yapp *et al*, 2000). Symptoms resolved on cessation of breastfeeding and no other cause for them was found on investigation. This case highlights the fact that preterm infants have immature metabolic systems.

Dodd *et al* (2000) reported two mothers who breastfed while taking nefazodone. There was interindividual variation in the amount of drug found in breast milk, unrelated to dose. One milk:plasma ratio was 3.17 and the other 0.14. Infant doses were 2.2% and 0.4%. There were no developmental difficulties in the infants.

Bupropion

There is one case report of a mother breastfeeding her 14-month-old son while taking bupropion. Neither the drug nor its metabolites were detectable in the single plasma sample taken from the infant (Briggs *et al*, 1993).

Similarly, assays in two mother–infant pairs found no detectable levels of bupropion and hydroxybupropion (its most active metabolite) in infant serum and no problems were reported (Baab et al, 2002).

Haas et al (2004) assessed the concentration of bupropion and all its active metabolites (hydroxybupropion, erythrobupropion and threohydrobupropion) in the milk of ten postpartum volunteers in an attempt to determine the average infant exposure. The calculated dose in breast milk was 6.75 microg/kg/day. Taking into account the metabolites, the total exposure to the infant would be 2% of the weight-adjusted maternal dose. There were no adverse events in the women. There is a report of a 6-month-old infant experiencing a seizure; however, no milk or plasma level of bupropion was taken at the time, so a causal relationship cannot be confirmed (Ginsberg, 2004). However, there are reports of seizures in adults taking bupropion.

Others

Hackett et al (2006) sampled four women taking reboxetine during pregnancy and their infants. The mean milk:plasma ratio was 0.06 and the relative infant dose 2.0%. One infant out of the four had developmental problems unrelated to reboxetine, the others met normal developmental milestones and no adverse events were reported.

St John's wort

Klier et al (2002) observed that hyperforin rather than hypericin was excreted into breast milk albeit in very small amounts (milk:plasma ratio <1) and undetectable in infant plasma. No side-effects were seen in either mother or infant. In 2003, Lee et al reported on a prospective cohort study of 33 women who were breastfeeding while taking St John's wort. Outcomes were compared with disease-matched controls on no medication and well women of a similar age and parity. There were more reports of colicky or drowsy infants in the St John's wort group but these did not require medical attention. There were no differences in reports of decreased milk production and infant weight gain over the first year between the groups.

Five women and two of their infants had breast milk, maternal and infant plasma sampled over an 18h period (Klier et al, 2006). Their hyperforin milk:plasma levels ranged from 0.04 to 0.13 and the percentages of infant plasma in relation to maternal dose were 0.17% and 0.15%. The relative mean dose per kg received by the infant was 0.9–2.5%. There were no maternal or infant adverse events. A systematic review (Dugoua et al, 2006) concluded that use of St John's wort during lactation 'appeared to be of minimal risk' but may cause side-effects. The authors also drew attention to the fact that taking it concomitantly with other psychotropics might lower their serum levels by St John's wort induction of CYP450 enzymes.

Systematic review data

Weissman *et al* (2004) undertook a systematic review pooling the available data relating to antidepressant exposure between 1966 and 2002. They concluded:

1   Nortriptyline, sertraline and paroxetine are the preferred choice for prescribing during lactation as they tend to produce low or undetectable levels in infant serum and are unlikely to develop elevated levels.
1   Fluoxetine does appear likely to produce elevated levels, particularly if there has been exposure during pregnancy. Citalopram may also give rise to elevated levels but the data are more limited.

Benzodiazepines and hypnotics

Benzodiazepines and their metabolites are excreted in breast milk. Some studies on benzodiazepines in breastfeeding mother–infant dyads have observed infant serum levels of a third to a sixth of maternal levels when mothers were taking high doses (Erkkola & Kanto, 1972). However, other studies have observed lower levels of benzodiazepines (e.g. Birnbaum *et al*, 1999) with clonazepam and lormetazepam (Humpel *et al*, 1982). The mean infant dose of alprazolam was reported as 3% in a study of eight women (Oo *et al*, 1995). Where higher concentrations do occur this is usually where there has also been *in utero* exposure. If benzodiazepines are required while breastfeeding then using a short half-life drug intermittently will reduce the risk of higher infant serum levels. However, there are reports of infants appearing restless and irritable (Anderson & McGuire, 1989) and drowsy (Ito *et al*, 1993) with alprazolam. Infants should be monitored for signs of CNS depression and apnoea. Iqbal *et al* (2002) have comprehensively reviewed the literature relating to diazepam, chlordiazepoxide, clonazepam, lorazepam and alprazolam and breastfeeding.

Lebedevs *et al* (1992) studied temazepam in ten breastfeeding mothers and their infants. The dose was 10–20mg at night and several of the mothers were taking other drugs in addition. The milk:plasma ratio ranged from <0.09 to <0.63 and the milk concentration was below the limit of detection for the assay in several samples. Zolpidem is excreted in breast milk in very small amounts (0.004–0.019% of the administered dose) and most of this takes place during 3h after the dose. The milk:plasma ratio at 3h was 0.13. No infant samples were taken (Pons *et al*, 1989).

Mood stabilisers

Lithium

Single case studies of lithium exposure via breastfeeding (seven cases in total) have given rise to estimates of concentrations in infant serum of between 30 and 200% of maternal levels (Tunnessen & Hertz, 1972; Schou & Amdisen, 1973; Sykes *et al*, 1976; Skausig & Schou, 1977). One infant is reported to have become cyanotic, floppy, lethargic and hypotonic, although it recovered. Another experienced an upper respiratory tract infection and developed a lithium level twice that of the maternal level. The infant recovered after breastfeeding was discontinued. Moretti *et al* (2003) reported 11 mothers with bipolar taking between 600 and 1500 mg lithium daily. There was wide variation in the dose the infant received via breast milk (0–30%) but no adverse events were reported. Lithium is therefore best avoided during breastfeeding due to the risk of toxicity in infants whose renal excretion will be immature at this stage. There are also risks of thyroid dysfunction, tremor, poor muscle tone and electrocardiogram changes. A further series of 10 mother–infant pairs was reported by Viguera *et al* (2007). They also observed a wide range in the dose received by the infant (25–92% of maternal serum level) with a mean of 24%. Although no development delays were reported by the sample, four infants had abnormalities of thyroid stimulating hormone, blood urea nitrogen or serum creatinine levels.

Anticonvulsants

Bar-Oz *et al* (2000) and Hägg & Spigset (2000) provide reviews of the use of anticonvulsants during breastfeeding, concluding that 'phenytoin, carbamazepine and valproic acid are generally considered safe for use during breastfeeding'. The focus will be on those anticonvulsants used as mood stabilisers.

Carbamazepine

Carbamazepine and its active metabolite 10,11-epoxide has been studied in over 25 cases; the vast majority of women with epilepsy were already on medication and additionally taking carbamazepine during pregnancy. Concentrations in breast milk range from 7 to 95% of the maternal serum level but most lie between 25–65%. Adverse events include hepatotoxicity (Frey *et al*, 1990; Merlob *et al*, 1992), a seizure (Brent & Wisner, 1998) and poor suckling (Froescher *et al*, 1984). It is classified by the American Academy of Pediatrics as safe to take while breastfeeding.

Valproate

There are over 90 reports of valproate in breast milk and only one has reported any adverse outcome so far, hence the American Academy of Pediatrics considers it safe to breastfeed. The infant of a mother taking sodium valproate 600 mg/day (and who had done so throughout pregnancy) developed thrombocytopenic purpura and anaemia (Stahl *et al*, 1997). The majority of reports have been on mothers with epilepsy, some of whom were also taking other anticonvulsants. However, there are two studies on mothers with bipolar.

Wisner & Perel (1998) reported two mothers who breastfed while taking valproate. When steady state had been achieved, the infant serum levels were 1.5 and 6% of maternal values. Two years later, Piontek *et al* (2000) assessed serum valproate levels in six mother–infant pairs. The mothers were taking doses of 750–1000 mg/day and all but one had serum levels within the therapeutic range of 56.2–79 microg/ml. The infant serum levels were 0.9–2.3% of maternal levels and none of th einfants experienced any adverse events.

Lamotrigine

Case reports suggest extensive passage of lamotrigine over the placenta and into breast milk (Rambeck *et al*, 1997; Tomson *et al*, 1997). Öhman *et al* (2000) monitored lamotrigine levels in nine pregnant women and their 10 infants through delivery and lactation. They confirmed extensive passage of lamotrigine over the placenta and into breast milk, but also noted a slow elimination in the neonate and a profound increase in maternal serum concentrations following delivery. Lamotrigine serum concentrations in the infant were 23–50% of maternal serum concentrations. It is metabolised by glucuronidation, a process that is immature in neonates, and which could lead to accumulation of the drug in the infant's system, although no adverse events were noted in this cohort. A further study adds to these concerns. Four women taking lamotrigine and their infants were studied; lamotrigine levels in the infants ranged from 20 to 43% of the maternal drug level. This had not declined by 2 months of age but no short-term adverse effects were reported (Liporace *et al*, 2004). In 2005, Gentile published a case report of a successful outcome in a mother who had taken lamotrigine throughout pregnancy and breastfeeding. The NICE guidelines on antenatal and postnatal mental health state that lamotrigine should not routinely be prescribed to breastfeeding women because of the risk of Stevens-Johnson syndrome in the infant (National Institute for Health and Clinical Excellence, 2007).

Gabapentin

Öhman *et al* (2005) reported five breastfeeding mother–infant pairs in which the mother had taken gabapentin during pregnancy and while breastfeeding. The milk:plasma ratio was 1.0 before nursing and the estimated dose of the infant was 1.3–1.8% of the maternal dose. When sampled 2–3 weeks after delivery, two of the infants had detectable concentrations of gabapentin but they were below the levels of the normal range of the assay and one had undetectable levels. No adverse events were reported. Kristensen *et al* (2006) report a further case in which the milk:plasma ratio was 0.86 and the estimated infant dose 2.34%. There were no adverse events.

Verapamil

The literature contains two reports of mothers breastfeeding while taking verapamil (Andersen, 1983). In the first, the infant was exposed to 240 mg *in utero* and during lactation. The infant's verapamil level was 2.1 ng/ml at 4 days postpartum. In the second case, the mother received 240 mg verapamil after delivery and no verapamil or its metabolite norverapamil could be detected in the infant's serum at 3 months postpartum. At typical doses, the neonatal intake of verapamil is estimated to be about a hundredth of the maternal dose.

Antipsychotics

Gentile (2008) systematically reviewed the literature published between 1950 and 2008 and stated that 'no conclusions can be drawn about the risk–benefit profile of the majority of antipsychotic medications' with two exceptions:

- clozapine should be contraindicated because of the possibility of inducing life-threatening events in the infant
- olanzapine is associated with an increased risk of extrapyramidal symptoms in breastfed babies.

Typical antipsychotics

Haloperidol is 90% protein bound, so limited amounts are available for absorption into breast milk. Whalley *et al* (1981) observed a milk:plasma ratio of around 0.6 and a low concentration of haloperidol in the infant's urine. No adverse events were reported and the child appeared to be developing normally at 6 months and again at 1 year. Yoshida *et al* (1998*b*) reported 12 breastfeeding mothers who were taking haloperidol, chlorpromazine or trifluoperazine. Nine of the women took haloperidol (five also took chlorpromazine and one imipramine) and the mean ratio of fore milk:plasma was 2.8 and of hind milk 3.6, i.e. a higher concentration in milk than plasma. One infant's mother in particular had high plasma and milk concentrations but no sample was taken from the baby, who had some developmental delay. Seven women took chlorpromazine and two trifluoperazine. Overall, the estimated infant dose for the drugs was 3% of the maternal dose/kg. There were some concerns about the infants of women who were prescribed both haloperidol and chlorpromazine but it is acknowledged that there may have been illness and other factors involved.

There is a report of two cases, the first in which a woman took flupenthixol and nortriptyline while breastfeeding and another in which a mother took zuclopentixol. Estimated daily infant dose of the antipsychotics was 0.5 and 0.3% respectively and 2.3% for nortriptyline (Matheson & Skjaeraasen, 1988).

Atypical antipsychotics

Olanzapine

Ernst & Goldberg (2002) and Patton *et al* (2002) reported a total of 21 infants exposed to olanzapine via breastfeeding. Five experienced adverse events including sedation, jaundice, cardiomegaly, cardiac murmur, shaking, poor feeding and lethargy, and an inability to roll from back to front at 7 months (development was normal by 11 months). A case report in 2000 (Kircheiner *et al*) gave an account of an infant whose plasma levels of olanzapine were a third of maternal levels but who appeared to experience no adverse events. Gentile (2004) summarised the milk:plasma ratios and infant doses in two studies of 12 infants and reported ratios of between 0.10 and 0.84 with relative infant doses from 0.22 to 2.5%.

Risperidone

Hill *et al* (2000) reported milk:plasma ratios of 0.42 for risperidone and 0.24 for 9-hydroxyrisperidone. The likely infant dose of the drug and metabolite was 0.84% and 3.46% respectively. A similar study of three breastfeeding women (Ilett *et al*, 2004) revealed milk:plasma ratios of <0.5% and relative infant doses were 2.3%, 2.8% and 4.7%. There were no adverse events reported. In 2005, Aichhorn *et al* reported a case in which milk levels were tenfold lower than maternal plasma levels and the infant dose was well below 10%. Again, there were no adverse events.

Quetiapine

Lee *et al* (2004) report a case in which a woman taking quetiapine during pregnancy also breastfed her infant. Levels of quetiapine in milk fell to almost the pre-dose levels by 2 h and the estimated infant dose was 0.09–0.43% of the maternal dose. The infant was followed up until 4.5 months of age and no problems were observed. Another mother breastfed for 12 weeks without any adverse events in the infant (Ritz, 2005), and Gentile (2006) reported a women who took quetiapine and fluvoxamine with 5 mg folic acid daily throughout pregnancy. A Caesarean section was performed because of pre-existing uterine myoma and she supplemented breastfeeding with formula. Her infant also experienced no problems. Rampono *et al* (2007) observed a milk:plasma ratio of 0.29 and a relative infant dose of 0.09% in a 3-month-old infant and also observed no adverse events.

Misri *et al* (2006) investigated the effects of adding quetiapine to antidepressant therapy in six postpartum women who had panic disorder or obsessive–compulsive disorder. In half the sample, medication was detected in breast milk: quetiapine was detected in only one woman who had been taking a dose of 400 mg/day. Two infants showed evidence of mild developmental delays.

Clozapine

There are reports of clozapine concentrations in breast milk being higher than in maternal serum (Barnas *et al*, 1994). The authors state that this is most likely due to the lipophilic nature of the drug. There are reports of sedation, agranulocytosis (Trixler &Tenyi, 1997) and cardiovascular instability (Dev & Krup, 1995), so breastfeeding is not advised. It has been noted that some might allow women with schizophrenia already on clozapine to continue the medication while breastfeeding but if this is the case it is essential that regular full blood counts are taken from the infant as well as the mother (Goodwin & Young, 2005).

Others

There are no human data related to ziprasidone or aripiprazole and breastfeeding.

Non-drug interventions

There are no published data on ECT, transcranial magnetic stimulation or light therapy and breastfeeding, but provided short-acting anaesthetic agents are used for ECT and any existing drugs the patient might be taking are not contraindicated, breastfeeding should be possible soon after treatment. If a mother needs to sleep for some time after each treatment, then expressing milk beforehand can enable someone else to feed the infant should this be needed before she wakes.

References

Aichhorn, W., Stuppaeck, C. & Whitworth, A. B. (2005) Risperidone and breast-feeding. *Journal of Psychopharmacology*, **19**, 211–213.

Aichhorn, W., Whitworth, A. B., Weiss, U., *et al* (2004) Mirtazapine and breast-feeding. *American Journal of Psychiatry*, **161**, 2325.

Altshuler, L. L., Burt, V. K., McMullen, M., *et al* (1995) Breastfeeding and sertraline: a 24-hour analysis. *Journal of Clinical Psychiatry*, **56**, 243–245.

Andersen, H. J. (1983) Excretion of verapamil in human milk. *European Journal of Clinical Pharmacology*, **25**, 279–280.

Anderson, P. O. & McGuire, G. C. (1989) Neonatal alprazolam withdrawal; possible effects of breast feeding. *Annals of Pharmacotherapy*, **23**, 614.

Baab, S. W., Peindl, K. S., Piontek, C. M., *et al* (2002) Serum bupropion levels in 2 breastfeeding mother–infant pairs. *Journal of Clinical Psychiatry*, **63**, 910–911.

Barnas, C., Bergant, A., Hummer, M., *et al* (1994) Clozapine concentrations in maternal and fetal plasma, amniotic fluid, and breast milk. *American Journal of Psychiatry*, **151**, 945.

Bar-Oz, B., Nulman, I., Koren, G., *et al* (2000) Anticonvulsants and breast feeding: a critical review. *Paediatric Drugs*, **2**, 113–126.

Begg, E. J., Duffull, S. B., Saunders, D. A., *et al* (1999) Paroxetine in human milk. *British Journal of Clinical Pharmacology*, **48**, 142–147.

Birnbaum, C. S., Cohen, L. S., Bailey, J. W., *et al* (1999) Serum concentrations of antidepressants and benzodiazepines in nursing infants: a case series. *Pediatrics*, **104**, e11.

Brent, N. B. & Wisner, K. L. (1998) Fluoxetine and carbamazepine concentrations in a nursing mother/infant pair. *Clinical Pediatrics*, **37**, 41–44.

Briggs, G., Samson, J., Ambrose, P., *et al* (1993) Excretion of bupropion in breast milk. *Annals of Pharmacotherapy*, **27**, 431–433.

Buist, A. & Janson, H. (1995) Effect of exposure to dothiepin and northiaden in breast milk on child development. *British Journal of Psychiatry*, **167**, 370–373.

Burch, K. J. & Wells, B. G. (1992) Fluoxetine/norfluoxetine concentrations in human milk. *Pediatrics*, **89**, 676–677.

Castberg, I. & Spigset, O. (2006) Excretion of escitalopram in breast milk. *Journal of Clinical Psychopharmacology*, **26**, 536–537.

Chambers, C. D., Anderson, P. O., Thomas, R. G., *et al* (1999) Weight gain in infants breastfed by mothers who take fluoxetine. *Pediatrics*, **104**, e61–e65.

Dev, V. & Krup, P. (1995) The side-effects and safety of clozapine. *Reviews in Contemporary Pharmacotherapy*, **6**, 197–208.

Dodd, S., Buist. A., Burrows. G. D., *et al* (1999) Determination of nefazodone and its pharmacologically active metabolites in human blood and breast milk by high-performance liquid chromatography. *Journal of Chromatography B: Biomedical Sciences and Applications*, **730**, 249–255.

Dodd, S., Maguire, K. P., Burrows, G. D., *et al* (2000) Nefazodone in the breast milk of nursing mothers: a report of two patients. *Journal of Clinical Psychopharmacology*, **20**, 717–718.

Dugoua, J. J., Mills, E., Perri, D., *et al* (2006) Safety and efficacy of St John's Wort (hypericum) during pregnancy and lactation. *Canadian Journal of Clinical Pharmacology*, **13**, e268–e276.

Epperson, N., Czarkowski, K. A., Ward-O'Brien, D., *et al* (2001) Maternal sertraline treatment and serotonin transport in breast-feeding mother–infant pairs. *American Journal of Psychiatry*, **158**, 1631–1637.

Epperson, C. N., Jatlow, P. J., Czarkowski, K., *et al* (2003) Maternal fluoxetine treatment in the postpartum period: effects on platelet serotonin and plasma drug levels in breastfeeding mother–infant pairs. *Pediatrics*, **112**, e425–e429.

Erkkola, R. & Kanto, J. (1972) Diazepam and breast-feeding. *Lancet*, **3**, 1235–1236.

Ernst, C. L. & Goldberg, J. F . (2002) The reproductive safety profile of mood stabilizers, atypical antipsychotics, and broad-spectrum psychotropics. *Journal of Clinical Psychiatry*, **63**, 42–55.

Frey, B., Schubiger, G. & Musy, J. P. (1990) Transient cholestatic hepatitis in a neonate associated with carbamazepine exposure during pregnancy and breast-feeding. *European Journal of Pediatrics*, **150**, 136–138.

Frey, O., Scheidt, P. & von Brennendorff, A. I. (1999) Adverse effects in a newborn infant breast-fed by a mother treated with doxepin. *Annals of Pharmacotherapy*, **33**, 690–692.

Froescher, W., Eichelbaum, M., Niesen, M., *et al* (1984) Carbamazepine levels in breast milk. *Therapeutic Drug Monitoring*, **6**, 266–271.

Gentile, S. (2004) Clinical utilization of atypical antipsychotics in pregnancy and lactation. *Annals of Pharmacotherapy*, **38**, 1265–1271.

Gentile, S. (2005) Lamotrigine in pregnancy and lactation. *Archives of Women's Mental Health*, **8**, 57–58.

Gentile, S. (2006) Quetiapine-fluvoxamine combination during pregnancy and while breastfeeding. *Archives of Women's Mental Health*, **9**, 158–159.

Gentile, S. (2008) Infant safety with antipsychotic therapy in breast-feeding: a systematic review. *Journal of Clinical Psychiatry*, **69**, 666–673.

Ginsberg, D. L. (2004) Bupropion-associated seizure in a breastfeeding infant. *Primary Psychiatry*, **11**, 26–27.

Goodwin, G. & Young, A. H. (2005) Using guidelines in real clinical situations: clozapine and breast feeding in bipolar disorder. *Journal of Psychopharmacology*, **19**, 317–318.

Haas, J. S., Kaplan, C. P., Barenboim, D., *et al* (2004) Bupropion in breast milk: an exposure assessment for potential treatment to prevent post-partum tobacco use. *Tobacco Control*, **13**, 52–56.

Hackett, L. P., Ilett, K. F., Rampono, J., *et al* (2006) Transfer of reboxetine into breastmilk, its plasma concentrations and lack of adverse events in the breastfed infant. *European Journal of Clinical Pharmacology*, **62**, 633–638.

Hägg, S. & Spigset, O. (2000) Anticonvulsant use during lactation. *Drug Safety*, **22**, 425–440.

Hägg, S., Granberg, K. & Carleborg, L. (2000) Excretion of fluvoxamine into breast milk. *British Journal of Clinical Pharmacology*, **49**, 286–288.

Hale, T. W., Shum, S. & Grossberg, M. (2001) Fluoxetine toxicity in a breastfed infant. *Clinical Pediatrics*, **40**, 681–684.

Heikkinen, T., Ekblad, U., Palo, *et al* (2002*a*) Pharmacokinetics of fluoxetine and norfluoxetine in pregnancy and lactation. *Clinical Pharmacology and Therapeutics*, **73**, 330–337.

Heikkinen, T., Ekblad, U., Kero, P., *et al* (2002*b*) Citalopram in pregnancy and lactation. *Clinical Pharmacology and Therapeutics*, **72**, 184–191.

Hendrick, V., Stowe, Z. N., Altshuler, L. L., *et al* (2001*a*) Fluoxetine and norfluoxetine concentrations in nursing infants and breast milk. *Biological Psychiatry*, **50**, 775–782.

Hendrick, V., Fukuchi, A., Altshuler, L., *et al* (2001*b*) Use of sertraline, paroxetine and fluvoxamine by nursing women. *British Journal of Psychiatry*, **179**, 163–166.

Hendrick, V., Altshuler, L., Wertheimer, A., *et al* (2001*c*) Venlafaxine and breast-feeding. *American Journal of Psychiatry*, **158**, 2089–2090.

Hendrick, V., Smith, L. M., Hwang, S., *et al* (2003) Weight gain in breastfed infants of mothers taking antidepressants. *Journal of Clinical Psychiatry*, **64**, 410–412.

Hill, R. C., McIvor, R. J., Wojnar-Horton, R. E., *et al* (2000) Risperidone distribution and excretion into human milk: case report and estimated infant exposure during breast-feeding. *Journal of Clinical Psychopharmacology*, **20**, 285–286.

Hipwell, A. E., Murray, L., Ducournau, P., *et al* (2005) The effects of maternal depression and parental conflict on children's peer play. *Child: Care, Health & Development*, **31**, 11–23.

Humpel, M., Stoppelli, I., Milia, S., *et al* (1982) Pharmacokinetics and biotransformation of the new benzodiazepine, lormetazepam, in man. III Repeated administration and transfer to neonates via breast milk. *European Journal of Clinical Pharmacology*, **21**, 421–425.

Ilett, K. F., Hackett, L. P., Dusci, L. J., *et al* (1998) Distribution and excretion of venlafaxine and O-desmethylvenlafaxine in human milk. *British Journal of Clinical Pharmacology*, **45**, 459–462.

Ilett, K. F., Kristensen, J. H., Hackett, L. P., *et al* (2002) Distribution of venlafaxine and its O-desmethyl metabolite in human milk and their effects in breastfed infants. *British Journal of Clinical Pharmacology*, **53**, 17–22.

Ilett, K. F., Hackett, L. P., Kristensen, J. H., *et al* (2004) Transfer of risperidone and 9-hydroxyrisperidone into human milk. *Annals of Pharmacotherapy*, **38**, 273–276.

Ilett, K. F., Hackett, L. P., Kristensen, J. H., *et al* (2005) Estimation of infant dose and assessment of breastfeeding safety for escitalopram use in postnatal depression. *Therapeutic Drug Monitoring*, **27**, 248.

Iqbal, M. M., Sobhan, T. & Ryals, T. (2002) Effects of commonly used benzodiazepines on the neonate, and the nursing infant. *Psychiatric Services*, **53**, 39–49.

Isenberg, K. E. (1990) Excretion of fluoxetine in human breast milk. *Journal of Clinical Psychiatry*, **51**, 169.

Ito, S., Blajchman, A., Stephenson, M., *et al* (1993) Prospective follow-up of adverse reactions in breastfed infants exposed to maternal medication. *American Journal of Obstetrics and Gynecology*, **168**, 1393–1399.

Jensen, P. N., Olesen, O. V., Bertelsen, A., *et al* (1997) Citalopram and desmethylcitalopram concentrations in breast milk and in serum of mother and infant. *Therapeutic Drug Monitoring*, **19**, 236–239.

Kent L. S. & Laidlaw J. D. (1995) Suspected congenital sertraline dependence. *British Journal of Psychiatry*, **167**, 412b–413b.

Kim, J., Riggs, K. W., Misri, S., *et al* (2006) Stereoselective disposition of fluoxetine and norfluoxetine during pregnancy and breast-feeding. *British Journal of Clinical Pharmacology*, **61**, 155–163.

Kircheiner, J., Berghofer, A. & Bolk-Weischedel, D. (2000) Healthy outcome under olanzapine treatment in a pregnant woman. *Pharmacopsychiatry*, **33**, 78–80.

Klier, C. M., Schäfer, M. R., Schmid-Siegel, B., *et al* (2002) St. John's wort (*Hypericum perforatum*): is it safe during breastfeeding? *Pharmacopsychiatry*, **35**, 29–30.

Klier, C. M., Schmid-Siegel, B., Schäfer, M. R., et al (2006) St. John's wort (Hypericum perforatum) and breastfeeding: plasma and breast milk concentrations of hyperforin for 5 mothers and 2 infants. Journal of Clinical Psychiatry, 67, 305–309.

Klier, C. M., Mossaheb, N., Lee, A., et al (2007) Mirtazapine and breastfeeding: maternal and infant plasma levels. American Journal of Psychiatry, 164, 348–349.

Koren, G., Moretti, M. & Kapur, B. (2006) Can venlafaxine in breast milk attenuate the norepinephrine and serotonin reuptake neonatal withdrawal syndrome. Journal of Obstetrics and Gynaecology Canada, 28, 299–302.

Kristensen, J. H., Ilett, K. F., Dusci, L. J., et al (1998) Distribution and excretion of sertraline and N-desmethylsertraline in human milk. British Journal of Clinical Pharmacology, 45, 453–457.

Kristensen, J. H., Ilett, L. P., Yapp, P., et al (1999) Distribution and excretion of fluoxetine and norfluoxetine in human milk. British Journal of Clinical Pharmacology, 48, 521–527.

Kristensen, J. H., Hackett, L. P., Kohan, R., et al (2002) The amount of fluvoxamine in milk is unlikely to be a cause of adverse effects in breastfed infants. Journal of Human Lactation, 18, 139–143

Kristensen, J. H., Ilett, K. F., Hackett, L. P., et al (2006) Gabapentin and breastfeeding: a case report. Journal of Human Lactation, 22, 426–428.

Kristensen, J. H., Ilett, K. F., Rampono, J., et al (2007) Transfer of the antidepressant mirtazapine into breast milk. British Journal of Clinical Pharmacology, 63, 322–327.

Lebedevs, T. H., Wojnar-Horton, R. E., Yapp, P., et al (1992) Excretion of temazepam in breast milk. British Journal of Clinical Pharmacology, 33, 204–206.

Lee, A., Woo, J. & Ito, S. (2004) Frequency of infant adverse events that are associated with citalopram use during breast-feeding. American Journal of Obstetrics and Gynecology, 190, 218–221.

Lee, A., Minhas, R., Matsuda, N., et al (2003) The safety of St. John's wort (Hypericum perforatum) during breastfeeding. Journal of Clinical Psychiatry, 64, 966–968.

Lepola, U., Penttinen, J., Koponen, H., et al (2000) Citalopram treatment and breast-feeding. Biological Psychiatry, 47, S149.

Lester, B. M., Cucca, J., Andreozzi, L., et al (1993) Possible association between fluoxetine hydrochloride and colic in an infant. Journal of the American Academy of Child and Adolescent Psychiatry, 32, 1253–1255.

Liporace, J., Kao, A. & D'Abreu. (2004) Concerns regarding lamotrigine and breast-feeding. Epilepsy and Behavior, 5, 102–105.

Lobo, E. D., Loghin, C., Knadler, M. P., et al (2008) Pharmacokinetics of duloxetine in breast milk and plasma of healthy postpartum women. Clinical Pharmacokinetics, 47, 103–109.

Mammen, O. K., Perel, J. M., Rudolph, G., et al (1997) Sertraline and norsertraline levels in three breastfed infants. Journal of Clinical Psychiatry, 58, 100–103.

Matheson, I. & Skjaeraasen, J. (1988) Milk concentrations of flupenthixol, nortriptyline and zuclopenthixol and between-breast differences in two patients. European Journal of Clinical Pharmacology, 35, 217–220.

Matheson, I., Pande, H. & Alertsen, A. P. (1985) Respiratory depression caused by N-desmethl doxepin in breast milk. Lancet, 16, 1124.

Merlob, P., Mor, N. & Litwin, A. (1992) Transient hepatic dysfunction in an infant of an epileptic mother treated with carbamazepine during pregnancy and breastfeeding. Annals of Pharmacotherapy, 26, 1563–1565.

Merlob, P., Stahl, B. & Sulkes, J. (2004) Paroxetine during breast-feeding: infant weight gain and maternal adherence to counsel. European Journal of Pediatrics, 163, 135–139.

Misri, S. & Sivertz, K. (1991) Tricyclic drugs in pregnancy and lactation: a preliminary report. International Journal of Psychiatry in Medicine, 21, 157–171.

Misri, S., Kim, J., Riggs, W., et al (2000) Paroxetine levels in postpartum depressed women, breast milk and infant serum. Journal of Clinical Psychiatry, 61, 828–832.

Misri, S., Corral, M., Wardrop, A. A., et al (2006) Quetiapine augmentation in lactation: a series of case reports. Journal of Clinical Psychopharmacology, 26, 508–511.

Moretti, M. E., Koren, G., Verjee, Z., *et al* (2003) Monitoring lithium in breast milk: an individualized approach for breastfeeding mothers. *Clinical Pharmacology and Therapeutics,* **25**, 364–366.

Murray, L. & Cooper, P. (1997) Postpartum depression and child development. *Psychological Medicine,* **27**, 253–260.

Murray, L., Sinclair, D., Cooper, P., *et al* (1999) The socioemotional development of 5-year-old children of postnatally depressed mothers. *Journal of Child Psychology and Psychiatry and Allied Disciplines,* **40**, 1259–1271.

National Institute for Health and Clinical Excellence (2007) *Antenatal and Postnatal Mental Health: Clinical Management and Service Guidance.* British Psychological Society & Royal College of Psychiatrists.

Öhman, I., Vitols, S. & Tomson, T. (2000) Lamotrigine in pregnancy: pharmacokinetics during delivery, in the neonate and during lactation. *Epilepsia,* **41**, 709–713.

Öhman, I., Vitols, S. & Tomson, T. (2005) Pharmacokinetics of gabapentin during delivery, in the neonatal period, and lactation: does a fetal accumulation occur during pregnancy? *Epilepsia,* **46**, 1621–1624.

Öhman, R., Hagg, S., Carleborg, L., *et al* (1999) Excretion of paroxetine into breast milk. *Journal of Clinical Psychiatry,* **60**, 519–523.

Oo, C. Y., Kuhn, R. J., Desai, N., *et al* (1995) Pharmacokinetics in lactating women; prediction of alprazolam transfer into milk. *British Journal of Clinical Pharmacology,* **40**, 231–236.

Patton, S. W., Misri, S., Corral, M. R., *et al* (2002) Antipsychotic medication during pregnancy and lactation in women with schizophrenia: evaluating the risk. *Canadian Journal of Psychiatry,* **47**, 959–965.

Perel, J. M., Wisner, K. L., Reiter, C., *et al* (2003) Sertraline therapy of postpartum depression, maternal therapeutic drug monitoring and infant exposure during breastfeeding. *Therapeutic Drug Monitoring,* **25**, 518.

Piontek, C. M., Baab, S., Peindl, K. S., *et al* (2000) Serum valproate levels in 6 breastfeeding mother–infant pairs. *Journal of Clinical Psychiatry,* **61**, 170–172.

Piontek, C. M., Wisner, K. L., Perel, J. M., *et al* (2001) Serum fluvoxamine levels in breastfed infants. *Journal of Clinical Psychiatry,* **62**, 111–113.

Pons, G., Francoui, C., Guillet, P. (1989) Zolpidem excretion in breast milk. *European Journal of Clinical Pharmacology,* **37**, 245–248.

Pons, G., Schoerlin, P., Tam, Y. K., *et al* (1990) Moclobemide excretion in human breast milk. *British Journal of Clinical Pharmacology,* **29**, 27–31.

Rambek, B., Cullman, G., Stories, S. R. G., *et al* (1997) Concentrations of lamotrigine in a mother on lamotrigine treatment and her newborn child. *European Journal of Clinical Pharmacology,* **51**, 481–484.

Rampono, J., Kristensen, J. H., Hackett, L. P., *et al* (2000) Citalopram and demethylcitalopram in human milk; distribution, excretion and effects in breast fed infants. *British Journal of Clinical Pharmacology,* **50**, 263–268.

Rampono, J., Kristensen, J. H., Ilett, K. F., *et al* (2007) Quetiapine and breast feeding. *Annals of Pharmacotherapy,* **41**, 711–714.

Ritz, S. (2005) Quetiapine monotherapy in post-partum onset bipolar disorder with a mixed affective state. *European Neuropsychopharmacology,* **15(Suppl. 3)**, S407.

Schmidt, K., Olesen, O. V. & Jensen, P. N. (2000) Citalopram and breast-feeding: serum concentration and side effects in the infant. *Biological Psychiatry,* **47**, 164–165.

Schou, M. & Amdisen, A. (1973) Lithium and pregnancy 3: lithium ingestion by children breast-fed by women on lithium treatment. *BMJ,* **2**, 138.

Skausig, O. B. & Schou, M. (1977) Breastfeeding during lithium treatment. *Ugeskr Laeger,* **139**, 400–401.

Spigset, O., Carleborg, L., Öhman, R., *et al* (1997) Excretion of citalopram in breast milk. *British Journal of Clinical Pharmacology,* **44**, 295–298.

Stahl, M., Neiderud, J. & Vinge, E. (1997) Thrombocytopenic purpura and anemia in a breast-fed infant whose mother was treated with valproic acid. *Journal of Pediatrics,* **130**, 1001–1003.

Stowe, Z. N., Owens, M. J., Landry, J. C., *et al* (1997) Sertraline and desmethylsertraline in human breast milk and nursing infants. *American Journal of Psychiatry*, **154**, 1255–1260.

Stowe, Z. N., Cohen, L. S., Hostetter, A., *et al* (2000) Paroxetine in human breast milk and nursing infants. *American Journal of Psychiatry*, **157**, 185–189.

Stowe, Z. N., Hostetter, A. L., Owens, M. J. *et al* (2003) The pharmacokinetics of sertraline excretion into human breast milk: determinants of infant serum concentrations. *Journal of Clinical Psychiatry*, **64**, 73–80.

Suri, R., Stowe, Z. N., Hendrick, V., *et al* (2002) Estimates of nursing infant daily dose of fluoxetine through breast milk. *Biological Psychiatry*, **52**, 446–451.

Sykes, P. A., Quarrie, J. & Alexander, F. W. (1976) Lithium carbonate and breast-feeding. *BMJ*, **2**, 1299.

Taddio, A., Ito, S., Koren, G. (1996) Excretion of fluoxetine and its metabolite norfluoxetine in human breast milk. *Pediatrics*, **36**, 42–47.

Tomson, T., Öhman, I. & Vitols, S. (1997) Lamotrigine in pregnancy and lactation: a case report. *Epilepsia*, **38**, 1039–1041.

Trixler, M. & Tenyi, T. (1997) Antipsychotic use in pregnancy. *What are the best treatment options? Drug Safety*, **16**, 403–410.

Tunnessen, W. W. & Hertz, C. G. (1972) Toxic effects of lithium in newborn infants: a commentary. *Journal of Pediatrics*, **81**, 804–807.

Verbeeck, R. K., Ross, S. G. & McKenna, E. A. (1986) Excretion of trazodone in breast milk. *British Journal Clinical Pharmacology*, **22**, 367–370.

Viguera, A. C., Newport, D. J., Ritchie, J., *et al* (2007) Lithium in breast milk and nursing infants: clinical implications. *American Journal of Psychiatry*, **164**, 342–345.

Weissman, A. M., Levy, B. T., Hartz, A. J., *et al* (2004) Pooled analysis of antidepressant levels in lactating mothers, breast milk, and nursing infants. *American Journal of Psychiatry*, **161**, 1066–1078.

Whalley, L. J., Blain, P. G. & Prime, J. K. (1981) Haloperidol secreted in breast milk. *BMJ*, **282**, 1746–1747.

Wisner, K. L. & Perel, J. M. (1991) Serum nortriptyline levels in nursing mothers and their infants. *American Journal of Psychiatry*, **148**, 1234–1236.

Wisner, K. L. & Perel, J. M. (1998) Serum levels of valproate and carbamazepine in breastfeeding mother–infant pairs. *Journal of Clinical Psychopharmacology*, **18**, 167–169.

Wright, S., Dawling, S. & Ashford, D. (1991) Excretion of fluvoxamine in breast milk. *British Journal of Clinical Pharmacology*, **31**, 209.

Yapp, P., Ilett, K. F., Kristensen, J. H., *et al* (2000) Drowsiness and poor feeding in a breast-fed infant: association with nefazodone and its metabolites. *Annals of Pharmacotherapy*, **34**, 1269–1272.

Yoshida, K. & Kumar, R. (1996) Breast feeding and psychotropic drugs. *International Review of Psychiatry*, **8**, 117–124.

Yoshida, K., Smith, B., Craggs, M., *et al* (1997*a*) Investigation of pharmacokinetics and of possible adverse effects in infants exposed to tricyclic antidepressants in breast-milk. *Journal of Affective Disorders*, **43**, 225–237.

Yoshida, K., Smith, B. & Kumar, R.C. (1997*b*) Fluvoxamine in breast milk and infant development. *British Journal of Clinical Pharmacology*, **44**, 210–211.

Yoshida, K., Smith, B., Craggs, M., *et al* (1998*a*) Fluoxetine in breast-milk and developments outcome of breast-fed infants. *British Journal of Psychiatry*, **172**, 175–178.

Yoshida, K., Smith, B., Craggs, M., *et al* (1998*b*) Neuroleptic drugs in breast-milk: a study of pharmacokinetics and of possible adverse effects in breast-fed infants. *Psychological Medicine*, **28**, 81–91.

Further reading

American Academy of Pediatrics (2006) The transfer of drugs and other chemicals into human milk. *Pediatrics*, **108**, 776–789.

American College of Obstetricians and Gynecologists (2008) ACOG Practice Bulletin: Clinical management guidelines for obstetrician–gynecologists number 92, April 2008. *Use of psychiatric medications during pregnancy and lactation. Obstetrics & Gynecology*, **111**, 1001–1020.

Gentile, S., Rossi, A. & Bellantuono, C. (2007) SSRIs during breastfeeding: spotlight on milk-to-plasma ratio. *Archives of Women's Mental Health*, **10**, 39–51.

Hale, T. W. & Ilett, K. F. (2002) *Drug Therapy and Breastfeeding*. Parthenon.

Yoshida, K., Smith, B. & Kumar, R. (1999) Psychotropic drugs in mothers' milk: a comprehensive review of assay methods, pharmacokinetics and of safety of breast-feeding. *Journal of Psychopharmacology*, **13**, 64–80.

Drugs and Lactation Database (LactMed)

A US peer-reviewed and fully referenced database of drugs to which breastfeeding mothers may be exposed. Among the data included are maternal and infant levels of drugs, possible effects on breastfed infants and on lactation, and alternative drugs to consider. For further information see their website http://toxnet.nlm.nih.gov/cgi-bin/sis/htmlgen?LACT

CHAPTER 10

Service provision

Service provision in the UK remains patchy and inadequate. Although the NICE guideline on antenatal and postnatal mental health (National Institute for Health and Clinical Excellence, 2007) states that there should be a multidisciplinary perinatal service in each locality, access to specialist expert advice, clear referral and management protocols, there remain many areas of the UK where there is no service at all and in others only some elements of a comprehensive service.

Less than half of the trusts in England provide any specialist perinatal service. Although 58% have protocols and documents related to the management of perinatal psychiatric disorders, over half of these are inadequate or outdated (Oluwatayo & Friedman, 2005). The number of dedicated in-patient mother and baby beds has fallen since the early 1990s, leaving 75% of trusts without a dedicated mother and baby unit. Twelve per cent of trusts still admit mothers and babies to beds in non-specialist (general adult) wards contrary to national recommendations, while just over a third have no specific services or arrangements in place for admitting mothers and their babies. Fewer than 25% provide the full range of in-patient and community perinatal services. Of those that do not, only 5% have plans for future development of perinatal services.

It is to be hoped that the proposed Managed Clinical Networks (NHS Scotland, 2002) will develop more equitable services and that the Royal College of Psychiatrists' Quality of Care Network might ensure that mother and baby unit standards are uniform. Services must take account of the fact that perinatal psychiatric disorders include new, chronic and recurrent illness in relation to pregnancy and childbirth across the whole range and severity of psychiatric disorders. There are adjustment disorders and distress, anxiety and depressive disorders of a severity below that requiring referral to secondary care, and which should be appropriately managed in primary care through to more severe and complex cases – women with comorbidity and severe and enduring mental illness who will require assessment and/or management by a specialist team.

The service provision for any defined area or population must relate to the epidemiology. This has been clearly defined and is based on the birth rate rather than the total population (Royal College of Psychiatrists, 2001). Care should be taken to note any possible increase in people of reproductive age in a given area, for example a new factory opening and attracting a young workforce to the area, or the arrival of migrant workers, refugees or asylum seekers who may be concentrated in a particular town or city. Such groups can elevate the birth rate in an area and might have specific needs that must be addressed.

Although services may be targeted at mothers, many of their partners will also be experiencing mental health problems (Ballard *et al*, 1994; Glangeaud-Freudenthal *et al*, 2004), and a mechanism of assessing and meeting their needs should also be considered. Closer relationships and joint working with child and adolescent services are essential because of the well-established links between parental mental illness and associated emotional and behavioural problems in children and teenagers. Maternal depression, for example, is associated not only with an increase in behavioural problems in children but also with a poorer response to treatment directed at the behaviour disorder (Rishel *et al*, 2006).

Primary care

The role of primary care services is to detect and treat mild and moderate mental health problems in relation to pregnancy and childbearing, and to detect and refer more severe problems and those at risk of more serious problems to secondary or tertiary services. When referring women with a history of mental health problems to maternity care, information regarding the psychiatric history must be included in the referral.

Health visitors can be trained in both non-directive counselling but also elements of CBT such as cognitive–behavioural counselling. Such additional skills can lead to not only more assessments of women's mental health being carried out and better recording of contacts, but also more referrals to mental health services (Appleby *et al*, 2003). Women with depression treated by health visitors trained in either a cognitive–behavioural or person-centred approach have better outcomes at 6 months than those treated with usual health visitor care (Morrell *et al*, 2007) and these interventions have proved cost-effective. However, some women, particularly those who are younger and of lower educational status, exclude themselves from healthcare (Murray *et al*, 2003) and primary care professionals must consider what additional input might be required to engage such vulnerable women whose infants have poorer outcomes. Educating women about perinatal depression using a case vignette enabled better recognition of depression and a better assessment of their own mental state (Buist *et al*, 2007), so this is a strategy that could be employed by the primary care team.

Training is available (Appendix IV) both for individual professionals and for those wishing to train others. However, trainers who had attended one course reported several barriers to implementing training in their own trust, including only having been trained themselves recently, lack of time allocated to training, lack of referral systems and health visitors declining training (Elliott *et al*, 2003).

There are also Sure Start (www.surestart.gov.uk) services which have projects in perinatal mental health, sometimes for specific groups such as adolescent mothers, and services such as Homestart (www.home-start. org.uk) which although not focused on perinatal mental health do work with many women suffering from perinatal mental illness. There are many support and information services provided by the voluntary sector, some of which are outlined in Chapter 2.

Secondary care

Maternity services

In England and Wales, NHS trusts consist of service provider organisations within secondary care and primary care trusts which both provide primary care and commission services from secondary care. All trusts providing maternity care should have guidelines for the management of women at risk of a mental illness relapse following delivery. Women with substance misuse should be managed according to national guidelines.

Midwives must make a systematic enquiry about current and past mental health and substance misuse at antenatal booking, but this should not be implemented until appropriate training has taken place and there is a mechanism in place for regular updating.

Psychiatric disorders must be identified as specific syndromes and the acronym 'PND' should not be used. Serious mental illness or problem drug and/or alcohol histories are high-risk pregnancies and should have their management supervised by an obstetrician. Obstetricians and midwives must be aware of the law in relation to child protection and when and whom to refer to if concerns arise.

Trusts should ensure that self-medication on maternity units is controlled by using secure lockers for storage to reduce the risk of overdose.

Mental health services

Psychiatric services must share information and management plans with maternity services, social services and other agencies involved in a woman's care. They must assess women at risk of puerperal illness even if they are well during pregnancy and must consider contraception in childbearing women, particularly if they are known not to attend primary care services for this. Referral can be made to the local family planning service.

Psychiatric health professionals must consider the possibility of serious physical illness in recently delivered women suffering from unusual symptoms and must not automatically attribute these to psychiatric disorder. A third of the psychiatric deaths reported in *Why Mothers Die*

(Lewis & Drife, 2004) were owing to physical causes and in 50% symptoms were misattributed to psychiatric disorder, resulting in a delay in diagnosis and effective treatment.

Specialist perinatal psychiatric services

These are justified by:

- the special needs of perinatal women and their infants
- the specialist knowledge, skills and understanding required of staff, especially the assessment and management of the mother–infant relationship, including the diagnosis and treatment of severe mother–infant relationship disorders
- the critical mass of patients required to afford adequate experience in developing and maintaining staff skills, and to justify the material and human resources
- the difficulty for general services of maintaining skills, and understanding and prioritising the needs of this group of patients in the face of competing demands.

Functions of a specialist service

- To assess and manage those suffering from puerperal psychosis and other severe postnatal mental illnesses.
- To provide a range of facilities for their management, including an in-patient mother and baby unit (or access to one), out-patient clinics, alternatives to admission (intensive home nursing and/or day hospital) and community treatment.
- To advise on and, if necessary, manage patients with continuing psychiatric disorder who become pregnant while under the care of other adult psychiatrists, and work closely with child and adolescent and learning disability services, jointly managing cases where necessary.
- To liaise with primary healthcare professionals to assist in the management of less serious psychiatric conditions.
- To provide an obstetric liaison service, assessing mental health problems associated with pregnancy and the postpartum period, and deal with emergencies.
- To provide prenatal counselling and high-risk management for women at risk of developing an illness postpartum owing to previous major mental illness.
- To undertake the assessment of women with severe chronic mental illness in respect of their ability to parent their child and provide expert medico-legal advice.

A multidisciplinary specialist perinatal mental health service will also be in a position to play a lead role in the development of services at all levels of healthcare provision, to contribute to the education and training of other healthcare professionals, and will function at different levels relating to primary care and providing specialist advice and management.

237

Community services

Day care and home treatment

Oates (1988) developed community-based treatment for puerperal psychosis that allowed some women to be entirely treated at home and reduced the length of stay for others. This might be achieved today with community-based specialist perinatal mental health staff working alongside home treatment teams. Home treatment teams are unlikely to have the skills and expertise to manage these women and their infants without such collaboration.

Day units may be situated alongside mother and baby units and share staff or be sited in the community. Oluwatayo & Friedman (2005) identified only two day-units in England. The first of these, the Parent and Baby Day Unit in Stoke-on-Trent has been well described in the literature and its cost-effectiveness established when compared with routine primary care of women with postnatal depression (Boath et al, 2003). It offers care delivered by a multidisciplinary team who provide individual and group psychological and social interventions, and nursery nurse support with psychiatric medical review and treatment.

Howard et al (2006) describe a mother and baby day hospital programme in the USA where a variety of individual and group interventions are offered. Most of the care is offered on a short-term basis (mean duration 5 days, range 1–22); the majority of patients are suffering from major depressive disorder and around three-quarters receive medication (Battle et al, 2006).

In-patient units

The first recorded admission of a mother and baby to a psychiatric hospital is credited to Main in 1948 (Main, 1948) and was arranged to avoid any detrimental effect on the baby or reduction in maternal confidence if they were separated. Since then, in the UK, France, Germany, Australia, and New Zealand in particular, several specialised mother and baby units have been established, and in recent years units in Geneva (Alberque et al, 2006) and Jerusalem (Maizel et al, 2005) have been described. However, in other parts of the world, for example the USA, there are none or very few.

Despite admission to a specialist mother and baby unit being recommended in the UK for all women requiring in-patient psychiatric care who have an infant under the age of 12 months (Royal College of Psychiatrists, 2001; National Institute for Health and Clinical Excellence, 2007), there remain an insufficient number of beds. They are not uniformly distributed throughout the country in relation to population centres but are concentrated in some regions with none in others.

The mean duration of admission in a more recent series of 100 consecutive admissions in the UK was 2 months (Kumar et al, 1995). Almost half were admitted under the Mental Health Act 1983. Most women had become ill within 2 weeks of delivery and admitted acutely. An

Australian unit reported their mean duration of admission as 21.7 days and the majority of their patients had schizophrenia, other psychoses or major depression (Milgrom et al, 1998). Salmon et al (2004) audited data from 1217 UK admissions between 1996 and 2002. The most common primary diagnoses were depressive illness (43%), schizophrenia (21%) and bipolar disorder (14%). The only predictor of self-harm was depressed mood and behavioural disturbance; self-harm and the age of the mother (16–25 years) were found to predict harm to the child. Mothers with schizophrenia were three times more likely to experience a poor outcome and were more likely to be separated from their infant on discharge. A similar audit in France and Belgium on a smaller number of mother–baby admissions ($n=176$), found that schizophrenia was the most common diagnosis and the majority (65%) of admissions resulted in a symptom-free or considerably improved maternal mental state (Glangeaud-Freudenthal et al, 2004). Problems related to risk of harm to the infant or poor emotional response were more common in mothers with schizophrenia, delusional disorders, personality disorder or learning disability than in mothers with bipolar disorder or bouffée délirante.

There are naturalistic follow-up studies of women who have been admitted to mother and baby units and the general wards, case reports and service descriptions, many dating from the 1960s and 1970s. These are comprehensively described in the final chapter of Brockington (1996). Only one controlled trial compares outcomes in 20 mothers admitted with their infant and 20 women admitted without their infant (Baker et al, 1961), but they were not randomised. All mothers admitted to the mother and baby unit were able to care for their infant on discharge, whereas 13 of the 20 admitted alone were not. The average duration of admission was 10 weeks in the mother and baby unit and 16 weeks on the general ward.

Specialist in-patient units should have between 6 and 12 beds and be staffed by specialist professionals who are able to care for both acutely ill mothers and their infants. Hence, there will be nursery nurses on the staff, nursery and play areas, and a milk preparation area, in addition to rooms for mothers, sitting and dining areas, offices and interview rooms. They should offer a range of therapeutic services and be closely linked to maternity, general medical, mental health and community services.

Initial nursing and psychiatric assessment should consider the needs and safety of the infant. The observation level required should take this into account, with infants sleeping in the nursery if the mother is too disturbed or any risk is posed. This should be reviewed regularly and observation levels may be reduced if the mother poses no risk and is able to engage in infant care with support. Treatment is likely to include medication, psychological therapy, mothering skills interventions, perhaps family or couple work, and there may be social needs such has housing and financial issues. Discharge planning should closely involve community services and include contraceptive advice and advice regarding the risk of recurrence of the illness after any future pregnancies.

Women admitted to mother and baby units appear to be satisfied with the care they receive and prefer them to general acute psychiatric wards (Neil *et al*, 2006). It is recommended that women who require acute psychiatric admission following childbirth are admitted to a specialist mother and baby unit (Royal College of Psychiatrists, 2001; Department of Health, 2002, 2004; Lewis & Drife, 2004; National Institute for Health and Clinical Excellence, 2007). None of the women whose death resulted from a severe postnatal illness in the 2000–2002 CEMD had been admitted to a specialist mother and baby unit, but the authors of a Cochrane review point out that there is no trial-based evidence for their effectiveness (Joy & Saylan, 2007).

Obstetric liaison

This involves not only assessing women referred by maternity services, whether they are pregnant or postpartum, but also being available for consultation and advice on specific problems, ensuring that screening at the time of booking for antenatal care is carried out, and educating midwifery and obstetric staff when required. Establishing good working relationships with local maternity services is essential. An understanding of the normal and abnormal pregnancy, delivery and postpartum period in addition to embryology, foetal and infant development not only aids communication with other professionals but enables the psychiatrist to detect problems and know when to refer for specialist opinion.

Child protection

In England and Wales, the Children Act 1989 was updated in 2004 and updated guidance 'Working Together to Safeguard Children' was issued in 2006 (HM Government, 2006). These documents together provided a framework which established local safeguarding children's boards, created actual or virtual 'children's trusts' under the auspices of local authorities and clarified the duty of all agencies to make arrangements to safeguard and promote the welfare of children (a child is defined as anyone who has not yet reached their 18th birthday). Section 11 of the Children Act 2004 (Office of Public Sector Information, 2004) places a duty on strategic health authorities, special health authorities, primary care trusts, NHS trusts and foundation trusts to ensure that they have regard to the need to safeguard and promote the welfare of children.

Clinical networks

These already exist in some UK areas and more should follow as the NICE guideline is implemented. Each network should be managed by a coordinating board of health professionals, commissioners, managers, service users and carers, and they should provide a multidisciplinary perinatal service in each locality which can provide the following functions.

- Direct services, consultation and advice to maternity, mental health and community services, both urgent and routine.

- Specialist expert advice on the risks and benefits of psychotropic medication during pregnancy and while breastfeeding.
- Clear referral and management protocols at all levels of care.
- Clear pathways of care for service users.
- Designated specialist in-patient services.

What skills do perinatal psychiatrists need?

Perinatal psychiatrists require knowledge and skill in managing mental disorders at all levels of severity and complexity in pregnant and postpartum women. Therefore, in addition to general psychiatric skills, they must have knowledge and awareness of normal pregnancy and postpartum psychological and physiological changes, embryology, foetal and infant development, and the organisation of maternity care in the UK. They should be aware of the pharmacodynamic and pharmacokinetic changes of pregnancy and the postpartum and have knowledge of psychopharmacology in relation to this.

Raphael-Leff (1991) explores the issues relating to psychotherapy with pregnant women and highlights the countertransference reactions in different types of therapists. These include envy in men or childless women, repressed elements from a non-pregnant therapist's own past pregnancies and 'powerful transference implants' from the patient which may induce the therapist to enact the parental role. She describes maternal therapists who may feel anxious about the patient nurturing their child and the difficulties that might surround a pregnant therapist whose own vulnerability and introspection may have increased.

Perinatal psychiatrists must be able to consult and liaise with psychiatric, maternity and obstetric staff and primary care services and have skills in multiagency working, particularly with childcare social services. They should ensure that they make themselves fully aware of local services for mothers in their area.

They should be familiar with policies and guidelines relating to perinatal mental health, both nationally and those developed in their local area.

Skills in the assessment of parenting may be required and are discussed in Chapter 4.

Medico-legal expertise

Perinatal psychiatrists should have knowledge of the legislation and guidance in relation to child protection. They will be asked by numerous bodies for reports including social services, Mental Health Act review tribunals and the courts. It is essential to develop skills in producing reports that will withstand the scrutiny of these agencies and cross-examination at tribunals and in court. Psychiatrists may be asked about parenting capacity but should not give expert opinion on this unless they are skilled in assessing it. Such assessment cannot be made on the basis of psychiatric interview and perusal of records alone, and must involve direct observation of parent–child interaction and interview of any others involved in childcare such as foster parents and/or other family members (Bass & Adshead, 2007).

Conclusion

It is to be hoped that service provision in the UK will improve to ensure a more equitable and comprehensive service is available to every woman who needs it, and that more collaborative working between services and agencies will improve the care and well-being of families.

References

Alberque, C., Robert, V. & Eytan, A. (2006) A peripartum inpatient psychiatric program for mothers and infants. *Psychiatric Services*, **57**, 721.

Appleby, L., Hirst, E., Marshall, S., *et al* (2003) The treatment of postnatal depression by health visitors: impact of brief training on skills and clinical practice. *Journal of Affective Disorders*, **77**, 261–266.

Baker, A. A., Morison, M., Game, J. A., *et al* (1961) Admitting schizophrenic mothers with their babies. *Lancet*, **ii**, 237–239.

Ballard, C. G., Davis, R., Cullen, P. C., *et al* (1994) Prevalence of postnatal psychiatric morbidity in mothers and fathers. *British Journal of Psychiatry*, **164**, 782–788.

Bass, C. & Adshead, G. (2007) Fabrication and induction of illness in children: the psychopathology of abuse. *Advances in Psychiatric Treatment*, **13**, 169–177.

Battle, C. L., Zlotnick, C., Miller, I. W., *et al* (2006) Clinical characteristic of perinatal psychiatric patients: a chart review study. *Journal of Nervous and Mental Disease*, **194**, 369–377.

Boath, E., Major, K. & Cox, J. (2003) When the cradle falls II: The cost-effectiveness of treating postnatal depression in a psychiatric day hospital compared with routine primary care. *Journal of Affective Disorders*, **74**, 159–166.

Brockington, I. (1996) *Motherhood and Mental Health*. Oxford University Press.

Buist, A., Speelman, C., Hayes, B., *et al* (2007) Impact of education on women with perinatal depression. *Journal of Psychosomatic Obstetrics and Gynaecology*, **28**, 49–54.

Department of Health (2002) *Women's Mental Health: Into the Mainstream: Strategic Development of Mental Health Care for Women*. TSO (The Stationery Office).

Department of Health (2004) *National Service Framework for Children, Young People and Maternity Services; Maternity Services*. TSO (The Stationery Office).

Elliott, S. A., Ashton, C., Gerrard, J., *et al* (2003) Is trainer training an effective method for disseminating evidence-based practice for postnatal depression? *Journal of Reproductive and Infant Psychology*, 21, 219–228.

Glangeaud-Freudenthal, N. M-C., & the MBU–SMF Working Group (2004) Mother–Baby psychiatric units (MBUs): national data collection in France and Belgium (1999–2000). *Archives of Women's Mental Health*, **7**, 59–64.

HM Government (2006) *Working Together to Safeguard Children*. TSO (The Stationery Office).

Howard, M., Battle, C. L., Pearlstein, T., *et al* (2006) A psychiatric mother–baby day hospital for pregnant and postpartum women. *Archives of Women's Mental Health*, **9**, 213–218.

Joy, C. B. & Saylan, M. (2007) Mother and baby units for schizophrenia. *Cochrane Database of Systematic Reviews*, **1**, CD006333.

Kumar, R., Marks, M., Platz, C., *et al* (1995) Clinical survey of a psychiatric mother and baby unit: characteristics of 100 consecutive admissions. *Journal of Affective Disorders*, **33**, 11–22.

Lewis, G. & Drife, J. (2004) *Why Mothers Die 2000–2002. The Sixth Report of the Confidential Enquiries into Maternal Deaths in the United Kingdom.* RCOG Press.

Main, T. F. (1948) Mothers with children in a psychiatric hospital. *Lancet*, **2**, 845–847.

Maizel, S., Kandel Katzenelson, S. & Fainstein, V. (2005) The Jerusalem psychiatric mother–baby unit. *Archives of Women's Mental Health*, **8**, 200–202.

Milgrom, J., Burrows, G. D., Snellen, M., *et al* (1998) Psychiatric illness in women: a review of the function of a specialist mother–baby unit. *Australian and New Zealand Journal of Psychiatry*, **32**, 680–686.

Morrell, C. J., Warner, R., Paley, G., *et al* (2007) The PONDER trial: something to think about. *Archives of Women's Mental Health*, **10**, 1.

Murray, L., Woolgar, M., Murray, J., *et al* (2003) Self-exclusion from healthcare in women at risk for postnatal depression. *Public Health Medicine*, **25**, 131–137.

National Institute for Health and Clinical Excellence (2007) *Antenatal and Postnatal Mental Health: Clinical Management and Service Guidance.* British Psychological Society & Royal College of Psychiatrists.

Neil, S., Sanderson, H. & Wieck, A. (2006) A satisfaction survey of women admitted to a psychiatric mother and baby unit in the northwest of England. *Archives of Women's Mental Health*, **9**, 109.

NHS Scotland (2002) *What are Managed Clinical Networks?* Hayward Medical Communications.

Oates, M. (1988) The development of an integrated community-orientated service for severe postnatal mental illness. In *Motherhood and Mental Illness: Causes and Consequences.* (eds R. Kumar & I.F. Brockington). Wright.

Office of Public Sector Information (2004) Arrangements to safeguard and promote welfare (Section 11). In *Children Act (2004).* TSO (The Stationery Office).

Oluwatayo, O. & Friedman, T. (2005) A survey of specialist perinatal mental health services in England. *Psychiatric Bulletin*, **29**, 177–179.

Raphael-Leff, J. (1991) Psychotherapy with pregnant women. In *Psychological Processes of Childbearing*, pp. 91–116. Chapman & Hall.

Rishel, C. W., Greeno, C. G., Marcus, S. C., *et al* (2006) Effect of maternal mental health problems on child treatment response in community-based services. *Psychiatric Services*, **57**, 716.

Royal College of Psychiatrists (2001) *Perinatal Mental Health Services: Recommendations for Provision of Services for Childbearing Women.* Royal College of Psychiatrists.

Salmon, M. P., Abel, K., Webb, R., *et al* (2004) A national audit of joint mother and baby admissions to UK psychiatric hospitals: an overview of findings. *Archives of Women's Mental Health*, **7**, 65–70.

Further reading

Royal College of Psychiatrists (2008) *Quality Network for Perinatal Mental Health Services: Standards for Mother and Baby In-patient Units.* Royal College of Psychiatrists (http://www.rcpsych.ac.uk/researchandtrainingunit/centreforqualityimprovement/perinatalqualitynetwork.aspx).

CHAPTER 11

Perinatal psychiatry in multi-ethnic societies

'In no known culture was pregnancy found to be ignored or treated with indifference, instead it elicited a gamut of emotions and feelings including responsibility and accountability by the parents as well as solicitude by social groups' (Mead & Newton, 1967).

Childbirth has been regarded by social anthropologists as a rite of passage with three phases: separation, a liminal in-between period when the mother is hospitalised for the birth and that of incorporation when she re-enters society in a new status. In modern secular Western societies, however, with rapid changes in family structure (increased likelihood of divorce and absent fathers), shorter stays in the maternity unit and an expectation of prompt return to work, this transition may be incomplete and the mother remains 'in limbo'. There is, for example, less attention than in traditional societies to marking the entry to the new parenting role, and to celebrating the birth with a public naming ceremony and family party. In the last three decades, the childbearing woman has a more ambiguous and possibly diminished status in society; the reaction it elicits from others may even include condolences and a questioning about who will look after the baby. A journalist for *The Guardian* newspaper (Bunting, 2006) has drawn attention to the fall of the birth rate in Europe with the headline 'Behind the baby gap lies a culture of contempt for parenthood'. She suggested that present-day culture values consumption, choice and independence, which may threaten the inherent demands of parenthood.

Thus, a sociocultural approach to understanding the stresses of childbirth is necessary for a comprehensive grasp of the causes and management of perinatal mental disorder in contemporary society. Familiarity with local values, priorities and culture (including language and religion), and the way these change over time is particularly important when developing a perinatal service for a multicultural society. Transcultural psychiatry begins 'at home', where the values of post-modern families (which may include excessive deference to biomedicine) are culturally based (see Littlewood, 1992).

This sociocultural approach to perinatal psychiatry, together with the theory and practice of dynamic/developmental psychiatry, is central to any working model for perinatal psychiatrists in present-day multi-ethnic, multifaith Britain (Cox, 1999). Furthermore, it is within a broad brain/mind context that the advances in the neuroscience of puerperal psychosis (Chapter 4) are best appreciated. The bio-psychosocial model popularised by Engel (1980) encourages exploration of the parents' personal narratives as well as the identification of ghosts and ancestors in the nursery (Fraiberg *et al*, 1987).

Low- and middle-income countries

In Africa, Collomb *et al* (1972) described Senegalese childbearing women as entering a world of worries and fears, and noticed that quite often anxiety 'wins out over veneration and contentment'. In many other low-income countries, childbirth and the associated mental disorders are times of great risk to the well-being and longevity of the mother and her infant. It is estimated that 1 in 16 mothers in some sub-Saharan African countries have a lifetime risk of dying in childbirth (World Health Organization, 2005), yet only recently in the United Nations Millennium Development Goals Report has this staggering statistic become at last an action call and an international public health priority (United Nations, 2005). Goal 5 has the target to reduce the maternal mortality ratio by three-quarters before 2015. Empowering women and promoting gender equality (Goal 3) are other tasks which, if achieved, will improve maternal and child health, as well as the well-being of the next generation.

Social support

A much-quoted paper by Stern & Kruckman (1983) described the sociocultural components that provided social support in traditional societies, and the authors suggested that the extent of this support may 'cushion or prevent the experience of postpartum depression'. The components they considered included:

- structuring of a distinctive postpartum time period
- protective measures and rituals reflecting the vulnerability of the mother
- social exclusion
- mandated rest
- assistance from relatives or a midwife
- social recognition through rituals, gifts, etc. of the new social status of the mother.

They pointed out that postnatal depression was infrequently described in traditional societies compared with Europe or the USA, and attributed this to the possibility that social support and higher status protected against maternal mental disorder. Their observation spurred on subsequent community studies, which indeed suggested that although depressive symptoms were readily identified in traditional societies, their impact and duration was different.

Transcultural study of postnatal depression

An international study led by Channi Kumar (Marks *et al*, 2004), for example, brought together research groups in Europe (France, UK, Sweden, Portugal, Italy, Switzerland and Austria) as well as Japan, USA and Uganda, with the aim to develop, harmonise and validate culturally sensitive research instruments for use in the perinatal field. Each research centre also used qualitative research methods (focus groups, key informant interviews) to explore whether or not postnatal depression was a recognised condition (see Oates *et al*, 2004). A morbid state of unhappiness postpartum was found in most of the cultures and countries studied, with symptoms similar to those commonly identified in postnatal depression; however, these symptoms were not universally regarded as a medical condition that required treatment by health professionals. In Uganda, for example, there was no folk disorder similar to postnatal depression familiar to local informants, although there was a traditional illness *Amakiro*, which included symptoms found in puerperal psychosis (Cox, 1979). The disability for a mother with depression was, however, considerable and included difficulty with household tasks (e.g. digging and carrying water) as well as problems with childcare. In a study from Malta by Felice *et al* (2006), low rates of depression postpartum were found in this cohesive Catholic island community. Likewise in Japan, where gender roles were more traditionally proscribed, and in Uganda where the status and social support from co-wives and tradition was clearly evident (Cox, 1983), the rates of depression were also less than that reported in urban areas in high-income countries.

It is likely, therefore, that social support available to mothers during pregnancy and in the year postpartum is an important variable that determines the duration of depression during pregnancy and postpartum – and its severity. A working knowledge of sociology (role change, gender tasks, family structure), psychology (personality traits, dependency, self-esteem) and social anthropology (values, meaning of symptoms and childbirth rituals) is important for a full understanding of the maintaining factors for perinatal mental health.

Psychoanalysts (e.g. Raphael-Leff, 2001) have described the unconscious identification that occurs between the mother and baby, as well as the problems that these processes cause if there were difficulties in these relationships and if the new mother herself had had an unhappy childhood, the mother–infant relationship being the vehicle through which knowledge and culture are passed on between generations. Thus, 'breaks in women's knowledge' (Fitzgerald, 1998) that occur in modern societies, because of increased mobility and more short-term relationships, can cause difficulty with parenting because of a lack of knowledge about childcare and familiarity with and access to supportive customs.

The benefits of health visitor 'listening visits' and of structured counselling postpartum may, therefore, best be explained by an understanding of these psychological mechanisms that are a component of any professional relationship. The health visitor (usually a woman), for example, provides advice, validation of status and specific practical knowledge about feeding and infant development that could have been available from the mother's own mother.

The anthropologist Lewis (1976) has said that if a mother does not know how to bring up her children, then the cultural heritage is in jeopardy. Present-day attempts by politicians to diminish the amount of challenging behaviour in adolescent boys and to help vulnerable families through programmes such as Sure Start may partially compensate for these 'breaks in women's knowledge' and, if successful, could enhance the neurodevelopmental processes of the infant and facilitate secure attachments.

Secular contemporary Western societies, in contrast to some traditional societies, are in general characterised by:

- delayed childbearing
- greater mobility of parents and financial independence of grandparents
- smaller families
- increased secularisation with decline in religious adherence
- breaks in the transmission of women's knowledge.

Public health considerations

Perinatal mental health problems and mental disorders are of increasing prominence to public health planners throughout the world. They impact on the viability of young families and may influence the extent to which the next generation of parents fulfil their responsibilities and maintain good mental health. There is also evidence that perinatal mental disorder can adversely affect attachment and cognitive development, particularly of boys in Western societies (see Chapter 6), and weight gain, including failure to thrive in the developing world (Patel *et al*, 2005). In a community study from Stoke-on-Trent (O'Brien *et al*, 2004) we found a twofold increase in the likelihood of clinical depression in mothers whose babies had non-organic failure to thrive. Possible explanations for this finding included feeding difficulties initiated by an irritable or crying baby, as well as the mother being unable to persist with feeding or having insufficient breast milk because of her depression.

The importance of the gender of the infant is a variable that has marked cultural assumptions; a female infant was found to be associated with maternal postnatal depression in the Sikh community in Wolverhampton (Clifford *et al*, 1997) and in studies in India (Chandran *et al*, 2002) and Nigeria (Abiodun, 2006). It is of interest that in Western Europe, in mostly

White populations, boys whose mothers had depression postpartum were more likely than girls to show behavioural disturbance as 15 year olds, and to have an elevated morning cortisol (Hay *et al*, 2001). The reason for this is unclear.

Grandparents

Transcultural research shows that grandparents are particularly useful in providing support in the immediate postpartum months, yet in almost all centres of the international study by Marks *et al* (2004), mothers-in-law were also found to be a possible source of unhappiness.

In modern Japan, the custom *Satogeri-bunben*, when a mother goes to her own mother's house for the birth and remains there for the first 40 days, is still practised but does not necessarily protect against postnatal depression (Yoshida *et al*, 2001). Likewise in China, 'doing the month' is still practised; after childbirth the new mother should not go outside or be blown by the wind, nor should she have sex with her husband. She should eat chicken and is supported during this month by her mother. These proscriptions clarify the responsibilities for the new mother and the expected practical and emotional support from the family. In Hong Kong, however, it has been shown by Lee *et al* (2004) that this practice is not always helpful and could heighten the conflict for the mother between her filial respect for her mother and her wish for autonomy. In Uganda, before the AIDS pandemic, the support for the new mother who was married was almost always available from co-wives or neighbours, and older children might also help with household tasks. The naming ceremony and baptism were particularly important and the name was usually chosen by the grandparent. A single parent, however, was severely ostracised, as the baby would have no name – and therefore no family.

Many traditional and modern societies are now in transition because of political unrest, urbanisation and globalisation, which increase mobility and the separation of the nuclear family. Single-parent families, serial marriages, as well as same-gender marriages, may suggest that the family into which an infant is born and within which the transition to parenthood occurs, is a vortex of change and innovation. The likelihood of increased levels of stress in the family, particularly in the mother, with the possibility of an adverse effect on infant development has therefore to be acknowledged. A recent qualitative study of same-gender parents identified lack of support from family of origin, challenges in negotiating parenting roles, and legal and policy barriers as stressors (Ross, 2005).

Refugees and asylum seekers

Women are particularly vulnerable to the stresses of migration and of cultural change. Those who have moved from their home country and become parents in a new country are particularly at risk for perinatal depression. Studies of immigrants from Cambodia and Vietnam to Australia (Matthey *et al*, 1997) find that such women are particularly vulnerable to postnatal depression.

There are additional stresses on immigrant parents as the father may be working away from home and absorbing the new culture and language, while the mother is less exposed to these influences and may become very isolated. Other difficulties include a conflict of values, as the mother and her baby socialise with local women with different attitudes towards childcare, as well as secular values different from the religious traditions of the immigrant.

Refugee families have often been exposed to very distinctive stressors. Asylum seekers arriving in the UK may have been traumatised and it can be a difficult task for the clinician to disentangle the symptoms of post-traumatic stress disorder from a comorbid depression or anxiety disorder. They may have experienced 'sequential traumatisation' and as a consequence have an increased risk of mental health problems. These stresses include: violence, torture and rape; poverty; stigma; uncertain legal status; and cultural bereavement.

Health workers in this field have identified a healing relationship, safety, remembrance and mourning, and reconnection as being important components of the refugees' recovery process. They also emphasise the stresses on the health professional working with vulnerable refugees, and the difficulties overcoming language and cultural handicaps, as well as the intrusion of their own feelings.

Drennan & Joseph (2005) have described the issues relevant for professional practice and identified the prioritisation of the mother's own basic needs, as well as the needs of the infant. The practical barriers and culturally determined barriers to care, which included limited access to services and language difficulties, as well as the fear of stigma and the lack of validation of depression by family and society, were other factors listed by Teng *et al* (2007).

The health professional working with immigrant groups may thus fear being de-skilled by cultural uncertainty and by language problems, as well as having inadequate assessment tools.

Edinburgh Postnatal Depression Scale: cultural issues

The EPDS (Cox *et al*, 1987), which was developed and validated in Scotland, has been translated into over 25 languages and validated for use in all continents (Cox & Holden, 2003; Henshaw & Elliott, 2005). The process of translating the Scale and using it in a non-English-speaking community brings the clinician face to face with the cultural components of perinatal mental disorders described and their satisfactory management. The issues of translation are fully discussed by Flaherty *et al* (1988), and each has to be addressed, i.e. the need to establish semantic validity, content validity, technical equivalence and construct validity.

Management issues

The development of a perinatal mental health service with appropriate referral pathways can only be established if there is a full awareness of sociocultural dimensions. Clinicians and managers are each required to be culturally competent, and so fully aware of their own cultural assumptions. It is also necessary for them to have hands-on experience of the assessment and an understanding of the psychology of refugees and their particular experience of stress. The provision of readily available trained interpreters, advocates and culture brokers is crucial in the modern world of increased migration. Awareness of the impact of changes in family structure on social support, familiarity with naming customs in ethnic minorities, understanding the values and beliefs of service users, as well as the pitfalls of superficial translation, are other examples of the required core skills and competencies.

References

Abiodun, O. A. (2006) Postnatal depression in primary care populations in Nigeria. *General Hospital Psychiatry*, **28**, 133–136.

Bunting, M. (2006) Behind the baby gap lies a culture of contempt for parenthood. *The Guardian*, Tuesday 7 March.

Chandran, M., Tharyan, P., Muliyil, J., *et al* (2002) Post-partum depression in a cohort of women from a rural area of Tamil Nadu, India: incidence and risk factors. *British Journal of Psychiatry*, **181**, 499–504.

Clifford, C., Day, A. & Cox, J. (1997) Women's health after birth. Developing the use of EPDS in a Punjabi-speaking community. *British Journal of Midwifery*, **5**, 616–619.

Collomb, H., Guena, R. & Diop, B. (1972) Psychological and social factors in the pathology of childbearing. *Foreign Psychiatry*, **1**, 77–89.

Cox, J. L. (1979) Amakiro: a Ugandan puerperal psychosis? *Social Psychiatry*, **14**, 49–52.

Cox, J. L. (1983) Postnatal depression: a comparison of African and Scottish women. *Social Psychiatry*, **18**, 25–28.

Cox, J. L. (1999) Perinatal mood disorder in a changing culture: a trans-cultural European and African perspective. *International Review of Psychiatry*, **11**, 103–110.

Cox, J. L. & Holden. J. (2003) *Perinatal Mental Health: A Guide to the Edinburgh Postnatal Depression Scale*. Gaskell.

Cox, J. L., Holden, J. M. & Sagovsky, R. (1987) Detection of postnatal depression. Development of the 10-item Edinburgh Postnatal Depression Scale. *British Journal of Psychiatry*, **150**, 782–786.

Drennan, V. M. & Joseph, J. (2005) Health visiting and refugee families: issues in professional practice. *Journal of Advanced Nursing*, **49**, 155–163.

Engel, G. (1980) The clinical application of the Bio-psycho-social model. *American Journal of Psychiatry*, **137**, 534–554.

Felice, E., Saliba, J., Grech, V., *et al* (2006) Validation of the Maltese version of the Edinburgh Postnatal Depression Scale. *Archives of Women's Mental Health*, **9**, 75–80.

Fitzgerald, M. H. (1998) *Hear Our Voices: Trauma, Birthing and Mental Health among Cambodian Women*. Sydney Transcultural Mental Health Centre.

Flaherty, J. A., Gaviria, F. M., Pathak D., *et al* (1988) Developing instruments for transcultural psychiatric research. *Journal of Nervous and Mental Disease*, **176**, 257–264.

Fraiberg, S., Adelson, E. & Shapiro, V. (1987) Ghosts in the nursery: a psychoanalytic approach to the problems of impaired infant–mother relationships. In *Selected Writings of Selma Fraiberg* (ed. L. Fraiberg), 100–136. Ohio State University Press.

Hay, D. F., Pawlby, S., Sharp, D., *et al* (2001) Intellectual problems shown by 11 year old children, whose mothers had postnatal depression. *Journal of Child Psychology and Psychiatry*, **42**, 871–889.

Henshaw, C. & Elliott, S. (eds) (2005) Appendix 2: Bibliography of translations and validation studies. In *Screening for Perinatal Depression*, pp. 205–211. Jessica Kingsley.

Lee, D. T. S., Yip, A. S. K., Leung, T. Y. S., *et al* (2004) Ethnoepidemiology of postnatal depression: prospective multivariate study of sociocultural risk factors in a Chinese population in Hong Kong. *British Journal of Psychiatry*, **184**, 34–40.

Lewis, I. M. (1976) *Social Anthropology in Perspective*. Penguin Books.

Littlewood, R. (1992) Russian dolls and Chinese boxes: an anthropological approach to the implicit models of comparative psychiatry. In *Transcultural Psychiatry* (ed. J. L. Cox). Croom Helm.

Marks, M., O'Hara, M., Glangeaud-Freudenthal, N., *et al* (2004) Transcultural study of postnatal depression: development of harmonised research methods. *British Journal of Psychiatry*, **184**(Suppl. 46).

Matthey, S., Barnett, B. E., & Elliott, A. (1997) Vietnamese and Arabic women's responses to the Diagnostic Interview Schedule (depression) and self-report questionnaires: cause for concern. *Australian and New Zealand Journal of Psychiatry*, **31**, 360–369.

Mead, M. & Newton, N. (1967) Cultural patterning of perinatal behaviour. In *Childbearing: Its Social and Psychological Aspects* (eds A.F. Richardson & S.A. Guttmacher). Williams & Wilkins.

Oates, M., Cox, J. L., Neema, S. *et al* (2004) Postnatal depression across countries and cultures: a qualitative study. *British Journal of Psychiatry*, **184** (suppl. 46), S10–S16.

O'Brien, I. M., Haycock, L., Hanna, P. *et al* (2004) Postnatal depression and faltering growth: a community study. *Pediatrics*, **113**, 1242–1247.

Patel, V., Desouza, N. & Rodrigues, M. (2005) Postnatal depression and infant growth and development in low income countries: a short study from Goa, India. *Archives of Diseases of the Child*, **88**, 34–37.

Raphael-Leff, J. (2001) *Psychological Processes of Childbearing*. University of Essex.

Ross, L. E. (2005) Perinatal mental health in lesbian mothers: a review of potential risk and protective factors. *Women and Health*, **41**, 113–128.

Stern, C. & Kruckman, L. (1983) Multi-disciplinary perspectives on post partum depression: an anthropological critique. *Social Science and Medicine*, **17**, 1027–1041.

Teng, L., Robertson Blackmore, E. & Stewart, D.E. (2007) Healthcare workers' perceptions of barriers to care by immigrant women with postpartum depression: an exploratory qualitative study. *Archives of Women's Mental Health*, **10**, 93–101.

United Nations (2005) *The Millennium Development Goals Report 2005*. United Nations Department of Public Information.

World Health Organization (2005) *Mothers and Children*. WHO.

Yoshida, K., Yamashita, H., Ueda, M. *et al* (2001) Postnatal depression in Japanese mothers and the reconsideration of 'Satogeri-bunben'. *Paediatrics International*, **43**, 189–193.

Further reading

Ingleby, D. (2004) *Forced Migration and Mental Health: Rethinking the Care of Refugees and Displaced Persons*. Springer-Verlag.

Wilson, J. P. & Drožek, B. (2004) *Broken Spirits: The Treatment of Traumatized Asylum Seekers, Refugees, War and Torture Victims*. Routledge.

Appendix I
Randomised controlled trials of interventions for postnatal depression

Study	Intervention	Country	Sample size, n	Inclusion criteria	Control group	Assessments	Maternal outcome(s)	Limitations
Holden et al, 1989	Non-directive counselling	UK	26	Research diagnostic criteria major/minor depression	Standard care	SPI, EPDS, research diagnostic criteria diagnoses	Intervention > control	Randomisation not described, health visitors trained in non-directive counselling also visited control group mothers, 12 mothers also had antidepressants
Meager & Milgrom, 1996	Group CBT	Australia	20	EPDS, BDI	Waiting list	EPDS, BDI, POMS, PSI, DAS, CSEI, SPS	Intervention > control	Randomisation unclear, 40% were on antidepressants, 40% terminated early
Wickberg & Hwang, 1996	Non-directive counselling	Sweden	41	DSM–III–R major depression	Standard care	SCID, HRSD, BDI, DAS, SAS–SR, IDD, PPAQ	Intervention > control	Possible selection bias, control group women could visit clinic where trained nurses worked
Appleby et al, 1997	Fluoxetine + 1 × CBC v. fluoxetine + 6 × CBC v. placebo + 1 × CBC v. placebo + 6 × CBC	UK	87	Research diagnostic criteria major/minor depression	None	EPDS, HRSD, CIS–R	Fluoxetine + CBC > placebo. No additive effect and 1 × CBC = 6 × CBC	No true control group, 54% declined to take part and take medication
O'Hara et al, 2000	Interpersonal psychotherapy	USA	120	DSM–IV major depression	Waiting list	SCID, HRSD, BDI, DAS, SAS–SR, IDD, PPAQ	Intervention > control ↓ depressive symptoms and ↑ social function	20% women withdrew from intervention group, assessors not masked

Study	Intervention	Country	Sample size, n	Inclusion criteria	Control group	Assessments	Maternal outcome(s)	Limitations
Prendergast & Austin, 2001	Early childhood nurse-delivered CBC	Australia	37	EPDS and clinical interview	Standard care	EPDS, MADRS	No significant group difference	Randomisation unclear, group differences in baseline EPDS scores, standard care could involve similar treatment to intervention
Honey et al, 2002	Health visitor-delivered groups with education, CBT and relaxation	UK	45	Depressive symptoms EPDS ≥12	Standard care	EPDS, DAS, WCC–R, FSSQ	Intervention > control for depressive symptoms but no difference for psychosocial functioning	Block randomisation method, intervention not manualised, unclear whether assessors were masked
Cooper et al, 2003	Non-directive counselling v. CBT v. dynamic therapy	UK	193	DSM–III–R depression	None	EPDS, SCID	All groups show improvement in depressive symptoms, only dynamic therapy reduced depressive disorder	Randomisation method open to bias, no true control group
Dennis, 2003	Individualised telephone-based peer support	Canada	42	Depressive symptoms EPDS ≥9	Standard care	EPDS, SES, CCSC, UCLA–Loneliness Scale, PSEI, PVEQ	Intervention > control	33% of those eligible declined, underpowered to detect differences in secondary outcomes

Study	Intervention	Country	Sample size, *n*	Inclusion criteria	Control group	Assessments	Maternal outcome(s)	Limitations
Misri *et al*, 2004	CBT + paroxetine *v*. paroxetine	Canada	35	DSM–IV depressive disorder and anxiety disorder	None	HRSA, HRSD, YBOCS, CGI	Both groups show improvements, no additional benefits from combining treatments	20% of eligible women did not complete, unclear how adherence assessed, no true control group
Milgrom *et al*, 2005	Group-based CBT *v*. group or individual counselling	Australia	159	DSM–IV major or minor depression	Standard care	BDI, BAI, SPS		Not individually randomised, 33% of those allocated treatments did not attend
Rojas *et al*, 2007	Psychoeducational group + treatment adherence support + medication if needed	Chile	226	DSM–IV major depression	Standard care	EPDS, SF–36	Intervention > control	Both groups on antidepressants
Morrell et al, 2006	Non-directive counselling *v*. CBT	UK	595	Depressive symptoms EPDS ≥11	Standard care	EPDS, general health, social support, life events, anxiety, parenting stress, and marital relations	Interventions > control Non-directive counselling = CBT	Randomisation unclear, some health visitors offered intervention to women they were concerned about irrespective of EPDS score

Abbreviations

BAI, Beck Anxiety Inventory; BDI, Beck Depression Inventory; CBC, cognitive–behavioural counselling; CBT, cognitive–behavioural therapy; CCSC, Child Care Stress Checklist; CGI, Clinical Global Impression; CIS–R, Clinical Interview Schedule – Revised; CSEI, Coopersmith Self-Esteem Inventory; DAS, Dyadic Adjustment Scale; EPDS, Edinburgh Perinatal Depression Scale; FSSQ, Duke–UNC Functional Social Support Questionnaire; HRSA, Hamilton Anxiety Rating Scale; HRSD, Hamilton Depression Rating Scale; IDD, Inventory to Diagnose Depression; MADRS, Montgomery–Åsberg Depression Rating Scale; POMS, Profile of Mood States; PPAQ, Postpartum Adjustment Questionnaire; PSEI, Peer Support Evaluation Inventory; PSI, Parenting Stress Index; PVEQ, Peer-Volunteer Perceptions of Peer Support; SAS–SR, Social Adjustment Scale – Self-Report; SCID, Structured Clinical Interview for DSM–IV (depression); SES, Self-Esteem Scale; SF–6, Short Form–36; SPI, Standardised Psychiatric Interview; SPS, Social Provisions Scale; WCC–R, Ways of Coping Checklist – Revised; YBOCS, Yale–Brown Obsessive Compulsive Scale

References

Appleby, L., Warner, R., Whitton, A., *et al* (1997) A controlled study of fluoxetine and cognitive–behavioural counselling in the treatment of postnatal depression. *BMJ*, **314**, 932–936.

Cooper, P. J., Murray, L., Wilson, A., *et al* (2003) Controlled trial of the short- and long-term effect of psychological treatment of post-partum depression: 1. Impact on maternal mood. *British Journal of Psychiatry*, **182**, 412–419.

Dennis, C. L. (2003) The effect of peer support on postpartum depression: a pilot randomized controlled trial. *Canadian Journal of Psychiatry*, **48**, 115–124.

Holden, J. M., Sagovsky, R. & Cox, J. L. (1989) Counselling in a general practice setting: controlled study of health visitor intervention in treatment of postnatal depression. *BMJ*, **298**, 223–226.

Honey, K. L., Bennett, P. & Morgan, M. (2002) A brief psycho-educational group intervention for postnatal depression. *British Journal of Clinical Psychology*, **41**, 405–409.

Meager, I. & Milgrom, J. (1996) Group treatment for postpartum depression: a pilot study. *Australian and New Zealand Journal of Psychiatry*, **30**, 852–860.

Milgrom, J., Negri, L. M., Gemmill, A. W., *et al* (2005) A randomized controlled trial of psychological interventions for postnatal depression. *British Journal of Clinical Psychology*, **44**, 529–542.

Misri, S., Reebye, P., Corral, M., *et al* (2004) The use of paroxetine and cognitive–behavioral therapy in postpartum depression and anxiety: a randomized controlled trial. *Journal of Clinical Psychiatry*, **65**, 1236–1241.

Morrell, C. J. (2006) Review of interventions to prevent or treat postnatal depression. *Clinical Effectiveness in Nursing*, **9**, e135–e161.

O'Hara, M. W., Stuart, S., Gorman, L. L., *et al* (2000) Efficacy of interpersonal psychotherapy for postpartum depression. *Archives of General Psychiatry*, **57**, 1039–1045.

Prendergast, J. & Austin, M. P. (2001) Early childhood nurse-delivered cognitive behavioural counselling for post-natal depression. *Australasian Psychiatry*, **9**, 255–259.

Rojas, G., Fritsch, R., Solis, J., *et al* (2007) Treatment of postnatal depression in low-income mothers in primary-care clinics in Santiago, Chile: a randomised controlled trial. *Lancet*, **370**, 1629–1637.

Wickberg, B. & Hwang, C. P. (1996) Counselling of postnatal depression: a controlled study on a population based Swedish sample. *Journal of Affective Disorders*, **39**, 209–216.

Appendix II
Organisations offering support and information

Source	Contact information	What's there
Association for Post-Natal Illness 145 Dawes Road Fulham London SW6 7EB	Helpline: 020 7386 0868 Email: info@apni.org Web: www.apni.org	Support and information for women with postnatal illness
Cry-sis BM Cry-sis London WC1N 3XX	Helpline: 08451 228 669 Web: www.cry-sis.org.uk	Support, help, advice and information for parents with a crying baby
Family Welfare Association 501–505 Kingsland Road London E8 4AU	Tel: 020 7254 6251 (South) 0161 684 2180 (North) Web: www.fwa.org.uk	Organisation that deals with complex and difficult issues facing families including domestic abuse, mental health problems, learning disabilities and severe financial hardship
Home-Start UK 2 Salisbury Road Leicester LE1 7QR	Information line: 0800 068 6368 Tel: 0116 233 9955 Email: info@home-start.org.uk Web: www.home-start.org.uk	Volunteers offer support, friendship and practical help in their own home to families with at least one child under 5 years of age who are having difficulties
Meet-a-Mum Association (MAMA) 7 Southcourt Road Linslade Leighton Buzzard Bedfordshire LU7 2TY	Helpline: 0845 120 3746 Web: www.mama.co.uk	Support and help for women with postnatal depressive illness, or who feel tired or isolated after having a baby or are simply in need of a friend
National Childbirth Trust Alexandra House Oldham Terrace London W3 6NH	Breastfeeding: 0870 444 8708 Pregnancy & birth: 0870 444 8709 Enquiries: 0870 444 8707 Web: www. nctpregnancyandbabycare.com	Information and support for expectant and new parents including antenatal classes, breastfeeding, counselling and postnatal support groups
Netmums 124 Mildred Avenue Watford WD18 7DX	Web: www.netmums.com	Support and information – a network of local websites, chat rooms and blogs
Perinatal Illness UK PO Box 49769 London WC1H 9WH	Enquiries: 07925 144411 Web: www.pni-uk.com	Support and information Message board, chat room and email support
Postpartum Support International PO Box 60931 Santa Barbara CA 93160 USA	Helpline: +1 800 944 4773[1] Enquiries: +1 805 967 7636 Email: PSIOffice@postpartum.net Web: www.postpartum.net	Provide information and advice, run support groups and are a network of professionals; most members are based in the USA

1. Toll-free helpline only operates within the USA.

Appendix III
Edinburgh Postnatal Depression Scale

The Edinburgh Postnatal Depression Scale was devised and validated in 1987 and should appear as follows. The copyright is held by the Royal College of Psychiatrists and must be reproduced in full and include the full reference as seen in the footnote.

Edinburgh Postnatal Depression Scale

Name ....

Address ....

Baby's age ....

As you have recently had a baby, we would like to know how you are feeling. Please <u>underline</u> the answer which comes closest to how you have felt in the past 7 days, not just how you feel today. Here is an example already completed:

I have felt happy:
Yes, most of the time
<u>Yes, some of the time</u>
No, not very often
No, not at all

This would mean: 'I have felt happy some of the time' during the past week. Please complete the other questions in the same way.

In the past 7 days

1. I have been able to laugh and see the funny side of things:
   As much as I always could
   Not quite so much now
   Definitely not so much now
   Not at all

2. I have looked forward with enjoyment to things:
   As much as I ever did
   Rather less than I used to
   Definitely less than I used to
   Hardly at all

3. I have blamed myself unnecessarily when things went wrong:
   Yes, most of the time
   Yes, some of the time
   Not very often
   No, never

4. I have been anxious or worried for no good reason:
   No, not at all
   Hardly ever
   Yes, sometimes
   Yes, very often

5. I have felt scared or panicky for no very good reason:
   Yes, quite a lot
   Yes, sometimes
   No, not much
   No, not at all

6. Things have been getting on top of me:
   Yes, most of the time I haven't been able to cope at all
   Yes, sometimes I haven't been coping as well as usual
   No, most of the time I have coped quite well
   No, I have been coping as well as ever

7. I have been so unhappy that I have had difficulty sleeping:
   Yes, most of the time
   Yes, sometimes
   No, not very often
   No, not at all

8. I have felt sad or miserable:
   Yes, most of the time
   Yes, sometimes
   No, not very often
   No, not at all

9.   I have been so unhappy that I have been crying:
Yes, most of the time
Yes, quite often
Only occasionally
No, not at all

10. The thought of harming myself has occurred to me:
Yes, quite often
Sometimes
Hardly ever
Never

Edinburgh Postnatal Depression Scale: scoring sheet

1. I have been able to laugh and see the funny side of things:
   As much as I always could   0
   Not quite so much now   1
   Definitely not so much now   2
   Not at all   3

2. I have looked forward with enjoyment to things:
   As much as I ever did   0
   Rather less than I used to   1
   Definitely less than I used to   2
   Hardly at all   3

3. I have blamed myself unnecessarily when things went wrong:
   Yes, most of the time   3
   Yes, some of the time   2
   Not very often   1
   No, never   0

4. I have been anxious or worried for no good reason:
   No, not at all   0
   Hardly ever   1
   Yes, sometimes   2
   Yes, very often   3

5. I have felt scared or panicky for no very good reason:
   Yes, quite a lot   3
   Yes, sometimes   2
   No, not much   1
   No, not at all   0

6. Things have been getting on top of me:
   Yes, most of the time I haven't been able to cope at all   3
   Yes, sometimes I haven't been coping as well as usual   2
   No, most of the time I have coped quite well   1
   No, I have been coping as well as ever   0

7. I have been so unhappy that I have had difficulty sleeping:
   Yes, most of the time   3
   Yes, sometimes   2
   No, not very often   1
   No, not at all   0

8. I have felt sad or miserable:
   Yes, most of the time   3
   Yes, sometimes   2
   No, not very often   1
   No, not at all   0

9. I have been so unhappy that I have been crying:
   Yes, most of the time   3
   Yes, quite often   2
   Only occasionally   1
   No, not at all   0

10. The thought of harming myself has occurred to me:
    Yes, quite often   3
    Sometimes   2
    Hardly ever   1
    Never   0

Appendix IV
Resources

For professionals

Antenatal Psychosocial Health Assessment (ALPHA)

This form is available from the Department of Family and Community Medicine, University of Toronto (http://dfcm19.med.utoronto.ca/research/alpha/.

HARP Mental Health and Well-being Resource

This website provides practical advice on working with interpreters, the kind of supports available for refugees and asylum seekers and some useful 'dos and don'ts' (www.mentalhealth.harweb.org/).

Postnatal depression training

Courses developed from investigations into the efficacy of different psychological interventions for postnatal depression (www.pndtraining. co.uk/). The first three ourses are commissioned by the client and delivered on the client site.

- A 4-day course aimed at practitioners and providing skills-based training to identify depression and to treat it. Treatment is based on a planned, structured and focused intervention using techniques derived from counselling and CBT.
- A 2-day course covering detection of depression and basic interventions.
- A 1-day workshop awareness and detection of perinatal mood disorders.

They also offer a residential course:

- Trainer's course. A 3-day course designed for those responsible for training primary healthcare workers. This course is delivered at the campus of the University of Reading, UK.

Postpartum Depression Screening Scale (PDSS)

This Scale is used to identify women at risk for postpartum depression and is published and distributed by Western Psychological Services (www.wpspublish.com).

The Royal College of Psychiatrists

The Royal College of Psychiatrists is developing online training modules entitled 'Parental mental health – keeping the family in mind', 'Managing pregnant substance misusers' and 'Infanticide', and has a completed module on 'Working through interpreters' (www.psychiatrycpd.co.uk/learningmodules.aspx).

Useful reading

Kelly, K & Little, B. (eds) (2001) Obstetrics for the non-obstetrician. In *Management of Psychiatric Disorders in Pregnancy*, pp. 17–63. Arnold.

For service users and carers

Community Practitioners' and Health Visitors' Association

'How Are You Feeling?' booklets for non-English speaking mothers can be obtained from www.amicus-cphva.org.

Mind

The booklet 'Understanding Postnatal Depression' can be viewed online or purchased from the online Mind shop and is likely to be helpful to those with postnatal depression (www.mind.org.uk/Information/Booklets/Understanding/Understanding+postnatal+depression.htm).

The Royal College of Psychiatrists

Leaflets for women with postnatal depression, and for carers and professionals. 'Mental Illness after Childbirth' contains useful information for anyone who wants to know more about mental illness after childbirth and is available in Chinese and Arabic. 'Postnatal Depression' is available in Chinese (www.rcpsych.ac.uk/mentalhealthinformation/mentalhealthproblems/postnatalmentalhealth.aspx).

Index

Compiled by Caroline Sheard

Modern Management of Perinatal Psychiatric Disorder

For my husband James and son Richard
Carol Henshaw

For my wife Karin, three daughters Christina, Ann-Marie and Susanne,
granddaughter Suzannah and grandson Joshua
John Cox

For my husband Flip
Joanne Barton